CRC SERIES IN AGING

Editors-in-Chief

Richard C. Adelman, Ph.D. George S. Roth, Ph.D.

VOLUMES AND VOLUME EDITORS

HANDBOOK OF BIOCHEMISTRY IN AGING
James Florini, Ph.D.
Department of Biology
Syracuse University
Syracuse, New York

HANDBOOK OF IMMUNOLOGY IN AGING
Marguerite M. B. Kay, M.D. and
Takashi Makinodan, Ph.D.
Geriatric Research Education and Clinical
Center
V.A. Wadsworth Medical Center
Los Angeles, California

SENESCENCE IN PLANTS
Kenneth V. Thimann, Ph.D.
The Thimann Laboratories
University of California
Santa Cruz, California

ALCOHOLISM AND AGING: ADVANCES IN RESEARCH
W. Gibson Wood, Ph.D.
Clinical Research Psychologist
Geriatric Research, Education, and Clinical
Center
VA Medical Center
St. Louis, Missouri
Merrill F. Elias, Ph.D.
Professor of Psychology
University of Maine at Orono
Orono, Maine

TESTING THE THEORIES OF AGING
Richard C. Adelman, Ph.D.
Executive Director
Professor of Biochemistry and Biology
Institute on Aging
Temple University
Philadelphia, Pennsylvania
George S. Roth, Ph.D.
Research Biochemist
Gerontology Research Center
National Institute on Aging
Baltimore City Hospitals
Baltimore, Maryland

HANDBOOK OF PHYSIOLOGY IN AGING
Edward J. Masoro, Ph.D.
Department of Physiology
University of Texas Health Science Center
San Antonio, Texas

IMMUNOLOGICAL TECHNIQUES APPLIED TO AGING RESEARCH
William H. Adler, M.D. and
Albert A. Nordin, Ph.D.
Gerontology Research Center
National Institute on Aging
Baltimore City Hospitals
Baltimore, Maryland

CURRENT TRENDS IN MORPHO-LOGICAL TECHNIQUES
John E. Johnson, Jr., Ph.D.
Gerontology Research Center
National Institute on Aging
Baltimore City Hospitals
Baltimore, Maryland

NUTRITIONAL APPROACHES TO AGING RESEARCH
Gairdner B. Moment, Ph.D.
Professor Emeritus of Biology
Groucher College
Guest Scientist
Gerontology Research Center
National Institute on Aging
Baltimore, Maryland

ENDOCRINE AND NEUROENDOCRINE MECHANISMS OF AGING
Richard C. Adelman, Ph.D.
Executive Director
Professor of Biochemistry and Biology
Institute on Aging
Temple University
Philadelphia, Pennsylvania
George S. Roth, Ph.D.
Research Biochemist
Gerontology Research Center
National Institute on Aging
Baltimore City Hospitals
Baltimore, Maryland

Additional topics to be covered in this series include Cell Biology of Aging, Microbiology of Aging, Pharmacology of Aging, Evolution and Genetics, Animal Models for Aging Research, Detection of Altered Proteins, Insect Models, and Lower Invertebrate Models.

Endocrine and Neuroendocrine Mechanisms of Aging

Editors

Richard C. Adelman, Ph.D.

Executive Director
Professor of Biochemistry and Biology
Institute on Aging
Temple University
Philadelphia, Pennsylvania

George S. Roth, Ph.D.

Research Biochemist
Gerontology Research Center
National Institute on Aging
Baltimore City Hospitals
Baltimore, Maryland

CRC Series in Aging

Editors-in-Chief

Richard C. Adelman, Ph.D.
George S. Roth, Ph.D.

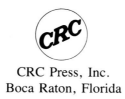

CRC Press, Inc.
Boca Raton, Florida

Library of Congress Cataloging in Publication Data
Main entry under title:

Endocrine and neuroendocrine mechanisms of aging

   (CRC series in aging)
   Bibliography: p.
   Includes index.
   1. Endocrinology.   2. Biological control
systems.   3. Aging.   4. Neuroendocrinology.
I. Adelman, Richard C., 1940–
II. Roth, George S., 1946–   III. Series.
[DNLM: 1. Endocrine glands—Physiology.
2. Hormones—Physiology.   3. Aging. WK 102 E54]
QP187.E52   612′.67   81-21736
ISBN 0-8493-5811-6   AACR2

   Direct all inquiries to CRC Press, 2000 Corporate Blvd. N.W., Boca Raton, Florida, 33431.

©1982 by CRC Press, Inc.

International Standard Book Number 0-8493-5811-6

Library of Congress Card Number
Printed in the United States

PREFACE

One of the most important and fastest growing areas of biogerontological research is that of neuroendocrine and endocrine regulation. This fact is not so surprising since such regulation concerns nearly all physiological functions, many of which exhibit decrement with increasing age. In addition, these studies help to bridge the gap in aging research between the molecular and the physiological. Sound bodies of data exist both with respect to the molecular bases of hormone action and the varied mechanisms by which neuroendocrine and endocrine factors regulate normal physiology.

It is the purpose of this volume to present a representative sampling of those neural and hormonal studies which have been the focus of the most intense interest in recent gerontological research. To this end we have been fortunate to enlist the aid of some of the most competent and innovative investigators in the field. More than this, however, an attempt has been made to provide detailed methodological as well as theoretical evaluation of the areas considered. It is our hope that those researchers interested in this area of regulation during aging will be able to utilize the information contained herein as a basis both for critical analysis as well as for the designing and execution of further experiments in this most important area.

Richard C. Adelman
George S. Roth

EDITORS-IN-CHIEF

Dr. Richard C. Adelman is currently Executive Director of the Temple University Institute on Aging, Philadelphia, Penn., as well as Professor of Biochemistry in the Fels Research Institute of the Temple University College of Medicine. An active gerontologist for more than 10 years, he has achieved international prominence as a researcher, educator, and administrator. These accomplishments span a broad spectrum of activities ranging from the traditional disciplinary interests of the research biologist to the advocacy, implementation, and administration of multidisciplinary issues of public policy of concern to elderly people.

Dr. Adelman pursued his pre- and postdoctoral research training under the guidance of two prominent biochemists, each of whom is a member of the National Academy of Sciences: Dr. Sidney Weinhouse as Director of the Fels Research Institute, Temple University, and Dr. Bernard L. Horecker as Chairman of the Department of Molecular Biology, Albert Einstein College of Medicine, Bronx, N.Y. His accomplishments as a researcher can be expressed in at least the following ways. He is the author and/or editor of more than 70 publications, including original research papers in referred journals, review chapters, and books. His research efforts have been supported by grants from the National Institutes of Health for the past 10 consecutive years, at a current annual level of approximately $300,000. He continues to serve as an invited speaker at seminar programs, symposiums, and workshops all over the world. He is the recipient of the IntraScience Research Foundation Medalist Award, an annual research prize awarded by peer evaluation for major advances in newly emerging areas of the life sciences. He is the recipient of an Established Investigatorship of the American Heart Association.

As an educator, Dr. Adelman is also involved in a broad variety of activities. His role in research training consists of responsibility for pre- and postdoctoral students who are assigned specific projects in his laboratory. He teaches an advanced graduate course on the biology of aging, lectures on biomedical aspects of aging to medical students, and is responsible for the biological component of the basic course in aging sponsored by the School of Social Administration. Training activities outside the University include membership in the Faculty of the National Institute on Aging summer course on the biology of aging; programs on the biology of aging for AAA's throughout Pennsylvania and Ohio; and the implementation and teaching of Biology of Aging for the Nonbiologist locally, for the Gerontology Society and other national organizations, as well as for the International Association of Gerontology.

Dr. Adelman has achieved leadership positions across equally broad areas. Responsibilities of this position include the intergration of multidisciplinary programs in research, consultation and education, and health service, as well as advocacy for the University on all matters dealing with aging. He coordinates a city-wide consortium of researchers from Temple University, the Wistar Institute, the Medical College of Pennsylvania, Drexel University, and the Philadelphia Geriatric Center, conducting collaborative research projects, training programs, and symposiums. He was a past President of the Philadelphia Biochemists Club. He serves on the editorial boards of the *Journal of Gerontology, Mechanisms of Ageing and Development, Experimental Aging Research,* and *Gerontological Abstracts.* He was a member of the Biomedical Research Panel of the National Advisory Council of the National Institute on Aging. He chairs a subcommittee of the National Academy of Sciences Committee on Animal Models for Aging Research. As an active Fellow of the Geronological Society, he is a past Chairman of the Biological Sciences section; a past Chairman of the Society Public Policy Committee for which he prepared Congressional testimony and represented the Society on the Leadership Council of the Coalition of National Aging Organizations; and is Secretary-Treasurer of the North American Executive Committee of the International Association of Gerontology. Finally, as the highest testimony of his leadership capabilities, he continues to serve on National Advisory Committees which impact on diverse key issues dealing with the elderly. These include a 4-year appointment as member of the NIH Study Section on Pathobiological Chemistry; the Executive Committee of the Health Resources Administration Project on publication of the recent edition of *Working with Older People—A Guide to Practice;* a recent appointment as reviewer of AOA applications for Career Preparation Programs in Gerontology; and a 4-year appointment on the Veterans Administration Long-Term Care Advisory Council responsible for evaluating their program on Geriatric Research, Education, and Clinical Centers (GRECC).

George S. Roth, Ph.D., is a research chemist with the Gerontology Research Center of the National Institute on Aging in Baltimore, Md., where he has been affiliated since 1972. Dr. Roth received his B.S. in Biology from Villanova University in 1968 and his Ph.D. in Microbiology from Temple University School of Medicine in 1971. He received postdoctoral training in Biochemistry at the Fels Research Institute in Philadelphia, Pa. Dr. Roth has also been associated with the graduate schools of Georgetown University and George Washington University where he has sponsored two Ph.D. students.

He has published more than 70 papers in the area of aging and hormone/neurotransmitter action, and has lectured, organized meetings, and chaired sessions throughout the world on this subject.

Dr. Roth's other activities include fellowship in the Gerontological Society of America, where he has served in numerous capacities, including chairmanship of the 1979 midyear conference on ''Functional Status and Aging.'' He is presently Chairman of the Biological Sciences Section and a Vice President of the Society. He has twice been selected as an exchange scientist by the National Academy of Sciences and in this capacity has established liasons with gerontologists, endocrinologists, and biochemists in several Eastern European countries. Dr. Roth serves as an editor of *Neurobiology of Aging* and is a frequent reviewer for many other journals including *Mechanisms in Aging and Development, Life Sciences, The Journal of Gerontology, Science,* and *Endocrinology.* He also serves as a grant reviewer for several funding agencies including the National Science Foundation. In 1981 Dr. Roth was awarded the Annual Research Award of the American Aging Association.

CONTRIBUTORS

Richard C. Adelman, Ph.D.
Executive Director
Professor of Biochemistry and Biology
Institute on Aging
Temple University
Philadelphia, Pennsylvania

Bennett J. Cohen, Ph.D., D.V.M.
Professor and Chairman
Unit for Laboratory Medicine
University of Michigan Medical School
Ann Arbor, Michigan

Arthur V. Everitt, Ph.D.
Associate Professor in Physiology
University of Sydney
Sydney, Australia

Nicola Fabris
Director
Center of Immunology
I.N.R.C.A. Research Department
Ancona, Italy

Charles R. Filburn, Ph.D.
Research Biochemist
Laboratory of Molecular Aging
Gerontology Research Center
Baltimore City Hospitals
Baltimore, Maryland

Philip W. Landfield, Ph.D.
Associate Professor
Department of Physiology and
Pharmacology
Bowman Gray School of Medicine
Winston-Salem, North Carolina

Joseph Meites, Ph.D.
Professor
Department of Physiology
Michigan State University
East Lansing, Michigan

Lucio Piantanelli
Center of Biochemistry
I.N.R.C.A. Research Department
Ancona, Italy

Eve P. Reaven, Ph.D.
Research Physiologist
Veterans Administration Medical Center
Palo Alto, California

Gerald M. Reaven, M.D.
Director, Geriatric Research
Education and Clinical Center
Veterans Administration Medical Center
Palo Alto, California

Gail D. Riegle, Ph.D.
Professor
Department of Physiology
Michigan State University
East Lansing, Michigan

George S. Roth, Ph.D.
Research Biochemist
Gerontology Research Center
National Institute on Aging
Baltimore City Hospitals
Baltimore, Maryland

Eva A. Sartin, D.V.M.
Resident in Pathology
School of Veterinary Medicine
University of Pennsylvania
Philadelphia, Pennsylvania

James L. Sartin, Ph.D.
Staff Biologist
Temple University Institute of Aging
Philadelphia, Pennsylvania

William E. Sonntag, Ph.D.
Neuroendocrine Research Laboratory
Department of Physiology
Michigan State University
East Lansing, Michigan

Richard W. Steger, Ph.D.
Assistant Professor
Department of Obstetrics and Gynecology
University of Texas Health Science Center
San Antonio, Texas

Jennifer Wyndham, B.Sc.
Department of Physiology
University of Sydney
Sydney, Australia

TABLE OF CONTENTS

Chapter 1

INSULIN AND GLUCOSE METABOLISM DURING AGING

Gerald M. Reaven and Eve P. Reaven

TABLE OF CONTENTS

I. INTRODUCTION

During the past several decades it has become clear that substantial changes occur in glucose and insulin metabolism during aging. Perhaps the most widely appreciated of these changes is the observation that glucose tolerance deteriorates with age. Indeed, the weight of evidence is so great, and the subject reviewed so frequently,[1-3] that it would not be useful to once again address the question whether or not aging is associated with a deterioration of glucose tolerance. Clearly it is. However, the significance of this statement is clouded by the fact that so many of the published studies of the effect of age on glucose and insulin metabolism do not consider certain methodological and theoretical questions. As a result, the authors of this chapter feel that there still exist two major unanswered questions relevant to the effect of age on glucose and insulin metabolism. The first of these is the most fundamental, and involves a decision as to whether the observed deterioration in glucose tolerance is due to age itself, or is secondary to a number of other factors which occur frequently in older individuals and may adversely modify carbohydrate homeostasis. A second, and related, question concerns the mechanism(s) responsible for the deterioration of glucose tolerance in older individuals. For example, is the observed glucose intolerance a function of an alteration in insulin secretion or of tissue sensitivity to insulin?

In this chapter, the authors will attempt to respond to the questions defined. They will review the available relevant literature, and, at the same time, point out the methodological and theoretical problems which make it difficult to come to definitive answers at this time. As such, the authors have not compiled an inclusive bibliography of experimental data related to the effect of aging on glucose and insulin metabolism. Instead, they have focused attention on what they believe to be the central issues.

The authors' inability to arrive at definitive conclusions at this time should not be discouraging. After all, experimentation on this subject has taken place over a period of many years with many different expressed goals. The utility of this presentation will be the degree to which it has successfully redefined the problems and pointed to possible experimental approaches to their solution.

II. AGE AND GLUCOSE METABOLISM

In this section the authors will attempt to review published data concerning the independent effect of age on glucose tolerance. In order to do this, it will be necessary to address two issues. The first problem will be to differentiate between the impact of age on glucose tolerance as distinguished from the effect of environmental factors well known to adversely modify carbohydrate metabolism. Once the initial distinction is made, it will still be necessary to determine if the observed changes in glucose tolerance are part of a normal and inevitable aging process, or are representative of an emerging population of individuals who develop diabetes as they age.

A. Effect of Age on Glucose Tolerance

Most of the available information concerning the effect of age on glucose tolerance is derived from studies of man. In order for such a study to be included in this evaluation, the authors of this chapter felt that certain criteria had to be fulfilled. In the first place, a substantial number of individuals had to be examined and the population studied had to cover a wide span of ages. For example, the demonstration that a group of old individuals (mean age of 70 years) had worse glucose tolerance than a group of young individuals (mean age of 30 years) is interesting, but by itself does not provide much insight as to whether or not age leads to a progressive deterioration of glucose tolerance. In order to answer this question there must be at least three groups of patients (young, middle, and old age) in the population studied. In addition, the authors felt that all groups (regardless of age) had to consist of healthy volunteers, all of whom were fully ambulatory. Although this latter consideration attempts to take into account the possibility that a decline in physical activity could be responsible for the deterioration of glucose tolerance that occurs with age, it should be pointed out that no published study has seriously analyzed this crucial factor. Finally, the authors felt that consideration had to be given to the effects of both obesity and inadequate carbohydrate intake on the changes in glucose tolerance that occur with age.

The application of these criteria greatly reduces the quantity of available information, but enough data remains to permit some consideration of the effect of age per se on glucose tolerance in man. There is considerably less information concerning the effect of age on carbohydrate metabolism in animals, and the authors' criterion for consideration of this information was less rigorous, i.e., the study had to include a substantial number of animals with one category of animals being at least 9 months of age.

1. Human Studies
a. Oral Glucose Tolerance

There are three studies which have attempted to determine the effect of age on the plasma glucose response to oral glucose in large numbers of healthy volunteers well matched for weight. Unfortunately, no consistent results were seen. The largest population was found in the study of Wingerd and Duffy,[4] who analyzed the results of oral glucose tolerance tests in 2248 females. The subjects were divided into three groups: ages 20 to 30 (711), 40 to 49 (974), and greater than 50 (567). The mean ages of the three groups were 32.5, 44.4, and 53.7 years, and the results indicated that there was a progressive rise in plasma glucose levels over this 20-year time span. The effect was most dramatic 1 hr after the oral glucose challenge, with a mean difference in plasma glucose of 32 mg/dℓ between the youngest and the oldest group. Although there was no formal attempt to stratify by degree of obesity, the relative weight of the three groups was comparable. However, this study has at least two important confounding variables; approximately 25% of the patient population was receiving sex hormone therapy of one kind or another and all of the patients had diabetic relatives. Although Wingerd and Duffy state that statistical analysis permitted the identification of age itself as a factor which led to worsening glucose tolerance, it would seem that this population may have not been an ideal one in which to estimate the effect of age itself on glucose tolerance.

The second largest study was that of Nolan et al.,[5] who performed oral glucose tolerance tests (1.75 g/kg body weight) in 707 nonobese and 479 obese females with nondiabetic glucose tolerance test results. The ages ranged from 20 to 60 years and the patients were divided into groups by decade. Fasting blood glucose levels were significantly lower in nonobese females ages 20 to 29, as compared to those aged 30 to 39. However, there was no progressive change in the successive decades. The plasma glucose level 30 min after the glucose challenge was also significantly lower in the 20 to 29 as compared to the 30 to 39 age group, and, as before, there was no further increase with successive decades. There were no significant differences at any other time point, and there were essentially no age-related changes in plasma glucose levels seen in the obese females. At first glance these data seem to indicate that the effect of age on glucose tolerance is minimal and that any deterioration that does take place occurs relatively early in life. However, there are two fundamental drawbacks to this conclusion. In the first place, patients over 60 years were not included, and it is certainly possible that changes in glucose tolerance could occur in those over 60. Second, patients with relatively minor degrees of glucose intolerance (using a series of criteria) were excluded from analysis. This maneuver results in what is almost a self-fulfilling prophecy; any deterioration of glucose tolerance that occurs with age is designated as the emergence of diabetes. This issue is an extremely important one, and will be discussed in detail in a subsequent section.

A third study of oral glucose tolerance in a large number of patients of all ages was carried out by Boyns et al.[6] These investigators determined the plasma glucose response of 220 healthy volunteers to a 50 g oral glucose load. The ages of the group ranged from 16 to 74, and they were selected by a stratification procedure in a manner that provided equal numbers in each age and sex group and an even distribution of body build in each of the groups. Known diabetics were excluded from the study population. In both sexes the mean blood glucose tended to rise progressively with age. In men there was a significant correlation between age and blood glucose before ($r = 0.24$), 30 ($r = 0.44$), 60 ($r = 0.54$), and 90 ($r = 0.36$) min after the glucose load. The effect of age was less dramatic in women, and significant correlations were only seen 30 ($r = 0.21$), and 60 ($r = 0.31$) min after oral glucose. The maximum quantitative effect of age was observed 60 min after the glucose challenge in both groups: mean blood glucose rose from 86 mg/dℓ in men less than 24 years to 136 mg/dℓ in males greater than 55 years, whereas the increment in females over the same age span was from 92 to 115 mg/dℓ.

Two other studies have attempted to assess the effect of age on oral glucose tolerance in a smaller number of subjects selected in order to minimize the effect of differences in degree of obesity. Kimmerling et al.[7] studied 100 volunteer subjects whose ages ranged from 22 to 69 years. They all had fasting plasma glucose levels less than 110 mg/dℓ, their relative body weights were between 0.75 to 1.20% of ideal body weight, and no correlation was noted between age and relative weight. These authors could find no correlation between age and plasma glucose, either in the fasting state or 120 min after an oral glucose challenge (40 g/m^2). The lack of correlation between age and plasma glucose level 120 min after oral glucose is consistent with the results of Boyns et al.,[6] but the two studies differ in that Boyns et al. could also show a small correlation ($r = 0.24$) between age and fasting glucose level.

Somewhat different results were found in a study by Rehfeld and Stadil[8] of 60 healthy volunteers, matched for height and weight. The group was subdivided into three subgroups of 20 subjects each (young, middle-aged, and old): ages 20 to 32 (mean = 27), 42 to 55 (mean = 48), and 65 to 81 (mean = 74). The mean plasma glucose response of the young and middle-aged groups to 50 g of oral glucose was essentially identical, suggesting that no change in glucose tolerance had occurred as patients aged from 20 to 55 years. However, there was a significant elevation in the mean plasma glucose level of the group of old subjects between 60 and 120 min after the oral glucose load.

There are several other studies in which the effect of age on glucose tolerance has been estimated in populations not matched for degree of obesity, but in which the investigators have attempted to take into account the potential effect of obesity by statistical analysis. Thus, Berger and colleagues[9] found a progressive rise in fasting plasma glucose from 91 mg/dℓ in the 3rd decade to 97 mg/dℓ in the 7th decade in a study of 263 healthy volunteers. There were statistically significant correlations between both age and fasting plasma glucose ($r = 0.25$), and age and percent of ideal body weight ($r = 0.15$). The authors state that when adjustments were made for adiposity the correlation of age with glucose persisted. Similarly, O'Sullivan and colleagues[10] found a "significant rise in blood glucose response of levels with advancing age" in approximately 150 volunteers of various ages. They also found that the degree of obesity increased with age. However, the authors state that "multiple regression analysis indicates that this rise in blood glucose levels with age remains significant." Unfortunately, they provide no further details as to the degree of correlation between glucose and age that existed either before or after taking degree of obesity into consideration. Thus, the reports of both Berger et al.[9] and O'Sullivan et al.[10] provide support for the notion that glucose tolerance deteriorates with age. On the other hand, it is difficult to ascertain from these data the quantitative nature of the changes that are due to age itself as distinguished from those related to obesity.

Finally, there are two other reports (which indicate that age affects oral glucose tolerance) in which it is even harder to evaluate the impact of obesity. Thus, Nilsson[11] described results which are similar to those of Boyns et al.[6] in that he noted a progressive deterioration of oral glucose tolerance with age in a large group of healthy volunteer subjects. However, Nilsson's data also indicate that the relative amount of body fat increases with age, and he also noted significant correlations between plasma glucose levels during the glucose tolerance test and degree of obesity. He presents data which suggest that these differences in degree of obesity cannot entirely account for the effect of age on glucose tolerance, but it is again difficult to quantitatively assess the relative impact of age itself, as distinct from obesity, on the deterioration of glucose tolerance. Similarly Vecchio and colleagues[12] found a positive correlation (r = 0.31) between age and total glycemic response to oral glucose (area under the glucose tolerance curve) in 166 volunteer male prisoners between 20 and 69 years. Although these authors indicate that there was no correlation between absolute body weight and glycemic response, they provide no data as to possible age-related differences in relative degree of obesity in the population studied.

b. Intravenous Glucose Tolerance

In two studies, appropriate design permits an estimate to be made of the effect of age, as distinguished from other metabolic variables, on intravenous glucose tolerance. Franckson et al.[13] estimated the glucose disappearance rate in 325 nonobese and in 150 obese subjects (>25% over their ideal weight). These authors suggest that there is a progressive deterioration in glucose tolerance as both obese and nonobese subjects from 15 to 85 years of age. This result is even more noteworthy in that the study excluded patients with minor impairments of glucose tolerance. On the other hand, inspection of the data suggests that the results of the study may not be so clear. Thus, the tests show that in a small number of very young subjects (less than 15 years) glucose was removed more efficiently than in a small number of very old subjects (above 75 years). On the other hand, it is not so evident that the glucose disposal rate was different in subjects between 25 to 65 years. Furthermore, all subjects were hospitalized patients convalescing from benign illnesses. The possibility that these findings might be a function of state of general health of the population must be considered. Furthermore, the potential impact of a decline in physical activity in the glucose tolerance of the hospitalized elderly is also a significant problem. For all these reasons, the significance of this study is questionable.

A more satisfactory methodological approach to the question of the effect of age on intravenous glucose tolerance is seen in the study by Dyck and Moorhouse.[14] These authors studied 61 volunteers, without known diabetic relatives, all of whom were within 10% of ideal body weight. Although there appeared to be a decrease in the ability of very old subjects to dispose of a glucose load (50 g/1.73 m^2), there was no obvious change up to the age of 50.

c. Tolbutamide Tolerance Tests

Two reports have dealt with the ability of tolbutamide to lower glucose concentrations in aging populations. These reports have described dissimilar results. First, Swerdloff et al.[15] showed that there was a progressive decline in the hypoglycemic effect of intravenous tolbutamide with age up to the 6th decade. These studies were carried out in 100 volunteers, aged 21 to 81 years, in whom there was no family history of diabetes, no known diabetes, nor evidence of inadequate carbohydrate intake. No analysis was made of differences in degree of obesity. On the other hand, only six subjects were more than 20% overweight, and the authors state that "within the weight limits of our study group there was no influence of obesity." In contrast, Vecchio et al.[12] determined blood glucose concentration 30 min after the oral administration of tolbutamide, and could find no correlation between the rate of fall of glucose levels and age in 166 male volunteers.

2. Animal Studies

The authors of this chapter could identify only three papers which provided data on animals studied for a time span of 12 months or more. Methodologically, the report of Klimas[16] was the most satisfactory. In this study, oral glucose tolerance tests (750 mg/kg) were performed on 24-hr fasted rats (20 rats each at 1, 3, 6, 10, 14, 18, 26, 30, and 34 months of age). Klimas stated that deterioration of oral glucose tolerance occurred within the first 6 months, but that there was no further change as rats lived to 34 months. The changes that did occur in the first 6 months were quantitatively modest, and upon inspection of the data it was possible to question if there was any real change in glucose tolerance beyond 3 months of age.

Gommers and DeGasparo[17] measured plasma glucose levels and intravenous glucose tolerance in 3-, 12-, and 24-month-old rats. There was no change in fasting glucose levels with age. However, the glucose levels 20 min after the intravenous glucose administration were significantly higher in the 12- and 24-month-old rats as compared to the 3-month-old rats. There appeared to be no significant difference between the 12- and 24-month-old rats. Unfortunately, these authors did not study rats between the ages of 3 to 12 months, and it is difficult to compare these results to those of Klimas who suggested that the changes in glucose tolerance that occur with age take place within the first 6 months of life. Furthermore, in this study rats received 1 g of glucose per kilogram body weight, which means that (on the average) 3-month-old rats received 213 mg of glucose and 12-month-old rats received 333 mg of glucose. It is certainly possible that this disparity in administered glucose could contribute to the differences in plasma glucose level attributed to the effect of age.

The third study which included rats greater than 1 year of age was that of Vranic and Pokrajac,[18] who determined plasma glucose levels in rats aged 20 days, 60 days, and 14 to 18 months. Random glucose levels following ad lib eating were similar in all age groups. At the end of a 24-hr fast the glucose level was higher in rats aged 14 to 18 months than in rats aged 60 days. On the other hand, glucose levels of 20-day-old rats and 14- to 18-month-old rats were comparable when measured at the same time point. Clearly, in order to see if there was age-associated progressive change in glucose tolerance, it would have been necessary to include a group of rats somewhere between 2 and 14 months of age.

Four other studies followed rats to 9 months of age with varying results. Thus, Hoffman et al.[19] found no change in plasma glucose levels (obtained between 9 and 10 A.M.) from rats aged 6 to 34 weeks of age, but did note that the disposal of an intravenous glucose load was impaired in 34-week-old rats as compared to 8- and 16-week-old rats. However, the number of animals was quite small, and the intravenous glucose load was administered on a per kilogram basis. Since the older rats were bigger, they received a greater challenge. As discussed earlier, the impact of differences in glucose load on the change in glucose tolerance is difficult to judge. This variable was controlled by Bracho-Romero and Reaven,[20] who compared the oral glucose tolerance of 3- and

9-month-old rats who had been matched for weight by controlling the dietary intake of the older rats as they aged. Glucose tolerance tests commenced at midday following 4 hr of food restriction. The results of this study showed a slight, but statistically significant, rise in plasma glucose response in older rats. On the other hand, Lavine and colleagues[21] found that the plasma glucose response to the intraperitoneal administration of glucose was constant from 6 to 34 weeks of age. Finally, Berdanier et al.[22] measured 16-hr fasting glucose levels in three different strains of rats at 50, 100, and 300 days of age with intriguing results. None of the three strains had a rise in fasting glucose level as rats aged from 50 to 100 days of age. However, one of the three strains had a significant rise in glucose level from 100 to 300 days of age, another had an intermediate elevation (of doubtful significance), while the third strain underwent trivial and clearly insignificant changes within the same duration of time.

These studies introduce the problem of comparing glucose tolerance in animals of varying sizes. It seems inappropriate to give animals of widely different sizes the same glucose load, but this is no *a priori* reason to assume that the administration of glucose on a per weight basis is any better. Studying animals of equal size by controlling the weight gain of the older ones introduces its own series of additional variables. Of even greater concern is the physical inactivity of small animals allowed to age in captivity, and this is a factor which must be taken into account in future studies.

It should be noted also that many of the described studies were carried out on animals fasted for 16 to 24 hr. This is a substantial fast for small animals, and one should consider the fact that prolonged fasting is accompanied by increased rates of gluconeogenesis which can alter plasma glucose levels. Finally, the possibility that different inbred strains of small animals may respond differently to the effect of age should receive further attention.

B. Age, Glucose Intolerance, and Diabetes Mellitus

The results reviewed so far provide some evidence for the notion that the deterioration of glucose tolerance that occurs with age is not entirely due to other variables such as obesity, chronic disease, etc. On the other hand, these data do not necessarily indicate that the observed changes represent a general phenomenon which is a simple function of age. Instead, it is possible that at least some portion of the decline in glucose tolerance seen with aging is due to the fact that an increased number of patients develop diabetes as a function of age.[23] Indeed, there is evidence that this may well occur. Both the Pima Indians of Arizona and the Nauruans of Micronesia have an extremely high incidence of diabetes, and in these populations it is possible to document bimodality of the plasma glucose response to oral glucose.[24,25] Demonstration of bimodality permits objective criteria to be used in the separation of patients at every age into two components: a lower component, presumed to consist of individuals with normal glucose tolerance, and an upper one, which includes patients with diabetes. In both of these populations, the proportion of individuals in the second component increased markedly with age. Furthermore, the magnitude of the deterioration in glucose tolerance that occurs with age was greatly attenuated when those individuals within the second component were removed from the analysis. Thus, in these populations there appear to be two factors which contribute to the glucose intolerance of aging. The first represents a generalized phenomenon which affects the majority of individuals as they age. The second factor is the development of a specific disease, diabetes, in many subjects, and it appears to be this latter event which primarily accounts for the observed deterioration of glucose tolerance that occurs in the whole of the two populations.

Bimodality of glucose tolerance has not been demonstrated in any Caucasian population studied to date, and this makes it much harder to assess the role that an age-related increase in the development of diabetes might play in the glucose intolerance of aging. On the other hand, there are some data which strongly suggest that this phenomenon may also contribute to the deterioration of glucose tolerance that has been noted in Caucasian populations. Kaufmann et al.[26] determined blood glucose values in 16,699 volunteers as part of a joint detection program for tuberculosis and diabetes. Blood was drawn on subjects who claimed to have been fasted for at least 90 min. Ages ranged from 21 to over 80, and the subjects were divided into 13 groups on the basis of age. The blood glucose values within each age group were broken down by percentile into 1, 5, 25, 50, 75, 95, and 99%. (The one percentile is that blood glucose level below which 1% and above which 99% of the values lie, whereas the 99 percentile is the converse.) These authors noted a distinct rise in glucose level of the 99 and 95 percentile with increasing age in both sexes. The increase in the 75 percentile was quite moderate, and there was little, if any, change with age in the other percentiles. These results indicate that there is not a uniform increase in blood glucose level with age throughout the population, and suggests that the observed change in glucose level noted with age may not be a simple function of age itself. As such, these results strongly resemble those described in the Pimas[24] and the Nauruans.[25] On the basis of these observations, it seems quite likely that at least part of the change in glucose tolerance noted with age in Caucasian populations is due to the development of a disease, diabetes mellitus, that occurs more frequently in older individuals.

III. AGE AND INSULIN

If glucose tolerance deteriorates with age, it is apparent that age must also have an effect on insulin secretion and/or action. In this section an attempt will be made to review the available evidence in this regard, while at the same time emphasizing the methodological issues that must be faced in an effort to define the effect of age on these two aspects of insulin metabolism.

A. Age and Insulin Secretion

The major effort to evaluate the effect of age on insulin secretion has consisted of measurements of plasma insulin levels, either fasting or in response to oral or intravenous glucose. Many such studies have been carried out, and it would not be useful to review these in detail. The results of the majority of these studies have been collated in recent reviews[1-3] and there is a surprising degree of unanimity in the published data. A small minority of these studies suggest that age might be associated with an absolute decrease in the concentration of plasma insulin. In contrast, the majority of available information indicates that insulin levels either remain constant or actually increase as individuals age, and this is true in the fasting state or in response to either oral or intravenous glucose. The simplest interpretation of these data is that insulin secretion is unimpaired with advancing age, and a decrease in insulin secretory response cannot account for the age-related deterioration of glucose tolerance. However, this interpretation has been challenged and the following argument has been proposed.[1] Older subjects have higher blood glucose levels, and it is the blood glucose concentration which is the major stimulus for insulin release. By implication, an insulin response which is unchanged with age may actually reflect a beta cell defect. In order to respond to this issue it is necessary to separate explicitly the question of the role of insulin secretion in the glucose intolerance of aging as distinguished from the effect of age on the beta cell response to glucose. As to the first question, the available evidence seems reasonably straightforward. The vast majority of the published data indicates that age is not associated with an absolute deficiency of insulin, and older individuals appear to have higher glucose levels at any given insulin levels than do younger subjects. Given this information, it seems very difficult to attribute the glucose intolerance of aging to a beta cell defect. The only caveat to this conclusion is the possibility that older individuals secrete a molecular species of insulin which is detected by the immunoassay in a normal manner, but which has less biological activity. For example, if older subjects secrete a greater proportion of proinsulin they could have higher levels of total immunoreactive insulin, but actually have a decline in the quantity of circulating insulin. This possibility has been examined by Duckworth and Kitabchi,[27] and their results suggest that this may be the case. They determined the total immunoreactive insulin and proinsulin-like material in the plasma of 68 nonobese subjects, divided into six groups by decade (15 to 24, 25 to 34, etc.). Subjects were given a 100-g oral glucose load, and plasma concentrations of total immunoreactive insulin and proinsulin were determined 60, 90, and 120 min later. The summed concentration of proinsulin-like material was similar in the 15- to 24-, 25- to 34-, and 35- to 44-year age groups. However, a significant elevation was noted in the 45- to 54-year age group, and the same level of increase persisted in the 55- to 64- and 65- to 74-year age groups. However, the relationship of these observations to the glucose intolerance of aging is questionable. In the first place, the number of patients was relatively small (i.e., 22 in the three age groups above 45 years). Second, the proportion of proinsulin-like material to total insulin was small, the differences seen with age were moderate, and the summed total insulin response after subtracting the value for proinsulin-like material was not decreased in the older subjects. Thus, these patients seemed to have adequate amounts of biologically active insulin even though increased levels of proinsulin were also present. Third, the assay used for proinsulin-like material was an indirect one, and this feature raises further questions as to the significance of the small changes noted. However, this is an important issue conceptually, and it is essential that further consideration be given to the possibility that older individuals may secrete a form of insulin which is biologically different than the insulin of younger individuals.

The question as to the effect of age on the insulin secretory response is more complicated. As Andres and Tobin point out,[1] in order to answer this question it is necessary to determine the ability of an identical stimulus to elicit insulin release from different aged subjects. Unfortunately, this is easier said than done. Andres and Tobin[1] suggest that this can be accomplished by use of the "hyperglycemic glucose-clamp" technique, in which the plasma glucose concentration is fixed at a predetermined steady level by rapid analysis of arterial glucose concentration and by appropriate adjustments of a continuous but variable intravenous glucose infusion rate. With this approach, they have maintained steady-state plasma glucose levels at 140, 180, 220, and 300 mg/dℓ in subjects of various ages, and they state that insulin secretion is diminished at the three lower glucose levels in older as compared to younger individuals.[1] Since they argue that the stimulus to insulin secretion is the same in all subjects, beta cell sensitivity must decrease with age. But is the stimulus to insulin secretion the same? Older subjects are relatively glucose intolerant, therefore they receive less glucose intravenously than do young subjects. Thus, young individuals get a bigger glucose load, and it has been shown[28,29] that larger glucose loads lead to increased insulin independently of measured changes in plasma glucose level. Thus, it could equally well be argued that the diminished insulin secretion in older subjects during the hyperglycemic glucose-clamp is simply a function of the fact that they receive less glucose. If both glucose load and glucose level are relevant variables in determining beta cell response, the insulin secretory response of old and young subjects can only be determined when both factors are held constant. Unfortunately this experimental situation can only be attained if the glucose tolerance of the individuals is essentially identical. The authors of this chapter do not know of any unequivocal way to assess the in vivo beta cell response of older individuals if they are glucose intolerant as compared to their younger counterparts.

However, it may be possible to gain some insight concerning the effect of age on insulin secretion by studying beta cell function in vitro in experimental animals of varying ages. This approach permits equalization of the insulinogenic stimulus, as well as avoiding other variables such as intestinal glucose absorption, gastrointestinal hormones which are insulin secretagogues, etc. The authors have used this method to study the effect of age on the ultrastructure and function of isolated incubated islets from rats 2 to 18 months of age.[30] These studies demonstrated that islet volume progressively increased with age, and that the increase in beta cell number was proportionate to the increase in total volume. Islet insulin content seemed to increase proportionately more than did total beta cell number. Despite this increase in beta cell number and insulin content per islet, the islet insulin secretory response to glucose stimulation decreased with age. The degree of this progressive decline in glucose-stimulated insulin release was especially dramatic when it was related to the estimated number of beta cells in the islet.

At first, demonstration of an age-related decline in glucose-stimulated insulin release by isolated rat islets seem to be at odds with the finding that insulin secretion is normal or increased in aging man. However, it must be remembered that the pancreas is bigger in older rats, and it is possible that total pancreatic insulin release could be normal or even elevated in the face of a decrease in insulin secretion per beta cell. Support for this view can be derived from the fact that a summary[1,3] of the results of studies of the effect of age on insulin secretion in the intact rat are similar to those described in man. However, it must be emphasized that rats grow as they age, and the administration of larger loads of glucose to older (and heavier) rats means that they are receiving a greater insulinogenic stimulus. This issue has been discussed in detail in a recent report[20] in which the plasma insulin response to the same oral glucose load (1.8 g/kg) in 3- and 9-month-old rats was compared. This could be done by restricting the dietary intake of the older rats by maintaining their weight from approximately 2 to 8 months of age. They were then allowed free access to food until studied at 9 months. Results indicated that both the plasma glucose and insulin response of the older rats were somewhat greater than that of the younger rats. However, it is impossible to ascertain the effect on insulin secretion of several months of caloric restriction and weight maintenance. It would seem the best way to define the effect of age on total pancreatic insulin secretion, as distinct from insulin secretion per beta cell, would be to study the effect of age on the insulin secretory capacity of the perfused intact pancreas. Good techniques exist for this procedure, and it offers many of the same advantages of the isolated islet.

B. Age and Insulin Action

The fact that the glucose intolerance of aging is associated with normal to elevated levels of circulating insulin led to the natural assumption that the cause of the glucose intolerance is resistance to the action of insulin. One possible explanation for the development of insulin resistance with age could be the secretion of a molecular species of insulin which is normally immunoreactive, but which has diminished biological activity. For example, older subjects could secrete more proinsulin, and this subject has been dealt with previously.

Another possibility is that the tissues of older individuals do not respond to their insulin as well as do the tissues of younger individuals. Attempts have been made to study this alternative in both man and animal, but the results to date are far from convincing. This is partly due to the fact that not much work has been done in this area, and partly to the methodological problems with the studies that have been conducted.

The report by Silverstone et al.[31] is most often quoted as demonstrating that age leads to a loss of normal insulin sensitivity, and it provides strong support for this notion. These authors studied the disappearance rate of an intravenous glucose load administered in conjunction with insulin. Selected for investigation were 35 male individuals age 23 to 86 years. They were divided into three age groups: young (mean age: 31), middle-aged (mean age: 49), and old (mean age: 79). The mean disappearance rate of intravenous glucose administered along with insulin was significantly higher (p < 0.01) in young (6.4%) as compared to old (2.5%) individuals. However, most of the loss of insulin sensitivity was already present in the middle-aged group, in whom the disappearance rate was 3.64%. The only drawbacks to the study are the relatively small number of patients examined (11 to 12 per age group), and the fact they were drawn from an inpatient population. Although all patients were said to be ambulatory, it is difficult to evaluate the effect of prior disease and physical activity on the results.

In contrast, three other studies have indicated that they were unable to demonstrate a loss of normal insulin sensitivity in man as a function of age. Martin et al.[32] determined the blood glucose response to intravenous insulin in 39 nonobese siblings of juvenile-onset diabetics. The patients' ages were between 21 and 64 years, and these authors could find no correlation between age and glucose tolerance or insulin sensitivity in this population. Similarly, Kalk et al.[33] found that the fall in blood glucose response to intravenous insulin in 30 older subjects (mean age: 76) was comparable to that seen in 26 young individuals (mean age: 38). Furthermore, the fasting plasma glucose levels of the two groups were similar. Recently, a somewhat more complicated approach has been used to answer the same question.[7] Insulin resistance was estimated as the steady-state plasma glucose value during a continuous infusion of epinephrine, propranolol, insulin, and glucose. Epinephrine and propranolol inhibit endogenous insulin release, and the infusion of insulin allows the same steady-state level of exogenous insulin to be attained in all subjects. Under these conditions, the height of the steady-state plasma glucose volume becomes a direct estimate of each patient's efficiency of insulin-stimulated glucose uptake. This technique was employed in 100 nonobese male volunteers, aged 21 to 69 years. No increase in insulin resistance with age in this population could be demonstrated, but the absence of an age-related increase in plasma glucose levels 2 hr after the patients received an oral glucose load was also noted.

The fact that none of the last three studies described could document an age-related loss of insulin sensitivity should not be too surprising since it appeared that none of these populations demonstrated a decline in glucose tolerance with aging in the first place. In contrast, Silverstone et al.[31] could document a loss of glucose tolerance in the same older subjects who were also less insulin sensitive. it would seem reasonable that future studies be aimed at quantitating the effect of age on insulin sensitivity in subjects who both have, and have not, shown a decline in glucose tolerance with age. In this regard, the "euglycemic clamp"[1] may provide the most useful approach. With this technique a priming dose of insulin is used to elevate plasma insulin level to a desired degree, and then a continuous insulin infusion is used to maintain the new level constant throughout the study. At the same time, glucose is infused in whatever amount is required to maintain the basal glucose concentrations. Under these conditions, the amount of infused glucose required to maintain euglycemia is a direct estimate of insulin sensitivity. By the use of this technique, and by varying the insulin level, it should be possible to construct an insulin-dose response curve in subjects of different ages. It is interesting in this regard that Andres and Tobin[1] state that this technique has indicated that there are no differences in insulin sensitivity as a function of age. In contrast, Davidson[3] quoted unpublished data from DeFronzo which demonstrate that insulin sensitivity decreases with age. Unfortunately, in neither case are the data published, and it is impossible to comment upon this apparent discrepancy. Indeed, what is really clear from the preceding discussion is the need for a serious evaluation of the effect of age on insulin sensitivity.

IV. CONCLUSIONS

On the basis of the data discussed in this presentation, it is apparent that the glucose intolerance of aging is not a simple phenomenon and that many factors contribute to the age-related changes that have been described. Of particular importance is the fact that older individuals frequently have chronic diseases, they are often overweight, and they are often not physically active. These factors all adversely modify glucose tolerance, and they have often been ignored in studies of the effect of age on glucose tolerance. There is no doubt that they are, at least partly, responsible for the dramatic changes in glucose tolerance that have been described in earlier reports. However, even if attention is confined to studies which have controlled for these variables, it is clear that considerable disagreement exists as to the effect of age on glucose tolerance. The problem is further compounded by the fact that the incidence of diabetes increases with age, and it seems quite likely that a significant portion of the deterioration in glucose tolerance attributed to aging is due to the development of diabetes. Indeed, one could take an extreme position and state that age itself, as differentiated from the effects of obesity, diabetes, etc., has a relatively trivial effect on glucose tolerance, and that even this effect is largely confined to patients over 60. The true effect of age on glucose tolerance probably lies somewhere between this estimate and one based on earlier studies where age-related variables were not controlled. Additional large-scale studies in man, in which every effort is made to control for various environmental variables, would certainly help clarify the situation.

On the other hand, the ability to approach this problem experimentally in man is greatly limited by the absence of any objective marker for diabetes, and in the absence of such a definition, the effect of age on glucose tolerance will always be overestimated. In this regard, the use of aging animals would appear to offer considerable advantage. Up to now, relatively little information has been derived from this approach. Although there are some methodological issues that need to be recognized in studying animals which are both growing and aging, these problems can be controlled, and valuable insights would be gained by well-conducted studies.

The question of the effect of age on insulin secretion and insulin action is less complex, and the major difficulty here appears to be lack of data. There is general agreement that the total insulin response to glucose does not decrease with age, and it appears that the glucose intolerance of aging is not due to insulin deficiency. However, information on the true impact of age on the glucose-induced insulin response is lacking; there are no published studies in which the glucose stimulation used was entirely comparable in young and old subjects. Similarly, information as to the effect of age on insulin action in man or animal is greatly limited. The methodological issues that must be faced in order to arrive at useful data on these subjects have been discussed in earlier sections and are not exessively demanding. As such, there is every reason to anticipate that relevant data will soon be available.

Finally, it should be pointed out that although age may have a less dramatic effect on glucose tolerance than previously believed, the changes that do occur are undeniably related to morbidity and mortality. Hopefully, the more learned about age-related changes in glucose and insulin metabolism, the more ability there will be to intervene at early time points to minimize the deleterious effect of these changes.

REFERENCES

1. **Andres, R. and Tobin, J. D.,** Endocrine systems, in *Handbook of Biology of Aging,* Finch, C. E. and Hayflick, L., Eds., Van Nostrand-Reinhold, New York, 1977, 357.
2. **Reaven, G.,** Does age affect glucose tolerance? *Geriatrics,* 32, 51, 1977.
3. **Davidson, M.,** The effect of aging on carbohydrate metabolism: a review of the English literature and a practical approach to the diagnosis of diabetes mellitus in the elderly, *Metabolism,* 28, 688, 1979.
4. **Wingerd, J. and Duffy, T. J.,** Oral contraceptive use and other factors in the standard glucose tolerance test, *Diabetes,* 26, 1024, 1977.
5. **Nolan, S., Thorsten, S., Chae, C., Vidalon, C., Gegick, C., Khurana, R. and Danowski, T. S.,** Age-related insulin patterns in normal glucose tolerance, *J. Am. Geriatr. Soc.,* 21, 106, 1973.
6. **Boyns, D. R., Crossley, J. N., Abrams, M. E., Jarrett, R. J., and Keen, H.,** Oral glucose tolerance and related factors in a normal population sample, *Br. Med. J.,* March 8, 595, 1969.
7. **Kimmerling, G., Javorski, W. C., and Reaven, G. M.,** Aging and insulin resistance in a group of nonobese male volunteers, *J. Am. Geriatr. Soc.,* 25, 349, 1977.
8. **Rehfeld, J. R. and Stadil, F.,** The glucose-induced gastrointestinal stimulation of insulin secretion in man: relation to age and gastrin release, *Eur. J. Clin. Invest.,* 5, 273, 1975.
9. **Berger, D., Crowther, R. C., Floyd, J. C., Pek, S., and Fajans, S. S.,** Effect of age on fasting plasma levels of pancreatic hormones in man, *J. Clin. Endocrinol. Metab.,* 47, 1183, 1978.
10. **O'Sullivan, J. B., Mahan, C. M., Freedlender, A. E., and Williams, R. F.,** Effect of age on carbohydrate metabolism, *J. Clin. Endocrinol. Metab.,* 33, 619, 1971.
11. **Nilsson, S. E., Lindhom, H., Bulow, S., Frostberg, N., Emilsson, T., and Steinkula, G.,** The Kristianstad survey, *Acta Med. Scand. Suppl.,* 428, 1, 1964.
12. **Vecchio, T. J., Oster, H. L., and Smith, D. L.,** Oral sodium tolbutamide and glucose tolerance tests, *Arch. Intern. Med.,* 115, 161, 1965.
13. **Franckson, J. R. M., Malaise, W., Arnould, Y., Rasio, E., Ooms, H. A., Balasse, E., Conard, V., and Bastenie, P. A.,** Glucose kinetics in human obesity, *Diabetologia,* 2, 96, 1966.
14. **Dyck, D. R. and Moorhouse, J. A.,** A high-dose intravenous glucose tolerance test, *J. Clin. Endocrinol. Metab.,* 26, 1032, 1966.
15. **Swerdloff, R. S., Pozefsky, T., Tobin, J. D., and Andres, R.,** Influence of age on the intravenous tolbutamide response test, *Diabetes,* 16, 161, 1967.
16. **Klimas, J. E.,** Oral glucose tolerance during the life span of a colony of rats, *J. Gerontol.,* 23, 31, 1968.
17. **Gommers, A. and DeGasparo, M.,** Variation de l'insulinemie en fonction de l'age chez le rat male non traite, *Gerontologia,* 18, 176, 1972.
18. **Vranic, M. and Pokrajac, N.,** The effect of age and fasting on blood sugar level in normal and adrenalectomized rats, *J. Gerontol.,* 16, 110, 1961.
19. **Hoffmann, C. C., Carroll, K. F., and Goldrick, R. B.,** Studies on lipid and carbohydrate metabolism in the rat: effects of diet on body composition, plasma glucose and insulin concentrations, insulin secretion in vitro and tolerance to intravenous glucose and intravenous insulin, *Austr. J. Exp. Biol. Med Sci.,* 50, 267, 1972.
20. **Bracho-Romero, E. and Reaven, G. M.,** Effect of age and weight on plasma glucose and insulin responses in the rat, *J. Am. Geriatr. Soc.,* 25, 299, 1977.
21. **Lavine, R. L., Chick, W. L., Like, A. A., and Makdisi, T. W.,** Glucose tolerance and insulin secretion in neonatal and adult mice, *Diabetes,* 20, 34, 1971.
22. **Berdanier, C. D., Marshall, M. W., and Moser, P.,** Age changes in the level of serum immunoreactive insulin in three strains of rats, *Life Sci.,* 10, 105, 1971.
23. **O'Sullivan, J. B.,** Age gradient in blood glucose levels, *Diabetes,* 23, 713, 1974.
24. **Rushforth, N. B., Bennett, P. H., Steinberg, A. G., Burch, T. A., and Miller, M.,** Diabetes in the Pima Indians, *Diabetes,* 20, 756, 1971.
25. **Zimmet, P. and Whitehouse, S.,** The effect of age on glucose tolerance: studies in a Micronesian population with a high prevalence of diabetes, *Diabetes,* 28, 617, 1979.
26. **Kaufmann, B. J., Grant, D. R., and Moorhouse, J. A.,** An analysis of blood glucose values in a population screened for diabetes mellitus, *Can. Med. Assoc. J.,* 100, 692, 1969.
27. **Duckworth, W. C. and Kitabchi, A. E.,** The effect of age on plasma proinsulin-like material after oral glucose, *J. Lab. Clin. Med.,* 88, 359, 1976.
28. **Peterson, D. T. and Reaven, G. M.,** Evidence that glucose load is an important determinant of plasma insulin response in normal subjects, *Diabetes,* 20, 729, 1971.
29. **Olefsky, J. M., Batchelder, T., Farquhar, J. W., and Reaven, G. M.,** Dissociation of the plasma insulin response from the blood glucose concentration during glucose infusions in normal dogs, *Metabolism,* 22, 1277, 1973.

30. **Reaven, E. P., Gold, G., and Reaven, G. M.,** Effect of age on glucose-stimulated insulin release by the beta cell of the rat, *J. Clin. Invest.,* 64, 591, 1979.

31. **Silverstone, F. A., Brandfonbrener, M., Shock, N. W., and Yiengst, M. J.,** Age differences in the intravenous glucose tolerance tests and the response to insulin, *J. Clin. Invest.,* 36, 504, 1957.

32. **Martin, F. I. R., Pearson, M. J., and Stocks, A. E.,** Glucose tolerance and insulin insensitivity, *Lancet,* 1, 1285, 1968.

33. **Kalk, W. J., Vinik, A. I., Pimstone, B. L., and Jackson, W. P. U.,** Growth hormone response to insulin hypoglycemia in the elderly, *J. Gerontol.,* 28, 431, 1973.

Chapter 2

AN IN VITRO SYSTEM FOR INVESTIGATION OF EFFECTS OF AGING ON THE REGULATION OF INSULIN SECRETION*

James L. Sartin, Eva A. Sartin, Bennett J. Cohen, and Richard C. Adelman**

TABLE OF CONTENTS

* Supported in part by grants AG-00368 and AG-00034 from the National Institutes of Health.
**Forward all inquiries to Dr. Adelman at the Institute on Aging, Temple University, 1601 N. Broad Street, Philadelphia, Pa., 19122.

I. INTRODUCTION

The impaired response by hepatic glucokinase activity to administration of glucose in aging rats[1] in large part reflects an altered pattern of glucose-stimulated secretion of insulin.[2,3] This was ascertained by isolating pancreatic islets of Langerhans from rats of different ages and challenging them in vitro by varying the concentration of glucose in the perifusion medium. Perifused, isolated islets provide a unique opportunity to study in an in vitro system, a phenomenon that characterizes intact organisms as they age. In order to do so appropriately, the system requires rigorous definition. As an in vitro system for the study of insulin secretion by young adults, perifused pancreatic islets are extremely well defined and in frequent use throughout the world. However, as the host from which the islet preparation is derived ages, there are important differences in functional behavior and methodological requirements, ignorance of which precludes the generation of valid data. The purpose of this article is to discuss the differences which characterize the perifused islet preparation as it is isolated and utilized from host rats of increasing age. Implications of experimental data were reviewed recently.[6]

II. METHODOLOGY

A. Materials

The enzyme used for digesting pancreas is a crude collagenase preparation which may be obtained from several companies. Collagenase type IV (Worthington®) and type V (Sigma®) were used successfully for digesting tissue from 24-month-old, male Sprague-Dawley rats. Collagenase is ordered in 100 mg batches and tested for its effectiveness. The activity of collagenase varies tremendously between batches. Therefore, each new order must be tested to determine the amount of enzyme per milliliter volume of tissue needed to effect a proper digestion. If a particular batch of collagenase proves suitable, a large quantity of the enzyme having the same lot number is obtained. Collagenase is stored frozen in dessicators in approximately 30 mg batches to insure long-term stability.

Hanks solution[4] is the buffer used to prepare and isolate the islets of Langerhans (see islet isolation procedure). The buffer is prepared fresh each day or may be purchased (GIBCO) and is adjusted to pH 7.4 with $NaHCO_3$ (7 g/100 mℓ). Buffer for room temperature washes is set aside and the remainder is refrigerated until use.

The perifusion media is Krebs ringer bicarbonate (KRB). Stock solutions of the salts are made fresh each week. Bovine serum albumen (BSA) is dialysed (higher quality BSA may be used without dialysis) against KRB and stored frozen. The buffer salts are added (except $CaCl_2$) and diluted with demineralized, distilled water to the final concentrations shown: NaCl (115 mM), $MgCl$ (1 mM), KH_2PO_4 (1.5 mM), KCl (5 mM), and Na HCO_3 (21 mM). $CaCl_2$ (2.0 mM) is added last and slowly to prevent formation of insoluble calcium salts. The KRB is gassed for 15 min with 95% O_2, 5% CO_2. BSA is added to a final concentration of 2%, the solution is filtered, and O_2 and CO_2 bubbled lightly through the buffer. This buffer is used to dissolve the test substances (i.e., glucose) which are placed in a 37° C water bath and gassed with 95% O_2, 5% CO_2 throughout the perifusion procedure. The perifusion chambers (Millipore®) are connected by tubing to a reservoir of KRB and a peristaltic pump. The perifusion chamber is submerged in a constant temperature water bath (37° C) and the perifusate is collected in 15 mℓ plastic tubes in a fraction collector (Figure 1).

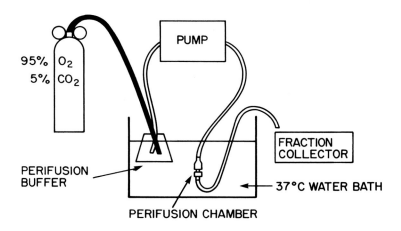

FIGURE 1. Simplified schematic of the perifusion system.

B. Isolation of Tissue

The rat is sacrificed by decapitation and a midline incision made with scissors. The rib cage is then removed to provide easy access to the bile duct with a syringe and needle. This is particularly useful in the larger sized old (24 month) rats. Before proceeding further, it is necessary to carefully check the pancreas for possible tumors (Figure 2). The 24-month-old male Sprague-Dawley rat, for example, has 18% incidence of pancreatic islet cell tumors.[5] Many of these tumors are insulin-secreting and in vitro data from the authors' laboratory indicate that the tumor tissue secretes insulin at a constant rate which is not under the influence of changes in glucose concentration. If a possible tumor is found, the pancreas is discarded. The possibility of microscopic islet cell tumors cannot be discounted and it is a good idea to clamp a section of pancreas so that it is not distended, place the tissue in 10% buffered formalin, and save for histologic examination. The final criterion will ultimately depend on the quality of the islet response to glucose. If the pancreas appears normal for an old rat, a 35 mm forcep is placed at the junction of the common bile duct and the duodenum so as to occlude the bile duct. A suture is placed around the bile duct between the pancreas and the branches of the bile duct leaving the liver. A slit is placed in the common bile duct above the suture and a blunted 22-gauge needle (a 25-gauge may be useful in the smaller 2-month-old rats) attached to a 30-cc syringe is inserted in the opening. The suture is tied around the bile duct and the needle. The pancreas is slowly distended with cold Hanks solution injected into the common bile duct. In young animals, 15 mℓ of Hanks is sufficient to completely inflate the pancreas, but 20 mℓ or more may be required for the older rat pancreas due to its larger size. It is sometimes difficult to completely distend the pancreas from a 24-month-old rat. If small areas of the pancreas are not distended, these may be carefully removed. Failure to distend portions of the pancreas may be partially avoided by slowly injecting the Hanks and by careful placement of the 35 mm forcep to occlude only the common bile duct.

The fat adhering to the pancreas is carefully trimmed and the pancreas removed by blunt dissection with scissors. Again, the old animal is more of a problem due to having a greater mass of fat. The pancreas from each of three young rats or two old rats provides sufficient volume of starting material for the digestion procedure. After removal, the pancreases are placed in a 50 mℓ plastic beaker, drained of excess fluid, and finely minced with scissors. After the mincing is complete, the beaker is filled with

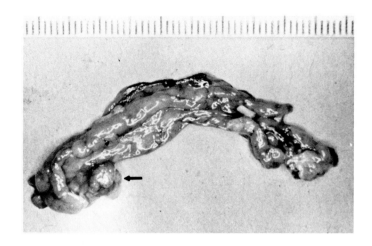

A

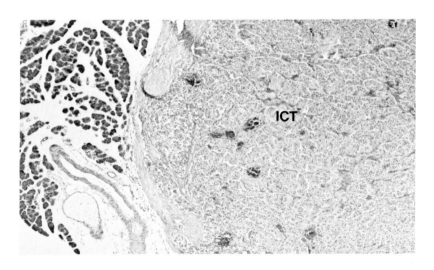

B

FIGURE 2. Gross appearance of an islet cell tumor in a pancreas from a 24-month-old Sprague-Dawley rat (A). Histologic sections of an islet cell tumor (B) and an abnormal islet (C) from 24-month-old Sprague-Dawley rats. (Hematoxylin-eosin.)

cold Hanks solution. Fat tissue will float to the top and may be removed by suction with a pasteur pipette. The remaining fluid is drained and the minced tissue is washed a second time. Equal portions of the minced pancreatic tissue are decanted into 15 mℓ graduated conical centrifuge tubes. Plastic tubes are used because islets may adhere to untreated glass. A volume of 2.0 mℓ of Hanks is maintained above the tissue. Collagenase (3 mg/mℓ of tissue; see previous section on collagenase) is added, the tubes are stoppered and mixed, and 95% O_2, 5% CO_2 is bubbled through the mixture for 30 sec. The tubes are stoppered, immersed in a water bath (37° C) and shaken vigorously by hand until the digestion is complete. With the collagenase now being used (Sigma®, type V) the time for digestion of the pancreatic material from young animals is 4 min.

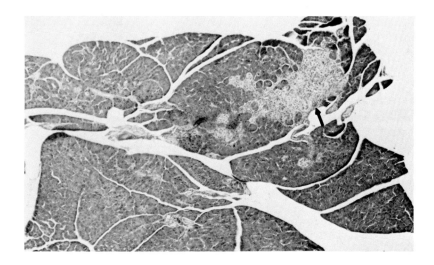

FIGURE 2C

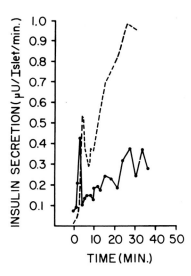

FIGURE 3. Patterns of insulin secretion in overdigested and normal islets
of Langerhans in perifusion. Solid line
indicates insulin secretion from overdigested islets.

The pancreas from older rats requires 0.5 to 1.0 additional minutes of digestion time
as compared to the young. The time and quality of the digestion will vary depending
on the age of donor animals, the activity of the collagenase preparation, amount of
collagenase used, and how vigorously the solutions are shaken.

Generally, if the digestion procedure is performed well, the perifusion will function
properly. A failure of the biphasic insulin response to occur probably results from an
overdigestion of the islets. The overdigestion of islets results in fewer islets present and
all of these are not completely intact islets. There also may be a near total lack of the
large-sized islets and the presence of islet tissue remnants (islet ghosts) which appear

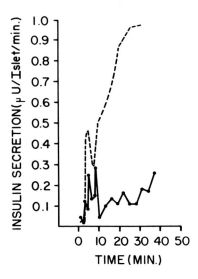

FIGURE 4. Patterns of insulin secretion from islets of Langerhans isolated in properly buffered Hanks solution and a Hanks solution with insufficient buffering capacity. Solid line indicates insulin release from poorly digested islets. The pH of the poorly buffered Hanks was adjusted with 1 M NaOH rather than 7% $NaHCO_3$.

as a fuzzy outline of an islet. The secretion pattern is blunter or there is a complete absence of the normal biphasic pattern of secretion (Figure 3). Likewise, an alteration in Hanks solution such as pH or lack of calcium may contribute to a poor digestion. If the pH of the Hanks solution is adjusted with NaOH rather than Na_2HCO_3, there is an insufficient buffering capacity for the digestion and the perifusion of these islets (Figure 4) results in a diminished second-phase secretion of insulin.

Islets may also appear underdigested. In this condition the full size range of islets appears in the field of view, however, most of the islets are surrounded by partially digested pancreatic tissue. Clean, intact islets may be chosen and these will respond properly to a glucose challenge. In the event that an insufficient number of islets are obtained, the partially digested islets and tissue may be recombined, centrifuged, excess Hanks removed, and the islets redigested. A second digestion should be performed with approximately 25% of the amount of collagenase used for the first digestion and for a duration of 15 sec.[9] This procedure will work for islets from old rats, although care must be taken in the digestion and selection of only intact islets.

At the end of the digestion, the solutions are diluted with approximately 9 mℓ Hanks solution at room temperature and centrifuged for 10 sec at 3000 rpm. The supernatant is decanted, replaced with fresh Hanks, mixed, and centrifuged for 15 sec at 2000 rpm. The pellet is again washed with fresh Hanks and centrifuged for 20 sec at 1000 rpm. The centrifugations are at room temperature and the times and speeds of centrifugation are easily altered with little effect on the islets. Following the third centrifugation, the islets are diluted with Hanks and mixed. A small amount of the digested material is decanted to plastic petri dishes with blackened bottoms and diluted with Hanks solution.

Islets appear in a wide range of sizes (Figure 5) and are selected by size using a

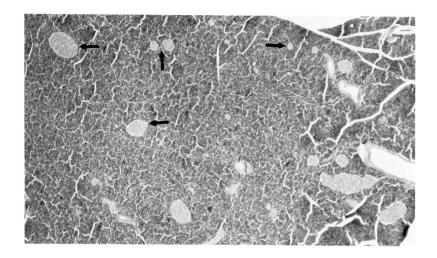

FIGURE 5. The presence of various sized isolated islets of Langerhans from 2-month-old Sprague-Dawley rats.

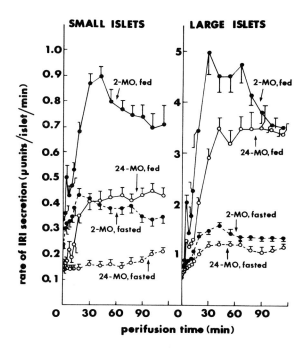

FIGURE 6. The rate of IRI secretion is calculated from the concentration of IRI in serially collected perifusates of islets of the indicated sizes isolated from rats of the indicated ages and nutritional status. Each value represents the mean ± standard error for four islet preparations. Each preparation consists of 50 to 100 islets collected and pooled from separate groups of 2 to 3 rats. (From Kitahara, A. and Adelman, R. C., *Biochem. Biophys. Res. Commun.*, 87, 1207, 1979. With permission.)

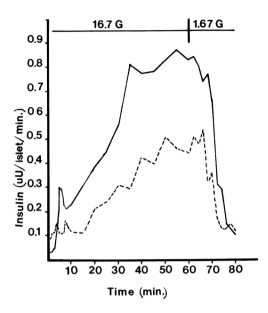

FIGURE 7. Reduction of insulin secretion after changing the glucose concentration from a stimulatory (16.7 mM) to a nonstimulatory (1.67 mM) level. Solid line indicates insulin secretion from islets isolated from young fed rats, dotted line represents secretion from islets from old fed rats.

calibrated eye-piece micrometer. When performing an aging study, the size of the islets chosen is crucial. The number of large islets increases as the animal ages[6,7] and large islets isolated from old rats are hypertrophied (Figure 2) and are larger than the largest sized islets from young rats.[3,7,8] Most importantly, the large islets secrete significantly greater quantities of insulin than do small islets[3] (Figure 6). Thus the use of randomly selected islets can confuse the data when comparing insulin secretion by islets from young vs. old rats. Suitable islets free of acinar tissue are transferred to a small petri dish using a pipette with a plastic tip. The islets are then transferred to a second petri dish (to minimize contamination with nonislet pancreatic tissue) containing KRB at room temperature plus 2.75 mM glucose which is kept oxygenated until needed. Three or four perifusions are performed from each digestion, so four groups of 100 small (50 large) islets are transferred 10 (or 5 for large islets) islets at a time to the second petri dish.

C. Perifusion of Isolated Islets

Filters (Millipore®; 5.0 μm-pore diameter, type SM) are wetted with KRB and seated on the perifusion chamber. A group of 100 islets is transferred to the filter, the chamber is sealed and filled with KRB (37° C) and the chamber attached to tubing from the peristaltic pump (after the pump is engaged). The chamber is inverted to clear air trapped in the chamber. The perifusion chamber is submerged in the water bath and collection of nonstimulated insulin secretion begins at 5-min intervals for 30 min and for 1-min intervals for 10 min. At the end of the control pre-perifusion, the concentration of glucose reaching the islets is raised to 16.7 mM (300 mg %). The perifusate is collected at 1.0-min intervals for 10 min to allow the detection of first-phase secretion which occurs at 4 to 5 min following the glucose change (1 to 2 min are required for the concentration of glucose bathing the islets to equilibrate at 16.7 mm) in islets from young rats and 5 to 6 min for islets from old rats.[3] After the first 10 min of stimulatory glucose, the collection interval is increased to 5 min. The total time for perifusion with 16.7 mm glucose is usually 30 to 60 min to achieve peak second-phase secretion. The perifusate is collected with a fraction collector in 15 mℓ plastic tubes containing 100 units of a protease inhibitor, Trasylol® (Calbiochem). The presence of Trasylol® is not critical for studies of insulin secretion, however samples should be kept on ice and frozen to insure stability of the samples.

Insulin content of the sample is assessed by a solid phase radioimmunoassay.[3]

An appropriate preparation of isolated, perifused small islets should respond to a stimulatory level of glucose (16.7 mM) with a biphasic pattern of insulin secretion, as well as a return to baseline secretion rates subsequent to reduction of the glucose concentration in the perifusion medium to 1.67 mM (Figure 7). Subsequent elevation of the glucose concentration in the perifusion medium to 16.7 mM should elicit the normal pattern of stimulated insulin secretion that was observed originally.

ACKNOWLEDGMENT

The authors would like to thank Dr. W. S. Zawalich, Yale University, for demonstrating his islet isolation and perifusion techniques.

REFERENCES

1. **Adelman, R. C.** An age-dependent modification of enzyme regulation, *J. Biol. Chem.*, 245, 1032, 1970.
2. **Gold, G., Karoly, K., Freeman, C., and Adelman, R. C.,** A possible role for insulin in the altered capability for hepatic enzyme adaption during aging, *Biochem. Biophys. Res. Commun.*, 73, 1003, 1976.
3. **Kitahara, A. and Adelman, R. C.,** Altered regulation of insulin secretion in isolated islets of different sizes in aging rats, *Biochem. Biophys. Res. Commun.*, 87, 1207, 1979.
4. **Lacy, P. E., Young, D. A., and Fink, C. J.,** Studies on insulin secretion in vitro from isolated islets of the rat pancreas, *Endocrinology*, 83, 1155, 1968.
5. **Cohen, B. J., Anver, M. R., Ringler, D. H., and Adelman, R. C.,** Age-associated pathological changes in male rats, *Fed. Proc. Am. Fed. Soc. Exp. Biol.*, 37, 2848, 1978.
6. **Sartin, J., Chaudhuri, M., Obenrader, M., and Adelman, R. C.,** The role of hormones in changing adaptive mechanisms during aging, *Fed. Proc. Am. Fed. Soc. Exp. Biol.*, 39, 3163, 1980.
7. **Remacle, C., Hauser, N., Jeanjean, M., and Gommers, G.,** Morphometric analysis of endocrine pancreas in old rats, *Exp. Gerontol.*, 12, 207, 1977.
8. **Reaven, R. P., Gold, G., and Reaven, G. M.,** Effect of age on glucose-stimulated insulin release by the B-cell of the rat, *J. Clin. Invest.*, 64, 591, 1979.
9. **Zawalich, W. S.,** personal communication.

Chapter 3

CYCLIC NUCLEOTIDE METABOLISM AND ACTION
DURING SENESCENCE

Charles R. Filburn

TABLE OF CONTENTS

I. INTRODUCTION

Identification of changes occurring during senescence in the capacity of various tissues to respond to external stimuli which are believed to act, at least in part, by elevating intracellular levels of cyclic AMP or cyclic GMP, has and continues to be an active and productive area of research. Trying to describe "state of the art" methodology that is appropriate for these studies represents a considerable task. A thorough study of factors involved in changes during senescence could necessitate assaying tissue levels of cyclic nucleotides, adenylate or guanylate cyclase, cyclic nucleotide phosphodiesterase, cyclic nucleotide dependent protein kinase, phosphoprotein phosphatase, and assessment of changes in phosphorylation of relevant proteins. The methodology involved in all of these areas has advanced considerably in the past decade, as reflected by an entire volume of the *Methods in Enzymology* series[2] and a later volume of *Advances in Cyclic Nucleotide Research*[1] devoted to these subjects. Since so much information is now available in this form, a detailed, recipe-like presentation of the methods needed for aging studies of cyclic nucleotide metabolism and action would be both redundant and prohibitively lengthy. In a review of the nature and size appropriate for the present volume, the approach taken will be first to establish a framework within which questions of altered responsiveness should be answered, and then to emphasize those points in the methods discussed which, from the author's viewpoint, are most relevant but may not have been mentioned or were not sufficiently emphasized in the two volumes mentioned above. The comments made reflect, in part, personal preferences resulting from the author's first-hand experience with some of the methods discussed. Equally acceptable, alternative procedures will be mentioned where appropriate.

Given that a physiological response to a stimulus acting via a cyclic nucleotide has changed during senescence, the immediate question to be answered is whether the stimulus induced the usual elevation in the intracellular cellular level of the cyclic nucleotide. Another indirect way of answering this is to assess the degree of in vivo activation of the cyclic nucleotide-dependent protein kinase. This approach is especially valuable in that it may more accurately reflect intracellular levels of the nucleotide, perhaps even within a compartment of the cell where the nucleotide is most active.

If changes in cyclic nucleotide level or protein kinase activation are found, cyclase and/or phosphodiesterase activities need to be assessed. If not, cyclic nucleotide-dependent protein kinase and/or phosphoprotein phosphatase activity levels must be measured. This basic recurring question in cases of altered responsiveness of changes in enzyme activity is usually answered in terms of "total activity," involving assays under optimal conditions for maximal activity. Frequently, the more relevent but less answered question is that of "functional activity," which necessitates assays simulating in vivo conditions of substrate and regulator concentrations. Since cytosolic protein "modulators" are now known for cyclases, phosphodiesterases, protein kinases, and phosphoprotein phosphatases, this additional complication must be considered. In the discussion of the assays that follow, each of these factors will be discussed in terms of the technical problems that exist in assessing functional activity.

Finally, the possibility exists that no changes in elevated cyclic nucleotide levels or enzyme activities will be associated with an altered response. Since cyclic nucleotides are considered to act principally, if not exclusively, through protein kinase-catalyzed phosphorylation of one or more proteins,[3] the key may be the level of the relevant endogenous protein substrate presumed to directly account for, as a consequence of altered activity, the physiological response. Assessing both the absolute level of such proteins and their state of phosphorylation before and after exposure to a stimulus may thus be necessary. This last question has now become more complicated by the observation that several of these phosphorylatable, regulatory proteins may have multiple sites of phosphorylation, and that both cyclic nucleotide-dependent and -independent protein kinases can phosphorylate some of these sites and effect changes in functional activity.[4] The increasing role of Ca^{2+}- and a Ca^{2+}-binding protein, termed calmodulin (CaM), in regulation of this class of protein kinase, in addition to regulatory roles in both synthesis and degradation of cyclic nucleotides, necessitates some consideration of the role of Ca^{2+} in mediating or modulating the physiological response(s) in question.

In addition, it is becoming increasingly apparent that hormones and neurotransmitters acting through cell surface receptors to stimulate cyclic nucleotide synthesis cannot be viewed in isolation. Other hormones acting through different receptors, or even the same hormone acting through a separate class of receptors, may have an inhibitory effect either at the level of cyclic nucleotide generation or at a point further along in the sequence of reactions regulating the response. A general scheme to illustrate this point and other points which will be made in discussing the enzymes and modulators involved is shown in Figure 1. Stimulus B is shown to interact with a receptor and to inhibit adenylate cyclase without necessarily generating an intracellular second messenger which itself produces this effect. Stimulus C is shown to be associated with a change in intracellular Ca^{2+} which may then act, alone or in concert with calmodulin, to modulate one or more of the cytosolic and/or membrane-bound enzymes involved in cyclic nucleotide metabolism or action. Although not shown, virtually all of these enzymes are found to some extent in the plasma membrane of most tissues. As will become evident in this review, the subcellular localization of these enzymes and substrates may play an important role in their functions and thus may need to be considered to fully assess their role(s) in changes in physiological responsiveness during senescence.

II. CYCLIC NUCLEOTIDE LEVELS

In measuring cyclic nucleotide levels of a tissue at a given point in time, the tissue is usually extracted with acid (perchloric acid or TCA), thus stopping further metabolism of nucleotides. Where this is difficult or too slow, freeze clamping or heat inactivation of enzymes by microwave radiation may be more useful (see Mayer et al.[5] for a discussion of these methods). In cases where homogenization of either fresh or frozen tissue can be done very quickly, a solution containing EDTA (10 mM) and a strong phosphodiesterase inhibitor (10 mM theophylline or 1 mM isobutylmethylxanthine) at neutral pH may accomplish the same thing, while still permitting assessment of protein kinase activation[6] (see section on protein kinase activation). To assure cessation of further metabolism, particularly if samples need to be stored, aliquots of these latter extracts may be heated or extracted with acid and then neutralized.

Assays of absolute levels of cyclic nucleotides are based upon the concentration-dependent inhibition by cyclic nucleotide containing extracts of binding of either ^{3}H-cyclic nucleotide to a partially purified binding protein[7] or of an ^{125}I-cyclic nucleotide analogue to an antibody.[8] The binding protein method was developed first and, though somewhat less sensitive than the radioimmunoassay, continues to be used where high sensitivity is not required and cost is a factor. Greater sensitivity and specificity is obtained with the radioimmunoassay technique as a consequence of acetylation or succinylation of extracted cyclic nucleotides. While this may permit considerable dilution of samples and results in fewer problems of interference by reagents or unknown contaminants, the possibility of interfering substances in extracts must still be checked.[9] This is done by determining that measured levels of cyclic nucleotide are proportional

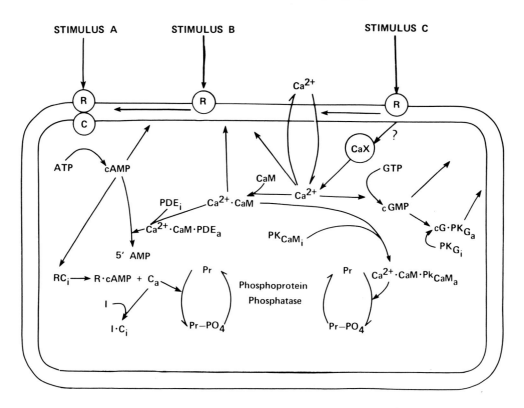

FIGURE 1. Generalized scheme of actions of interactions and stimuli regulating intracellular levels of cyclic nucleotides and Ca^{2+}. R, receptor; C, catalytic component of adenylate cyclase; RC_i, inactive cyclic AMP-dependent protein kinase; C_a, active catalytic subunit; I, protein inhibitor of catalytic subunit; PK_{CaM_i}, $Ca^{2+} \cdot CaM \cdot PK_{CaM_a}$ inactive and active $Ca^{2+} \cdot CaM$-dependent protein kinase, respectively; P_r, protein kinase substrate; CaM, calmodulin; $cG \cdot PK_{G_i}$, $cG \cdot PK_{G_a}$, inactive and active cyclic GMP-dependent protein kinase, respectively; PDE_i, $Ca^{2+} \cdot CaM \cdot PDE_a$, inactive and active $Ca^{2+} \cdot CaM$-dependent cyclic nucleotide phosphodiesterase; CaX, intracellular Ca^{2+} store.

to the amount of extract used, i.e., that the slope or shape of the inhibition curve is the same as that of a standard curve based on a pure solution of cyclic nucleotide. Where it occurs, interference may depend upon the concentration of the extract, the type of tissue extracted, or the extraction reagents. The problem is usually resolved by purification of extracts through one or a combination of chromatographic steps.[10,11] Purification may be accomplished with[11] or without neutralization of acid extracts,[10] depending on the method chosen. When the radioimmunoassay method is used, the dilution of extract occurring at this step may present no problem and alleviate the need for lyophilization and redissolution in small volumes. Analysis of the actual data may be facilitated and performed more accurately by linearization of the data, perhaps best done with a curve-fitting program described by Brooker et al.[8]

As with all of the other measurements to be discussed, the choice of denominator in expression of data may affect the outcome regarding detection of changes during senescence. The choice, whether it be wet weight, dry weight, protein, DNA, etc., should be based on the most functionally meaningful base for the tissue and/or response in question.

III. CYCLIC NUCLEOTIDE SYNTHESIS

A. Assay of Adenylate Cyclase

Measurement of adenylate cyclase activity in homogenates or membrane preparations usually entails detection of very low levels of conversion of ATP to cyclic AMP, thus necessitating use of a radioactive isotope, $[^{32}P]$-α-ATP, to detect picomole amounts of product. While use of a radioimmunoassay to measure absolute amounts offers greater sensitivity and can be used for this purpose,[8] it suffers from lack of linearity and uncertainty about product degradation. Use of $[^{32}P]$-α-ATP together with a regenerating system for maintenance of ATP concentration (creatine phosphate plus creatine phosphokinase or phosphoenolpyruvate plus pyruvate kinase), and a phosphodiesterase inhibitor (theophylline or isobutylmethylxanthine) plus an excess of unlabeled cyclic AMP to minimize degradation of newly synthesized ^{32}P-cyclic AMP, has become the method of choice. The problem of removal of substrate and metabolites during isolation of product has been solved most effectively by two-step chromatography of samples, first through a cation-exchange resin, then alumina.[12,13] Very low blanks and high recovery of product, plus the ability to reuse columns, makes this procedure the method of choice.

The use of regenerating systems to maintain ATP concentrations is not without its problems. Metal chelation by phosphoenolpyruvate may result in inhibition if excessively high levels are used, and commercial preparations of creatine phosphate may contain inhibitors of the cyclase.[14] In both cases the level of ATP and/or guanine nucleotide used may influence these effects and, thus, must be evaluated and controlled where age-related differences are suspected.

Certain other points of technique merit emphasis. To monitor recovery of ^{32}P-cyclic AMP during chromatography, ^{3}H-cyclic AMP is usually added after the incubation is stopped. This later addition fails to monitor phosphodiesterase-catalyzed degradation of newly made product, which may be appreciable despite the presence of a large amount of unlabeled cyclic AMP in the reaction mixture, when assaying homogenates or assessing the effect of cytosolic factors on membrane cyclase activity. Including the ^{3}H-labeled monitor in the reaction mixture allows assessment of cumulative losses over the entire assay and yields a more accurate estimate of activity. A ^{14}C-adenosine monitor may be added to distinguish degradation loss from column loss,[15] but this results in additional calculations and usually is unnecessary.

In some cases addition of EDTA has been found useful in obtaining reproducible, hormonally sensitive membrane preparations of adenylate cyclase. This effect may result from chelation of inhibitory, multivalent metal ions or their removal from nucleotide pyrophosphatase.[14] Since Ca^{2+} at relatively low concentrations may be inhibitory, this chelating function can be served for both purposes equally well, perhaps even better, by EGTA, which binds Ca^{2+} and other multivalent metal ions, but does not interfere significantly with the Mg^{2+} required for cyclase activity. Thus, inclusion of EGTA may serve to give a more reproducible basal activity which can then be assessed as to sensitivity to Ca^{2+} using a Ca^{2+}-EGTA buffer,[16] particularly in those systems where regulation by calmodulin and micromolar levels of Ca^{2+} is suspected.

B. Functional Considerations of Adenylate Cyclase Activity

The major aspects of adenylate cyclase activity that must be evaluated in aging studies include (1) basal activity, (2) sensitivity to hormones and/or guanine nucleotides, and (3) responsiveness to hormones and/or guanine nucleotides. Basal activity, when measured on membrane preparations, is at least partially dependent on the level of residual guanine nucleotide, which may be difficult to completely remove. In addition, the presence of pyrophosphatase may cause substrate and guanine nucleotide depletion, while any 5' nucleotidase present may cause production of adenosine, which inhibits some cyclase preparations.[17] Inclusion of myokinase and adenosine deaminase may eliminate these problems.[14] In cases where the effects of adenosine itself are of interest, 2'-deoxyATP may be substituted for ATP.[17] Since the metabolite 2'-deoxyadenosine does not intereact with adenosine receptors, this effectively circumvents the complications arising from generation of adenosine during the course of the assay.

Extensive washing of membranes to remove guanine nucleotides may be undesirable in some cases. Thus, comparison of GTP-stimulated activities may be preferable and, in fact, is probably closer to the in vivo basal condition. Unless it can be shown that intracellular GTP levels change with age, the most meaningful comparisons then become "basal activity" in the presence of a physiological level of GTP and the effect of a particular hormone or neurotransmitter at various concentrations. In this regard, it is important to point out that GTP may not always be stimulatory. A variety of hormones and neurotransmitters are known to decrease intracellular cyclic AMP or to attenuate increases caused by stimulatory agents. It is now clear that some of these agents inhibit adenylate cyclase, and require GTP and/or Na^+ for this effect. Since these stimulatory and inhibitory effects can occur over a relatively narrow range of GTP concentration,[18] great attention must be paid to GTP concentration when assessing the effects of regulatory agents (for discussions of GTP and Na^+ effects see reviews by Abramowitz et al.,[19] Jakobs,[20] and Rodbell[21]).

The evaluation of the dose-response relationship of various agonists and adenylate cyclase activity answers two equally important questions: (1) sensitivity, or the threshold concentration at which an increase occurs, usually a simple function of the K_a for half-maximal stimulation; and (2) responsiveness, the V_{max} or size of the stimulation produced at a maximal concentration. A change in either value during senescence is likely to translate into a change in the amount of cyclic AMP being made at submaximal, physiological levels of many agonists and may result in an altered response. Thus, both values are needed for a full understanding of any age changes that may occur.

Recently stimulation of both basal and hormone-stimulated adenylate cyclase has been observed by two factors not usually considered in aging studies of membrane preparations: (1) physiological levels of NaCl, and (2) cytosolic factor(s), some of which are apparently protein in nature and present in a variety of tissues. Physiological levels of NaCl and/or KCl also have marked effects on phosphodiesterase and protein kinase activities (see following), and thus should be viewed as important elements in assessing the activities of all the enzymes of cyclic nucleotide metabolism and action. Regarding adenylate cyclase, differential effects of NaCl may be observed on basal compared to hormone-stimulated activity.[15] While some of these effects are attributable to the Cl^- ion, Na^+ also plays a role, along with GTP.[20,21] Thus, assessing the effects of physiological levels (extracellular) of NaCl may be useful, even essential, in eliciting age-related changes in regulation.

The cytosolic factors causing stimulation may be a combination of guanine nucleotides and one or more proteins.[22–24] Assessing homogenates cyclase activities, but in the presence of sufficient added GTP to satisfy the requirements of the guanine nucleotide regulatory component(s), may help to meet these dependencies and give better estimates of activity. It is possible that some of this stimulation is indirect, due only to substrate sparing or prevention of adenosine inhibition by cytoplasmic myokinase or adenosine deaminase, respectively.[14] Inclusion of these enzymes in reaction mixtures, or at least assessing their effects when added, should avoid this uncertainty. Since adenylate cyclase activity in the presence of F^- is often, though questionably, used as an index of maximal or total activity, and since cytosolic proteins now appear to be involved in this stimulation, the same comments regarding GTP effects and the value of using homogenates in studying F^- activated cyclase apply.

Another factor which may influence adenylate cyclase activity (as well as protein kinase and phosphodiesterase) in broken cell preparations is proteolysis. Mild proteolysis can activate adenylate cyclase in many cell types[25-27] and in some cases is evident or more pronounced in the presence of GTP.[25,26] Regardless of whether this effect involves destruction of a GTP-dependent inhibitory protein or some other component interacting with the cyclase, the extent to which this occurs as a consequence of the release of proteases during homogenization of tissues represents an artifactual change from a basal condition and complicates assessment of changes during senescence. Homogenization under isotonic conditions plus the addition of appropriate protease inhibitors may be necessary with some tissues to alleviate this concern. Some caution is required in the use of protease inhibitors since inhibition of stimulated cyclase activity has been observed with some inhibitors.[28,29]

C. Assay of Guanylate Cyclase

Many of the comments made regarding assay of adenylate cyclase apply equally to guanylate cyclase. In some cases less assay sensitivity may suffice, which may partly explain the use of [^{3}H]-GTP as well as [^{32}P]-α-GTP in many studies. Purification of [^{3}H]-cyclic GMP is accomplished by precipitation of most of the substrate and metabolites by zinc acetate-sodium carbonate, followed by chromatography on PEI-cellulose columns and monitoring of recovery by absorbance at 252 nm.[30] Purification of [^{32}P]-cyclic GMP is accomplished by zinc carbonate-sodium acetate precipitation followed by chromatography on alumina columns, with absorbance monitoring of recovery,[30] or by sequential ion-exchange, alumina chromatography, with added ^{3}H-cyclic GMP used to monitor recovery.[31] This latter method, similar to the procedure used for adenylate cyclase assay, appears to offer the greatest sensitivity, i.e., lowest blanks in an assay using labeled GTP as substrate. With either isotopic substrate, it is essential to include a regenerating system (creatine phosphate plus creatine phosphokinase) along with a cyclic GMP trap and a phosphodiesterase inhibitor. In cases where even greater sensitivity is needed, unlabeled GTP may be used and cyclic GMP determined by radioimmunoassay. The same limitation on linearity and the problem of product degradation mentioned previously obtain here, but can be assessed if the method must be used.

D. Functional Considerations of Guanylate Cyclase Activity

In discussing the regulation of cyclase activity in the action of hormones or neurotransmitters believed to act through cyclic nucleotides, a sharp contrast exists between adenylate and guanylate cyclase. While many agents are known to stimulate adenylate cyclase, and while the list of physiologically relevant proteins known to be regulated by cyclic AMP-mediated phosphorylation continues to grow (see Krebs and Beavo[4] for a review), no hormones or neurotransmitters have been shown convincingly in an in vitro cyclase assay to activate guanylate cyclase, and virtually no protein has been found with a demonstrated function related to a physiological response to agents which elevate intracellular cyclic GMP. Nevertheless, the ability of cyclic GMP analogues to mimic the actions of some of these agents, plus the antagonism that exist in some cases with agents known to stimulate adenylate cyclase, argues for some discussion of the regulation of cyclic GMP synthesis in the present context. A more extensive discussion of the properties and subcellular distribution of guanylate cyclase can be found in reviews by Kimura and Murad[32] and Murad et al.[33,34]

In assessing total guanylate cyclase activity, attention must be given to the fact that in many tissues activity is both cytosolic and membrane bound, but usually in a tissue-specific fashion.[31] Furthermore, the distribution observed may be markedly dependent upon the assay conditions, i.e., much latent particulate activity is observed when a nonionic detergent (Lubrol® PX or Triton® X-100) is included in the assay, resulting in a large proportion of total activity being membrane bound. In addition, kinetic properties of the soluble and particulate activities appear to be distinctly different and in a tissue-specific fashion. While maximal activity with both forms require Mn^{2+}, in some tissues cytosolic activity may be unaffected by high Mn^{2+}, stimulated by addition of Ca^{2+} to a low concentration of Mn^{2+}, and exhibit classical Michaelis-Menten kinetics with a relatively low K_m, while particulate activity may be inhibited by high Mn^{2+} or the addition of Ca^{2+} to low Mn^{2+} and may exhibit positive cooperativity with a relatively higher level of GTP needed to elicit maximal activity.[33,34] Consequently, any assessment of total activities and subcellular distribution of cyclase activity during aging should give careful consideration to these properties in establishing assay conditions. Since changes in subcellular distribution have been observed in liver during regeneration following partial hepatectomy and during neonatal development[35] as well as in neoplasms,[36] such studies during postmaturational development may prove fruitful.

The question of functional guanylate cyclase activity is much more difficult to address. While no hormones have been shown convincingly to activate guanylate cyclase in a cyclase assay using broken-cell preparations, various other agents have been shown to increase activity substantially. The list includes detergents, bile salts, fatty acids and lipids, H_2O_2, NaN_3, $NaNO_2$, nitroprusside, and other agents containing or convertible to NO.[34] Many of these effects appear to involve oxidation-reduction reactions, although the effects of unoxidized fatty acids may be different and possibly of some physiological significance.[37] In addition, various endogenous substances,[38,39] as well as a heat stable enterotoxin from *Escherichia coli*[40] increase activity, while heme proteins may be inhibitory,[33,34] particularly where NaN_3 activation is being measured. In some cases, activation by one or more of these agents produces changes in the cation and GTP requirements of the cyclase.[33] Thus the "state of activation" of guanylate cyclase may be reflected in the ratio of activity with Mg^{2+} compared to Mn^{2+}, which is low under "basal" conditions but approaches one at least with redox-mediated activation.[41] Assessment of this ratio may serve to elicit changes during senescence in guanylate cyclase that might otherwise be missed. One other approach worth considering is use of low, more physiological levels of Mn^{2+}, or higher levels of Mg^{2+}, and assessing the effect of micromolar levels of Ca^{2+} where a role for Ca^{2+} in cyclic GMP synthesis is known or suspected. More meaningful approaches to measuring functional activity of guanylate cyclase must await a better understanding of the mechanisms of regulation of the membrane-bound and cytosolic enzyme(s).

IV. CYCLIC NUCLEOTIDE DEGRADATION

A. Assay of Cyclic Nucleotide Phosphodiesterase

Degradation of cyclic nucleotides by phosphodiesterase results in production of 5'-nucleotides, which may then be converted by phosphatases and deaminase to various nucleosides. This complication of product conversion, plus the need for methods sensitive enough to allow assay at and below the micromolar concentrations typically found in most tissues, necessitates use of radioactive substrates. Both [3H]- and [32P] cyclic nucleotides have been used, with the [3H] cyclic nucleotides used most frequently. All of the methods in use are basically similar in using 5'-nucleotidase to assure conversion of product to nucleosides, but differ in the method used to separate products ([3H] nucleosides or [32P] inorganic phosphate) from unhydrolyzed substrate. This separation may involve the simple addition of an anion-exchange resin directly to the reaction mixture,[42] chromatography of part or all of the reaction mixture on columns of anion-exchange resin,[43,44] polyacrylamide-boronate gel,[45] alumina,[46,47] PEI cellulose thin-layer plates[48] or paper,[49] or isolation of inorganic phosphate with molybdate plus isobutanol[50] or charcoal.[51] The relative advantages and disadvantages of most of these methods have been discussed recently.[45] Sensitivity, simplicity, speed, and reproducibility characterize column methods,[44–46] with the relatively low blanks providing a decided advantage. Use of [^{32}P] cyclic nucleotides and simple charcoal separation may be the simplest and most sensitive method,[51] but the relative availability and cost of [^{3}H]-substrates makes them most useful.

When assayed at 1 μM cyclic nucleotide, homogenates or extracts from most tissues contain quite high levels of phosphodiesterase activity, necessitating considerable dilution to avoid excessively high rates of hydrolysis and to assure proportionality to amount of material assayed. Since such large dilutions may result in enzyme instability, it is advisable to perform incubations at 30° C and to include added protein (0.1 to 0.5% bovine serum ablumin) in the reaction mixture. The dilution required for proportionality must be checked for the tissue in question since tissue specific levels of activators and inhibitors may be present (see following). Blanks may be minimized by stopping the initial incubation with acid[47,51] followed by neutralization prior to the second nucleotidase step.[47] Since some nucleotidase preparations may also contain proteases which are known to activate some forms of phosphodiesterases,[52] a two-step assay with a denaturation step between the initial incubation and the nucleotidase incubation is preferable. Where relatively high concentrations of sample protein are used, effects of endogenous proteases should be guarded against. As described for adenylate cyclase, this may be accomplished by judicious choice of homogenization conditions and/or use of protease inhibitors.

B. Functional Considerations of Phodphodiesterase Activity

Evaluating changes in cyclic nucleotide phosphodiesterase activity, whether measured as total activity or activity at physiological substrate concentration (≤ 1 μM), is somewhat more complicated than assessing cyclase activities. In most mammalian tissues three or more forms of phodphodiesterase have been described, each differing both in kinetic properties and subcellular distribution (for reviews see Appleman et al.[53] and Wells and Hardman[54]). Because of substantial differences in V_{max} and K_m of the different forms, maximal, total activity for a tissue may be attained only at very high, unphysiological substrate concentrations, while measurements at low substrate concentrations may be a composite of activities of the different forms determined by their relative, tissue-specific levels. Consequently, a first approach in assessing activities in homogenates or in subcellular fractions must entail assay conditions that take advantage of the differences in regulatory properties or subcellular distribution of the multiple forms, thus achieving at least some discrimination in relative activity levels. Suggestions of age-related changes might then be examined further using one or more separation techniques (anion-exchange chromotography, gel filtration, isoelectric focusing, polyacrylamide gel electrophoresis, sucrose density-gradient centrifugation, affinity column chromatography) under conditions in which quantitative recoveries can be obtained.

The three forms of phosphodiesterase that are often found in mammalian tissues and are readily separated by DEAE-cellulose column chromatography[55] differ markedly in their regulatory properties. One form that is predominantly cytosolic is activated at least five- to tenfold by the Ca^{2+}·CaM complex and is several-fold more active with cyclic GMP than with cyclic AMP at 1 μM substrate (see Wolff and Brostrom[115] for more details). It is important to note that basal activity of this enzyme may be increased by certain proteinases[56] or may be decreased by normal intracellular levels of K^+.[57] Thus, having taken the usual precautions to minimize proteolysis, measuring the increase in activity obtained with 100 μM or more free Ca^{2+} plus excess calmodulin over that observed with EGTA, in both cases with 150 mM KCl and 1 μM cyclic GMP as substrate, should serve as a good index of the activity of the $Ca^{2+} \cdot CaM$-dependent phosphodiesterase. Cyclic AMP may also be used as substrate, particularly where effects of Ca^{2+} on cyclic AMP degradation are of most concern, but the $Ca^{2+} \cdot CaM$-independent activity due to the other forms of phosphodiesterase may be somewhat greater than with cyclic GMP.

A second form of phosphodiesterase observed in many tissues is characterized by positive cooperativity, comparable activity with the two cyclic nucleotides, cyclic GMP stimulation of cyclic AMP hydrolysis, and distribution in both cytosolic and particulate fractions of some tissues.[54,58] It should be noted that the membrane-bound component of this activity may be localized to one region of the plasma membrane in polar cells, e.g., the basolateral membrane of the proximal tubule cell of the renal cortex.[59] Optimal conditions for assay of this activity appear to be with 1 μM cyclic AMP substrate ±1 to 3 μM cyclic GMP, under conditions where $Ca^{2+} \cdot CaM$-dependent phosphodiesterase activity is minimal (EGTA, 150 mM KCl). Further discrimination may be achieved by adding the inhibitor Ro 20-1724, which, unlike theophylline and isobutylmethylxanthine, inhibits other phosphodiesterases but does not block the cyclic GMP stimulation.[60] Since this enzyme appears to play some role in the ability of acetylcholine to attenuate hormonal elevation of cyclic AMP levels,[60] particular attention should be given to this component of total activity in tissues where similar interactions involving cyclic AMP-elevating and cyclic GMP-elevating stimuli occur.

A third form of phosphodiesterase commonly found in mammalian tissues is relatively specific for cyclic AMP with a "low K_m" in the micromolar or submicromolar range, is usually localized to the plasma membrane and may undergo changes in activity in response to various hormones or changes in the intracellular level of cyclic AMP.[54] Some of these hormonal effects are acute, e.g., insulin,[61] epinephrine, and ACTH effects[62] on fat cells, while other involve longer exposure, e.g., thyroid hormone effects on fat cells.[63] Thus, this enzyme may be especially interesting in age-related comparisons intended to elucidate changes in hormonal responsiveness. The fact that the enzyme is relatively active at submicromolar concentrations of cyclic AMP and is usually membrane bound affords some discrimination from other forms of phosphodiesterase, but otherwise there is no way, other than sucrose density centrifugation or solubilization and chromatographic separation, to be sure that this activity is being exclusively measured in homogenates or crude preparations.

It should be apparent that any attempt to relate changes in phosphodiesterase activity in homogenates or crude extracts to changes in the level of one or more of the forms of the enzyme must be based on further separation of the enzyme from other forms, using methodology that permits quantitative recovery of the sample applied. Gel filtration, anion-exchange chromatography, and isoelectric focusing have proven very useful for this purpose.[44] As long as assays are performed under conditions where the effects of endogenous activators or inhibitors are diluted out (see section on assay techniques) the stability of most forms of the enzyme should permit meaningful assessment of the relative levels of the different forms in a tissue at different stages of postmaturational development.

V. CYCLIC NUCLEOTIDE ACTION

A. Assay of Cyclic Nucleotide-Dependent Protein Kinase Activity

Measurement of the transfer of the γ-phosphate group of ATP to an amino acid residue (usually serine or threonine) on a protein, where relatively little nucleotide substrate may be consumed, requires [^{32}P]-γ-ATP for sensitivity and complete separation of the labeled protein from residual [^{32}P]-γ-ATP and ^{32}Pi produced during the incubation. This may be accomplished by TCA precipitation of the protein, addition of carrier protein (bovine serum albumin), followed by collection and washing on a glass fiber filter[64] or, alternatively, by adsorption of protein onto filter paper disks followed by washing in TCA, ethanol, and ethyl ether.[65,66] Where the possibility of significant acyl phosphate formation exists (in homogenate or membrane preparations containing high levels of ATPase), these nonkinase generated counts may be eliminated by dissolution of the precipitated protein in cold 1 N NaOH followed by reprecipitation in TCA and collection on a filter. Complete precipitation and recovery of substrate protein may require use of a TCA-tungstate reagent when highly basic substrates are used.[66]

In order to achieve linearity of activity with time and amount of protein, it is necessary to include ATPase inhibitors (F$^-$, oubain) and phosphoprotein phosphatase inhibitors (F$^-$, PO$_4^{-2}$), particularly when homogenates or membrane preparations are assayed. Since Ca^{2+} inhibits cyclic nucleotide-dependent protein kinases, EGTA should also be included, as well as a phosphodiesterase inhibitor, to minimize degradation of added cyclic nucleotides. Considerable dilution may be necessary to achieve proportionality due to phosphatase activity and/or appreciable levels of a protein inhibitor of cyclic AMP-dependent protein kinase activity.[67] Use of histone H2B may be necessary to accurately measure activity at high dilutions. As with phosphodiesterase assays using low levels of protein, dilutions should be made with and incubations carried out with an added, stabilizing protein (0.5 mg/mℓ bovine serum albumin), in this case one that is not a protein kinase substrate.[67]

Assaying cyclic AMP- or GMP-dependent protein kinase activity in a homogenate or crude extract that contains both forms, as well as other cyclic nucleotide-independent forms, is accomplished by taking advantage of the regulatory properties of the two forms. Cyclic AMP-dependent protein kinase is activated by cyclic AMP at 100-fold lower concentrations than by cyclic GMP and can be inhibited by a protein inhibitor as well as high concentrations of Mg^{2+}. Cyclic GMP-dependent protein kinase shows a comparable 100-fold specificity for cyclic GMP and is unaffected by this inhibitor, and, at least in a test tube, requires high Mg^{2+} for maximal activity. Gill and Walton[66] have shown that by using appropriate combinations of concentrations of cyclic nucleotides, protein inhibitor, and Mg^{2+}, each protein kinase can be assayed in a mixture of the two with good specificity. Inclusion of a protein modulator of cyclic GMP-dependent protein kinase[68] may give additional specificity as long as histones are used as substrates. It is important to note, however, that many mammalian tissues appear to contain much more cyclic AMP-dependent than cyclic GMP-dependent protein kinase, thus compromising use of the method where the ratio is very high. Additionally, cyclic AMP-dependent protein kinase, though active towards the commonly used substrate protamine, is not inhibited by the protein inhibitor when this substrate is used. It should be avoided and histones, preferably H2B, used for measurements of total activity.

Use of specific histones as substrates may give the impression for some tissues that most of the protein kinase activity present is cyclic AMP-dependent.[69] Simply using a different substrate, e.g., protamine or casein, and changing assay conditions slightly can change this picture appreciably. The catalytic subunit of cyclic AMP-dependent protein kinase has four- to sixfold more activity with histone H2B than with protamine at low ionic strength, but addition of 150 mM KCl or NaCl inhibits activity with histone and increases activity with protamine.[70] This appears to be an ionic strength effect and not related to the nature of either cation of anion.[71] The importance of ionic strength in assay conditions is further evident from the fact that cyclic nucleotide-independent forms of protein kinase are stimulated by physiological or higher levels of NaCl or KCl. This effect may be due in part to a salt-induced change in the substrate, but must be considered and controlled when distinctions between cyclic nucleotide-dependent and independent protein kinase activities are made.

Although many examples of cyclic nucleotide-independent forms of protein kinase are known (see reviews by Walsh and Ashby,[72] Rubin and Rosen,[73] and Nimmo and Cohen[74]) the Ca^{2+}·CaM-dependent form(s) are of particular interest in the context of regulation by hormones or neurotransmitters which alter levels of intracellular Ca^{2+} (Figure 1). Phosphorylation of myosin light chain,[75] glycogen phosphorylase,[76] and glycogen synthase[77] is regulated by apparently different kinases, all Ca^{2+}·CaM-dependent, and can be used as measures of these respective activities. A "multifunctional" kinase with activity towards various substrates, including histones, has also been described.[78] Some caution is required in measuring this activity, however, since calmodulin, a rather acidic protein, is now known to bind to basic proteins, including histones.[79,80] Careful attention must be paid to concentrations of both histone substrate and calmodulin to observe the Ca^{2+}-dependent, stimulatory effect of added calmodulin.

B. Functional Considerations of Protein Kinase Activity

Two forms of cyclic AMP-dependent protein kinase, differing in their cyclic AMP-binding regulatory subunits but sharing the same catalytic subunit, are usually found in mammalian tissues, are present in species and tissue-specific levels,[74] and may be differentially distributed between membranes and cytosol.[74,81] A particulate form of the kinase with properties distinctly different from these two forms has been reported for some tissues.[81,82] Many minor differences have also been reported for the cytosolic forms, but it remains unclear to what extent this is due to varying degrees of proteolysis of the regulatory subunits and subsequent changes in the cyclic AMP-binding and catalytic subunit-inhibitory properties of the subunits.[74,83]

Irrespective of these differences, the basic considerations regarding functional activity of the catalytic subunit are (1) the total tissue level of catalytic activity, (2) the state of activation of the enzyme(s) under basal and stimulated conditions, (3) the level of membrane-bound kinase where this localization appears to be important to cyclic AMP-mediated changes in membrane function, and (4) the susceptibility of endogenous substrates to further phosphorylation. Measurement of total activity has been discussed. The distribution of this activity between different forms of the enzyme can be assessed, as with phosphodiesterases, with DEAE-cellulose column chromatography.[74,81] Again, procedures to minimize proteolysis must be used to avoid ambiguities in any age-related comparisons, with care being taken to use inhibitors which do not interact with the catalytic subunit.[84]

Since the in vivo cyclic AMP-dependent protein kinase activity is a function of the degree of cyclic AMP-induced activation of the total activity present, as well as the degree to which this level of activity exceeds that of the heat-stable protein inhibitor,[72] measurement of activity ratios (−cyclic AMP/+cyclic AMP) in stimulated tissue can be very useful in understanding mechanism(s) of altered responsiveness. In making such measurements, it is important that tissue extractions and assays be done under conditions that avoid or minimize further dissociation or reassociation of the protein kinase subunits. In addition, subtraction of cyclic AMP-independent activity, determined by measuring activity sensitive to excess protein inhibitor in −cyclic AMP assay tubes, should be done where this activity is appreciable. Use of histone H2B instead of mixed histones may facilitate this measurement, but conditions for homogenization and assay, e.g., ionic strength of medium, percent homogenate, range of dilution of sample, and histone concentration, may vary depending on the relative levels of the two cyclic AMP-dependent protein kinases present.[85,86] Some compromise may be necessary where both forms are present in approximately equal levels, and it may be impossible to achieve conditions that freeze the intracellular equilibrium that exists between the kinase subunits.[87] Nevertheless, the activity ratio measurement remains a sensitive reflection of an in vivo event, particularly where compartmentalization may preclude detection of increases in cyclic AMP at threshold concentrations of hormones.[88,89]

An alternate, indirect monitor of activation of cyclic AMP-dependent protein kinase is measurement of the level of bound cyclic AMP, presumably to the regulatory subunit of the enzyme. Regulatory and catalytic subunits appear to be present in equal amounts in mammalian tissues[67] and, in fact, bound cyclic AMP has been shown to correlate with a hormonally induced, cyclic AMP-mediated response.[90] This method appears more cumbersome than determination of kinase activity ratios and offers no advantages over that technique. Both should be used with an appreciation for the fact that the changes being measured may take place with some agents under conditions where no physiologic response occurs,[90,91] presumably due to compartmentalization within some cell types or to the presence of multiple, differentially responsive cell types in a tissue or organ.

A change in the dose-response relationship of cyclic AMP and of cyclic AMP-dependent protein kinase(s) could result in altered tissue responsiveness where threshold levels of a stimulus are being studied. Thus, comparison of the binding characteristics, or the "K_D" of regulatory subunits and the "K_a" for activation by cyclic AMP of the protein kinase, in differentially responsive tissues would appear to be essential. It must be realized, however, that even under conditions where artifacts of proteolysis following homogenization have been avoided, the values measured for these two constants have only limited meaning. Swillens et al.[92] have pointed out quite correctly that such apparent K_as are not true dissociation constants, since the protein kinase itself dissociates upon binding of cyclic AMP. Such measured values vary with enzyme concentration,[93] as has been shown by the marked increase observed when the protein kinase was assayed at a physiological, i.e., in vivo, concentration.[94] Such measurements may not be practical with the limited amounts of tissue available for studies of senescence. Comparison of K_as may still be useful, however, as long as the protein kinase activity used is adjusted to the same maximal level while determining dose-response relationships.

The measurement of in vivo activation of cyclic GMP-dependent protein kinase is much more difficult than with cyclic AMP-dependent protein kinase because of the relatively rapid dissociation of the cyclic GMP·G-kinase complex[95] and the relatively high levels of cyclic AMP-dependent activity that may be present. Such assays are possible, however, and the fact that activation can be observed with a stimulus (acetylcholine) that both increases cyclic GMP and causes a physiological response, but not with one (nitroprusside) that increases cyclic GMP but fails to elicit a physiological response[96] (again emphasizing the importance of compartmentalization), indicates the value of the technique. Better methodology may be necessary before the method can be applied routinely in aging studies.

In addition to the protein inhibitor specific for the catalytic subunit of cyclic AMP-dependent protein kinase, other proteins have now been identified which inhibit cyclic GMP-dependent and cyclic nucleotide-independent protein kinases.[97,98] The apparent ability of the "Walsh inhibitor" to regulate in vivo kinase activity under basal conditions,[72] plus the fact that the inhibitor level in a cell or tissue may change as a function of diet[72] or hormonal state,[72,98] indicates that assessment of the level of this and other inhibitors is necessary in cases of altered hormonal responsiveness. If basic proteins are used to assay these levels, assay conditions, particularly protein kinase and histone concentrations, must be precisely controlled since the acidic inhibitor protein(s) may bind to the basic protein(s) used as substrate.[99]

VI. PHOSPHOPROTEIN PHOSPHATASE

A. Assay of Phosphoprotein Phosphatase Activity

Much of the methodology used in protein kinase assays is applicable to phosphoprotein phosphatase determinations, except that now acid soluble ^{32}Pi is measured instead of acid insoluble ^{32}P protein. Where a phosphorylated enzyme serves as substrate, e.g., glycogen phosphorylase or synthase, a change in activity may serve as the index of phosphorylation, but greatest sensitivity is usually attained with ^{32}P-labeled substrates. These are normally prepared just prior to use with commercially available preparations of protein kinase and histones or other proteins.[100] As with protein kinases, endogenous protein inhibitors exist which may cause low estimates of activity unless diluted out or removed. A divalent metal ion (Mn^{2+} or Mg^{2+}) may be required for activity,[101] but this should be determined for the tissue or extract being studied and the particular phosphatase activity being assayed.

B. Functional Considerations of Phosphoprotein Phosphatase Activity

Compared to the voluminous literature on protein kinases, very little work has been done towards characterizing phosphoprotein phosphatase(s) in different tissues. Only recently was it appreciated that what was previously considered to be a small, multifunctional enzyme actually exists in multiple forms of higher molecular weight.[74,102,103] Again, as with cyclases, phosphodiesterases, and protein kinases, proteolysis confuses the picture obtained thus far. Rabbit muscle phosphorylase phosphatase can be degraded by a Ca^{2+}-dependent protease from a less active, high molecular weight form to be more active, lower molecular weight forms.[104] These phosphatases appear to be regulated differentially by protein inhibitors and activators,[105,106] one inhibitor of which is active only after being phosphorylated by cyclic AMP-dependent protein kinase.[107] The extent to which these effectors are present in various mammalian tissues is not known. Much additional basic work and a better understanding of the regulation and specificity of phosphoprotein phosphatases is needed before changes in their activities that may occur during senescene can be put into a meaningful, functional perspective.

VII. PHOSPHORYLATION OF ENDOGENOUS PROTEINS

A. Detection of Phosphorylation of Endogenous Proteins

The most commonly used method of detecting specific protein phosphorylation involves separation of ^{32}P-labeled proteins by polyacrylamide gel electrophoresis and quantitation by slicing and counting or autoradiography and densitometry. Labeling may be done by incubation of tissue with phosphate-free media containing carrier-free ^{32}Pi, followed by treatment with the appropriate stimulus, or by incubation of homogenates or subcellular fractions with [^{32}P]-γ-ATP of high specific activity in the presence and absence of a cyclic nucleotide or Ca^{2+}. In either case, incubations are terminated as quickly as possible, usually by heating with added sodium dodecyl sulfate (SDS).[108] Some distinction between particulate and cytosolic proteins can be made by homogenizing labeled tissue with a buffered solution containing sucrose, NaF (50 mM), NaHPO$_4$ (10 mM), EDTA (10 mM), and protease inhibitors to preserve states of phosphorylation. A major problem incurred with intact cells exists in the ^{32}P-RNA that is generated and appears as a high background in the gels, thus interfering with measurement of low level phosphorylation of minor proteins. Extraction with the above solution of inhibitors plus NP-40, a detergent which does not readily solubilize nuclear but does solubilize plasma membranes, and removal of nuclei by centrifugation may partially alleviate this problem. Alternatively, treatment of samples with an RNAse that remains active in 0.3% SDS and mercaptoethanol may also help to reduce this background.[109]

Two additional techniques that may facilitate detection of changes in phosphorylation involve the use of ^{33}Pi and ^{35}S-labeled ATP-γ-S. By using ^{33}Pi or [^{33}P]-γ-ATP to phosphorylate proteins in one sample and ^{32}Pi or [^{32}P]-γ-ATP in another, and then combining equal aliquots of the samples prior to electrophoresis, a ^{32}P/^{33}P ratio can be determined in gel slices which, when measured on individual slices and compared to the total sample, is very sensitive to relatively small changes in phosphorylation of specific bands. Phosphoprotein phosphatases do not readily dephosphorylate thiophosphorylated proteins.[110,111] Thus, substituting recently available [^{35}S]ATP-γ-S for ATP can result in a higher degree of phosphorylation than could otherwise be obtained, permitting a more accurate assessment of the maximum degree of phosphorylation that can be attained for a particular protein in preparations containing a mixture of protein kinase and phosphoprotein phosphatase activities.

While the techniques available for separation of proteins, particularly two-dimensional polyacrylamide gel electrophoresis, permit the detection and quantitation of phosphorylation of a large number of proteins, it must be appreciated that these measurements usually do not indicate moles of phosphate per mole of protein. Expression of data as increase in cpm or in arbitrary units of area determined from densitometric tracings gives no information regarding the actual state of phosphorylation of the protein in question. In cases where the protein of interest is readily identified on gels, isoelectric focusing may be used to separate the phosphorylated from the dephosphorylated form of the protein and compare the relative levels of each.[112] Otherwise, involved purification procedures or preparation of an antibody against the protein and isolation from other proteins by antibody precipitation appear to be the only other ways of obtaining this information. Of course when the protein in question is a well characterized enzyme, for which the relationship of state of phosphorylation and activity is known, measurement of activity should indirectly give the same information.

B. Functional Considerations of Protein Phosphorylation

Since the physiological responses mediated by cyclic nucleotides and, to some extent, Ca^{2+} are believed to relate ultimately to a change in the state of phosphorylation of one or more proteins, quantitation of specific protein phosphorylation is the single, most meaningful measurement that can be made in understanding the mechanism of an altered physiological response and the actual relevance of any changes observed in cyclase, phosphodiesterase, kinase, or phosphatase activities. It must be emphasized, however, that while numerous examples exist in the literature of cyclic nucleotide- and Ca^{2+}-mediated changes in protein phosphorylation, the number of identified proteins with functions known to be regulated by the state of phosphorylation of the protein is limited.[4] Fortunately, the list of enzymes regulated by phosphorylation-dephosphorylation continues to grow,[4] though still at a much faster pace for cytosolic than for membrane proteins. Nearly all of these well characterized protein kinase substrates are cytosolic, with still very few membrane-associated proteins. Since many of the effects of hormonal and neurotransmitter stimuli involve changes in membrane permeability properties, this lack of understanding of the significance of phosphorylation of specific membrane proteins limits the value of quantitation of these phosphorylations in aging systems. As knowledge in this area accumulates, particularly regarding endogenous substrates of cyclic GMP-dependent protein kinase, more complete explanations of the mechanism(s) underlying altered responsiveness during senescence will be possible.

VIII. CALMODULIN

As mentioned earlier, the actions and interactions of cyclic nucleotides and Ca^{2+} in mediating the effects of a multitude of extracellular stimuli make it virtually impossible in many systems to consider one without the other. The general scheme presented in Figure 1 is only a simplistic attempt to describe relationships that have been discussed in more detail for specific tissues by Berridge[113] and Rasmussen and Goodman[114] as well as many others. It now appears that the Ca^{2+}-dependent regulatory protein termed calmodulin, plays a pervasive role in many tissues in mediating the regulatory effects of intracellular Ca^{2+} (for recent reviews see Wolff and Brostrom,[115] Klee et al.,[116] and Wang and Waisman[117]). Acting through calmodulin, Ca^{2+} is known to regulate adenylate cyclase, a cyclic nucleotide phosphodiesterase, and protein kinases in an increasing number of tissues. In addition, the Ca^{2+}·CaM-dependent myosin light-chain kinase of smooth muscle is itself subject to regulation by phosphorylation by cyclic AMP-dependent protein kinase.[118] Furthermore, cyclic AMP-dependent and Ca^{2+}·CaM-dependent protein kinases are now known to act on some of the same endogenous substrates, but are able to phosphorylate different sites on the same protein.[119,120] Thus, it is inevitable that studies of altered responsiveness to hormones and neurotransmitters during senescence will be concerned with the roles and tissue levels of calmodulin.

At present, calmodulin levels in tissue extracts have been measured either by its stimulatory effect on the Ca^{2+}·CaM-dependent phosphodiesterase or by radioimmunoassay.[121,122] The phosphodiesterase activation assay requires Ca^{2+} and suffers from interference by CaM-binding proteins known to exist in many tissues,[116] whereas the radioimmunoassay is done in the presence of EGTA and avoids possible underestimations of tissue levels.[121,122] The simplicity and sensitivity of the radioimmunoassay makes it preferable in any comparative studies, but until the recently produced antibodies, particularly the more sensitive antibody of Chafouleas et al.,[122] become generally available the phosphodiesterase activation assay may suffice for assay of tissues for which interference by heat-stable CaM-binding proteins does not occur. The same comments made for radioimmunoassay of cyclic nucleotides apply for calmodulin assays, whichever one is used, in that activity should be proportional to volume of extract when compared to standard curves generated with purified calmodulin, showing the same slope. Partial purification may be necessary to remove interfering substances.

IX. MECHANISM(S) OF ALTERED RESPONSIVENESS DURING SENESCENCE

Of the many reports showing "age-dependent" changes in some component of cyclic nucleotide-mediated hormone or neurotransmitter action, only a limited number have identified changes that occur during the postmaturational, senescent stage of the life span. In these reports, the bulk of the information to date is concerned with regulation of cyclic nucleotide synthesis, with progressively less known proceeding to the last step (protein phosphorylation) in cyclic nucleotide action. Decreases in stimulation of cyclic AMP synthesis have been observed in specific regions of the brain with dopamine[123–127] and norepinephrine[123,126] and with ACTH in fat cells,[128] while an increase was observed in the liver with epinephrine.[129,130] Some of these studies were done with homogenates and some with membrane preparations, but only in the case of epinephrine and glucagon stimulation of liver adenylate cyclase was the importance of cytosolic constituents determined.[130] Interestingly, an even greater age-dependent difference was observed by assaying homogenate activity compared to particulate activity, presumably due in part to the presence of cytosolic protein factors.[131]

Although some uncertainty exists as to whether the decrease observed in dopamine stimulation of striatal adenylate cyclase is maturational or postmaturational[126] and may be species dependent,[127] the potential significance of this change in senescent changes in brain function make it particularly interesting for further study. Further study is needed since no report to date has attempted to assess during senescene the additional roles and interactions of adenosine,[132] Ca^{2+} and calmodulin,[132–134,136] and GTP,[135,136] [all now known to participate in regulation of striatal adenylate cyclase(s)] with dopamine in mature and senescent striata. The complexity of adenylate cyclase and of dopamine receptors in this region of the brain is only now becoming apparent, and as more information is obtained additional, more meaningful studies of both cyclic nucleotide and Ca^{2+} metabolism and action should be possible.

The role of guanyl nucleotides was investigated in a study of hormone regulation of adenylate cyclase in the rat fat cell,[128] a cell for which a cyclic AMP-regulated function, lipolysis, is known to decline during senescence. Assays of membrane preparations showed parallel decreases in both basal and hormone-activated activity with or without the analogue GMPP(NH)P; stimulation by glucagon decreased drastically during maturation, by ACTH substantially during both maturation and senescence, and by epinephrine only modestly.[128] The role of the natural endogenous nucleotide GTP, now known to both stimulate and inhibit this cyclase, was not studied. Another study reported a decline in catecholamine responsiveness of fat-cell adenylate cyclase during senescence which was accompanied by a marked reduction in β-receptors in the membranes.[137]

Regardless of whether these different cyclase results reflect differences in methodology, additional studies relating lipolysis to cyclic AMP accumulation suggest that some change distal to cyclic AMP generation may be involved.[138] Senescent fat cells were found to achieve their maximal rate of lipolysis, which was 50% lower than mature cells when expressed on per cell basis, and their maximal rate of cyclic AMP accumulation, which was similar in the two groups, at a much lower dose of epinephrine than mature cells. This change did not appear to be due to decreased levels of either cytosolic or particulate phosphodiesterase activity.[138] Analogous studies with ACTH and dibutyryl cyclic AMP in mouse fat cells showed a decrease in glycerol released/ cell, but no change when the data were based on cell surface area or triglyceride content.[139] Dependence of lipolytic rate on cell size, which may diminish during senescence, is a complication in these studies. However, the observation that rates of lipolysis at threshold doses of hormone correlate much better with protein kinase activity ratio than with cyclic AMP levels[140] points to a need for this measurement in such studies. Even more meaningful would be the measurement of triglyceride lipase content, activity, and state of phosphorylation at both low and high doses of hormone. Of additional interest in this system is the observation that dietary restriction of older, mature rates increases responsiveness of fat-cell adenylate cyclase to epinephrine, glucagon, and ACTH,[141] as well as the lipolytic response to epinephrine.[142,143] A full understanding of the mechanism for this effect may require many of these same measurements.

Relatively little has been done in relating protein kinase activity to changes in responsiveness during senescence. Schmidt and co-workers have examined the level and characteristics of cyclic AMP-dependent protein kinase in the rat hippocampus and cerebral cortex[144] and human cerebral cortex[145] during senescence, but observed no changes. Careful studies of the number and staining density of proteins and of cyclic AMP stimulation of phosphorylation of specific proteins in synaptosomes and synaptic membranes of various regions of the rat brain, including the caudate nucleus, also failed to reveal any changes during senescence.[144] No attempt has yet been made to assess the effect of Ca^{2+} and calmodulin, which stimulate the phosphorylation of some of the same proteins as cyclic AMP, albeit at different sites on these proteins,[120] as well as other membrane proteins. Since the functional significance of the phosphorylation of the synaptic membrane proteins identified so far is unknown, the choice of which proteins to quantitate remains arbitrary and limits the value of such studies until these questions are answered.

The role of cyclic AMP-dependent protein kinase has also been examined, although indirectly, in the decreased stimulation of testosterone production observed in isolation Leydig cells in response to gonadotropin.[146] Senescent Leydig cells contained 23% fewer gonadotropin receptors than mature cells and achieved maximal testosterone production at a lower dose of hormone. However, the increases in both total intracellular cyclic AMP and protein-bound cyclic AMP (presumably bound to the regulatory subunit of the protein kinase) were similar in both age groups.[146] Since cyclic AMP binding capacity has been shown to equal cyclic AMP-dependent protein kinase activity in many tissues,[67] the reduced level of testosterone production in stimulated cells appears to be due to a change distal to protein kinase activity. Changes in the levels of protein kinase inhibitor(s) or of phosphoprotein phosphatase or its effectors could account for this diminished response. Quantitation of the level and state of phosphorylation of the protein(s) involved in the secretory response, which at present are not known, may eventually serve to elucidate the nature of the defect. The fact that prolonged in vivo pretreatment with gonadotropin can restore senescent cells to a responsive state comparable to mature cells provides an additional tool with which to answer these questions.[147]

One other senescent system for which the role of cyclic AMP-dependent protein kinase has been examined is the isolated, perfused septum of the rat heart.[148,149] Upon exposure to isoproterenol, septa from senescent rats exhibit a diminished inotropic response compared to mature septa. No difference was observed in β-receptor number or characteristics in the two groups. Increases in total cyclic AMP and in protein kinase activity ratio were the same for both groups, as were the levels of total cytosolic and particulate cyclic AMP-dependent protein kinase. No difference was seen in the level of cyclic AMP producing half-maximal activation of cytosolic and particulate kinase activities. In addition, perfusion with dibutyryl cyclic AMP failed to restore the decreased contractile response of the senescent septa to the level of mature septa. A modest increase in the total tissue level of heat-stable inhibitors(s) of the catalytic subunit of cyclic AMP-dependent protein kinase was detected, along with a comparable increase in particulate phosphoprotein phosphatase activity.[149] Cumulatively, these latter two changes could serve to reduce the cyclic nucleotide-induced increase in phosphorylation of the protein(s) presumed to mediate the inotropic response. As yet, however, phosphorylation of proteins has not been studied using mature and sensecent septa.

One of the well studied targets of cyclic AMP action in the myocardium, the sarcoplasmic reticulum, is the subject of ongoing studies on the mechanism of the reduced inotropic response. The uptake of Ca^{2+} by the sarcoplasmic reticulum, which can be stimulated by cyclic AMP-dependent protein kinase, decreases during senescence.[150] Treatment of preparations of sarcoplasmic reticulum from mature and senescent hearts with cyclic AMP-dependent protein kinase, Mg^{2+}, ATP, and cyclic AMP stimulates uptake in both preparations, but still leaves the senescent preparation with a lower level of uptake than that from mature rats. Virtually all of the cyclic AMP-dependent phosphorylation occurs in "phospholamban," the small protein for which the state of phosphorylation correlates with the rate of Ca^{2+} uptake in myocardial sarcoplasmic reticulum from other species.[151] In canine sarcoplasmic reticulum, this protein is also phosphorylated at a second site by a Ca^{2+}·CaM-dependent protein kinase present in the sarcoplasmic reticulum, and phosphorylation at this site may be critical for the stimulatory effect of Ca^{2+} uptake associated with cyclic AMP-dependent phosphorylation.[119] Knowledge of the effect of calmodulin on phospholamban phosphorylation, of the level of phospholamban, and of the level of endogenous phosphatase(s) active on phosphorylated phospholamban in mature and senescent preparations of rat sarcoplasmic reticulum should shed considerable light on the nature of the defect in the senescent heart.

X. PERSPECTIVES FOR FUTURE STUDIES ON AGING

Studies of responsiveness of various tissues during senescence to stimuli acting through cyclic AMP indicate that changes may occur at the first step in the sequence, synthesis, as well as steps beyond protein kinase activation. Very little has been done so far in assessing the interactions of different stimuli or the regulatory role(s) of Ca^{2+} and calmodulin and their interactions with cyclic nucleotides in regulating these senescencing systems. Further identification and characterization of endogenous substrates of cyclic nucleotide- and Ca^{2+}·CaM-dependent protein kinases, particularly those substrates localized in cellular membranes and believed to have central roles in the regulation of membrane permeability, should facilitate elucidation of specific changes underlying altered responsiveness. The existence of multiple forms of the various enzymes involved in the metabolism and action of cyclic nucleotides, of an increasing number of effectors of these enzymes, both stimulatory and inhibitory, and of multiple sites of phosphorylation in some protein kinase substrates makes possible a wide range of specific, perhaps subtle molecular changes which could account for the observed changes in responsiveness. A wider range of methods than have been used to date will have to be applied to various systems to fully understand the mechanism(s) that underlie the changes that occur during senescence.

REFERENCES

1. **Brooker, G., Greengard, P., and Robison, G. A.,** *Advances in Cyclic Nucleotide Research,* Vol. 10, Raven Press, New York, 1979.
2. **Hardman, J. G., and O'Malley, B. W.,** *Methods in Enzymology,* Vol. 38 (Part C), Academic Press, New York, 1974.
3. **Greengard. P.,** Phosphorylated proteins as physiological effectors, *Science,* 199, 146, 1978.
4. **Krebs, E. G. and Beavo, J. A.,** Phosphorylation-dephosphorylation of enzymes, *Annu. Rev. Biochem.,* 48, 923, 1979.
5. **Mayer, S. E., Stull, J., and Wastila, W. B.,** Rapid tissue fixation and extraction techniques, *Methods Enzymol.,* 28, 3, 1974.
6. **Keely, S. L., Corbin, J. D., and Park, C. R.,** Regulation of adenosine 3':5'-monophosphate-dependent protein kinase, *J. Biol. Chem.,* 250, 4832, 1975.
7. **Gilman, A. G. and Murad, F.,** Assay of cyclic nucleotides by receptor protein binding displacement, *Methods Enzymol.,* 38, 49, 1974.
8. **Brooker, G., Harper, J. F., Terasaki, W. L., and Moylan, R. D.,** Radioimmunoassay of cyclic AMP and cyclic GMP, *Adv. Cyclic Nucleotide Res.,* 10, 1, 1979.
9. **Albano, J. D. M., Barnes, G. D., Maudsley, D. V., Brown, B. L., and Etkins, R. P.,** Factors affecting the saturation assay of cyclic AMP in biological systems, *Anal. Biochem.,* 60, 130, 1974.
10. **Schultz, G., Bohme, E., and Hardman, J. G.,** Separation and purification of cyclic nucleotides by ion-exchange resin column chromatography, *Methods Enzymol.,* 38, 9, 1974.

11. **Mao, C. C. and Guidotti, A.,** Simultaneous isolation of adenosine 3′,5′-cyclic monophosphate (cAMP) and guanosine 3′,5′-cyclic monophosphate (cGMP) in small tissue samples, *Anal. Biochem.,* 59, 63, 1974.

12. **Salomon, Y., Londos, C., and Rodbell, M.** A highly sensitive adenylate cyclase assay, *Anal. Biochem.,* 58, 541, 1974.

13. **Salomon, Y.,** Adenylate cyclase assay, *Adv. Cyclic Nucleotide Res.,* 10, 35, 1979.

14. **Johnson, R. A.,** Stimulatory and inhibitory effects of ATP-regenerating systems on liver adenylate cyclase, *J. Biol. Chem.,* 255, 8252, 1980.

15. **Katz, M. S., Kelly, T. M., Pineyro, M. A., and Gregerman, R. I.,** Anions and cations as stimulators of liver adenylate cyclase, *Biochim. Biophys. Acta,* 632, 11, 1980.

16. **Bartfai, T.,** Preparation of metal-chelate complexes and the design of steady-state kinetic experiments involving metal nucleotide complexes, *Adv. Cyclic Nucleotide Res.,* 10, 219, 1979.

17. **Cooper, D. M. F. and Londos, C.,** Evaluation of the effects of adenosine on hepatic and adipocyte adenylate cyclase under conditions where adenosine is not generated endogenously, *J. Cyclic Nucleotide Res.,* 5(4), 289, 1979.

18. **Cooper, D. M. F., Schlegel, W., Lin, M. C., and Rodbell, M.,** The fat cell adenylate cyclase system. Characterization and manipulation of its bimodal regulation by GTP, *J. Biol. Chem.,* 254, 8927, 1979.

19. **Abramowitz, J., Iyengar, R., and Birnbaumer, L.,** Guanyl nucleotide regulation of hormonally-responsive adenylyl cyclases, *Mol. Cell. Endocrinol.,* 16, 129, 1979.

20. **Jakobs, K. H.,** Inhibition of adenylate cyclase by hormones and neurotransmitters, *Mol. Cell. Endocrinol.,* 16, 147, 1979.

21. **Rodbell, M.,** The role of hormone receptors and GTP-regulatory proteins in membrane transduction, *Nature (London),* 284, 17, 1980.

22. **Bhat, M. K., Iyengar, R., Abramowitz, J., Bordelon-Riser, M. E., and Birnbaumer, L.,** Naturally soluble component(s) that confer(s) guanine nucleotide and fluoride sensitivity to adenylate cyclase, *Proc. Natl. Acad. Sci. U.S.A.,* 77, 3836, 1980.

23. **Crawford, A., MacNeil, S., Amirrasooli, H., and Tomlinson, S.,** Properties of a factor in cytosol that enhances hormone-stimulated adenylate cyclase activity, *Biochem. J.,* 188, 401, 1980.

24. **Omrani, G. R., Gammon, D. E., and Bilezekian, J. P.,** Regulation of catecholamine-responsive adenylate cyclase activity in rat reticulocyte membranes by endogenous factors. General characteristics and resolution into protein and nucleotide components, *Biochim. Biophys. Acta,* 629, 455, 1980.

25. **Anderson, W. B., Jaworski, C. J., and Vlakakis, G.,** Proteolytic activation of adenylate cyclase from cultured fibroblasts, *J. Biol. Chem.,* 253, 2921, 1978.

26. **Anderson, W. B., Mukku, V. R. and Johnson, G. S.,** Enhanced GTP-dependent activities of the adenylate cyclase system: bases for increased hormonal responsiveness, *Arch. Biochem. Biophys.,* 197, 599, 1979.

27. **Stengel, D., Lad, P. M., Nielsen, T. B., Rodbell, M., and Hanoune, J.,** Proteolysis activates adenyl cyclase in rat liver and AC⁻ lymphoma cell independently of guanine nucleotide regulatory site, *FEBS Lett.,* 115, 260, 1980.

28. **Partington, C. R. and Daly, J. W.,** Effect of proteases and protease inhibitors on adenylate cyclase activity in rat cerebral cortical membranes, *Arch. Biochem. Biophys.,* 198, 255, 1979.

29. **McIlroy, P. J., Richert, N. D., and Ryan, R. J.,** Effects of proteinase inhibitors of adenylate cyclase, *Biochem. J.,* 188, 423, 1980.

30. **Garbers, D. L. and Murad, F.,** Guanylate cyclase assay methods, *Adv. Cyclic Nucleotide Res.,* 10, 57, 1979.

31. **White, A. A. and Karr, D. B.,** Improved two-step method for the assay of adenylate and guanylate cyclase, *Anal. Biochem.,* 85, 451, 1978.

32. **Kimura, H. and Murad, F.,** Subcellular localization of guanylate cyclase, *Life Sci.,* 17, 837, 1975.

33. **Murad, F., Mittal, C., Arnold, W. P., Ichihara, K., Braughler, M., and Mahmoud, E. Z.,** Properties and regulation of guanylate cyclase: activation by azide, nitro compounds and hydroxyl radicals and effects of heme containing proteins, *Molecular Biology and Pharmacology of Cyclic Nucleotides*: Proceedings of the NATO Advanced Study Institute on Cyclic Nucleotides held in Tremazzo, Italy, September 1977, Vol. 1, Folco, G. and Paoletti, R., Eds., Elsevier, Amsterdam, 1978, 33.

34. **Murad, F., Arnold, W. P., Mittal, C. K., and Braughler, J. M.,** Properties and regulation of guanylate cyclase and some proposed functions for cyclic GMP, *Adv. Cyclic Nucleotide Res.,* 11, 175, 1979.

35. **Kimura, H. and Murad, F.,** Increased particulate and decreased soluble guanylate cyclase activity in regenerating liver, fetal liver, and hepatoma, *Proc. Natl. Acad. Sci. U.S.A.,* 72, 1965, 1975.

36. **Criss, W., Murad, F., Kimura, H., and Morris, H. P.,** Properties of guanylate cyclase in adult rat liver and several Morris hepatomas, *Biochim. Biophys. Acta,* 445, 500, 1976.

37. **Ichihara, K., El-Zayat, M., Mittal, C. K., and Murad, F.,** Fatty acid activation of guanylate cyclase from fibroblasts and liver, *Arch. Biochem. Biophys.,* 197, 44, 1979.

38. **Asakawa, T., Johnson, C., Ruiz, J., Scheinbaum, I., Russell, T. R., Ho, R., and Sutherland, E. W.,** Activation by "feedback" regulator and some properties of guanylate cyclase of plasma membrane of epididymal fat cells, *Biochem. Biophys. Res. Commun.,* 72, 1335, 1976.

39. **Deguchi, T.,** Endogenous activating factor for guanylate cyclase in synaptosomal-soluble fraction of rat brains, *J. Biol. Chem.,* 252, 7617, 1977.

40. **Field, M., Graf, L. H., Laird, W. J., and Smith, P. L.,** Heat-stable enterotoxin of *Escherichia coli*: *in vitro* effects on guanylate cyclase activity, cyclic GMP accumulation and ion transport in small intestine, *Proc. Natl. Acad. Sci. U.S.A.,* 75, 2800, 1978.

41. **Kimura, H., Mittal, C. K., and Murad, F.,** Appearance of magnesium guanylate cyclase activity in rat liver with sodium azide activation, *J. Biol. Chem.,* 251, 7769, 1976.

42. **Thompson, W. J. and Appleman, M. M.,** Multiple cyclic nucleotide phosphodiesterase activities in rat brain, *Biochemistry,* 10, 311, 1971.

43. **Thompson, W. J., Terasaki, W. L., Epstein, P. M. and Strada, S. J.,** Assay of cyclic nucleotide phosphodiesterase and resolution of multiple molecular forms of the enzyme, *Adv. Cyclic Nucleotide Res.,* 10, 69, 1979.

44. **Bauer, A. C. and Schwabe, U.,** An improved assay of cyclic 3',5'-nucleotide phosphodiesterases with QAE-Sephadex columns, *Naunyn Schmiedebergs Arch. Pharmacol.,* 311, 193, 1980.

45. **Davis, C. W. and Daly, J. W.,** A simple direct assay of 3',5'-cyclic nucleotide phosphodiesterase activity based on the use of polyacrylamide-boromate affinity gel chromatography, *J. Cyclic Nucleotide Res.,* 5, 65, 1979.

46. **Filburn, C. R. and Karn, J.,** An isotopic assay of 3',5'-nucleotide phosphodiesterase with aluminum oxide columns, *Anal. Biochem.,* 52, 505, 1973.

47. **Filburn, C. R., Colpo, F., and Sacktor, B.,** Regulation of cyclic nucleotide phosphodiesterase of cerebral cortex by Ca^{2+} and cyclic GMP, *J. Neurochem.,* 30, 337, 1978.

48. **Rangel-Aldao, R., Schwartz, D., and Rubin, C. S.,** Rapid assay of cyclic AMP and cyclic GMP phosphodiesterase, *Anal. Biochem.,* 87, 367, 1978.

49. **Nakai, C. and Brooker, G.,** Assay of adenylate cyclase and cyclic nucleotide phosphodiesterases and the preparation of high specific activity ^{32}P-labeled substances, *Biochim. Biophys. Acta,* 391, 222, 1975.

50. **Schonhofer, P. S., Skidmore, J. F., Bourne, H. R., and Krishna, G.,** Cyclic 3',5'-AMP phosphodiesterase in isolated fat cells. Simple and sensitive methods for the assay of phosphodiesterase activity in fat cells and studies of the enzyme inhibition by theophylline, *Pharmacology,* 7, 65, 1972.

51. **Johnson, R. A. and Walseth, T. F.,** The enzymatic preparation of $[\alpha\text{-}^{32}P]ATP$, $[\alpha\text{-}^{32}P]GTP$, $[^{32}P]cAMP$, and $[^{32}P]cGMP$, and their use in the assay of adenylate and guanlate cyclases and cyclic nucleotide phosphodiesterases, *Adv. Cyclic Nucleotide Res.,* 10, 135, 1979.

52. **Strewber, G. J. and Manganiello, V. C.,** Purification and characterization of phosphodiesterase activator from kidney-lysosomal protease, *J. Biol. Chem.,* 254, 1891, 1979.

53. **Appleman, M. M., Thompson, W. J., and Russell, T. R.,** Cyclic nucleotide phosphodiesterases, *Adv. Cyclic Nucleotide Res.,* 3, 65, 1973.

54. **Wells, J. N. and Hardman, J. G.,** Cyclic nucleotide phosphodiesterases, *Adv. Cyclic Nucleotide Res.,* 8, 119, 1977.

55. **Russell, T. R., Terasaki, W. L., and Appleman, M. M.,** Separate phosphodiesterases for the hydrolysis of cyclic adenosine 3',5'-monophosphate and cyclic guanosine 3',5'-monophosphate in rat liver, *J. Biol. Chem.,* 248, 1334, 1973.

56. **Sakai, T., Yamanaka, H., Tanaka, R., Makino, H., and Kasai, H.,** Stimulation of cyclic nucleotide phosphodiesterases from rat brain by activator protein, proteolytic enzymes, and a vitamin E derivative, *Biochim. Biophys. Acta,* 483, 121, 1977.

57. **Davis, C. W. and Daly, J. W.,** Calcium-dependent 3':5'-cyclic nucleotide phosphodiesterase. Inhibition of basal activity at physiological levels of potassium ions, *J. Biol. Chem.,* 253, 8683, 1978.

58. **Terasaki, D. W. L. and Appleman, M. M.,** The role of cyclic GMP in the regulation of cyclic AMP hydrolysis, *Metabolism,* 24, 311, 1975.

59. **Filburn, C. R., Liang, C. T., and Sacktor, B.,** Cyclic nucleotide phosphodiesterase of the renal cortex. Characterization of basal-lateral membrane activities, *J. Membr. Biol.,* 37, 29, 1977.

60. **Erneux, C., van Sande, J., Dumont, J. E., and Boeymaems, J. M.,** Cyclic nucleotide hydrolysis in the thyroid gland. General properties and key role in the interrelations between concentrations of adenosine 3':5'-monophosphate and guanosine 3':5'-monophosphate, *Eur. J. Biochem.,* 72, 137, 1977.

61. **Kono, T., Robinson, F. W., and Sarver, J. A.,** Insulin-sensitive phosphodiesterase: its localization, hormonal stimulation and oxidative stabilization, *J. Biol. Chem.,* 250, 7826, 1975.

62. **Paulson, L. G., Lowell-Smith, C. J., Mangoniello, V. C., and Vaughan, M.,** Effects of epinephrine, adrenocorticotraphic hormone, and theophylline on adenosine 3',5'-monophosphate phosphodiesterase activity in fat cells, *Proc. Natl. Acad. Sci. U.S.A.,* 71, 1639, 1974.

63. **van Inwegen, R. G., Robison, G. A., Thompson, W. J., Armstrong, K. J., and Stouffer, J. E.,** Cyclic nucleotide phosphodiesterases and thyroid hormones, *J. Biol. Chem.,* 250, 2452, 1975.

64. **Miyamats, E., Kuo, J. F., and Grungard, P.,** Cyclic nucleotide-dependent protein kinases, *J. Biol. Chem.,* 244, 6395, 1969.

65. **Corbin, J. D. and Reimann, E. M.,** Assay of cAMP-dependent protein kinases, *Methods Enzymol.,* 38, 287, 1974.

66. **Gill, G. N. and Walton, G. M.,** Assay of cyclic nucleotide-dependent protein kinases, *Adv. Cyclic Nucleotide Res.,* 10, 93, 1979.

67. **Hofmann, F., Bechtel, P. J., and Krebs, E. G.,** Concentrations of cyclic AMP-dependent protein kinase subunits in various tissues, *J. Biol. Chem.,* 252, 1441, 1977.

68. **Kuo, W. N. and Kuo, J. F.,** Isolation of stimulatory modulator of guanosine 3':5'-monophosphate-dependent protein kinase from mammalian heart devoid of inhibitory modulator of adenosine 3':5'-monophosphate-dependent protein kinase, *J. Biol. Chem.,* 251, 4283, 1976.

69. **Traugh, J. A., Ashby, C. D., and Walsh, D. A.,** Criteria for the classification of protein kinases, *Methods Enzymol.,* 38, 290, 1974.

70. **C. Filburn,** unpublished observations.

71. **Moll, G. W. and Kaiser, E. T.,** Ionic inhibition of catalytic phosphorylation of histone by bovine brain protein kinase, *J. Biol. Chem.,* 252, 3007, 1977.

72. **Walsh, D. A. and Ashby, C. D.,** Protein kinases: aspects of their regulation and diversity, *Recent Prog. Horm. Res.,* 29, 329, 1973.

73. **Rubin, C. S. and Rosen, O. M.,** Protein phosphorylation, *Annu. Rev. Biochem.,* 44, 831, 1975.

74. **Nimmo, H. G. and Cohen, P.,** Hormonal control of protein phosphorylation, *Adv. Cyclic Nucleotide Res.,* 8, 145, 1977.

75. **Drabowska, R., Sherry, J. M. F., Aromatorio, D., and Hartshorne, D. J.,** Modulator protein as a component of the myosin light chain kinase, *Biochemistry,* 17, 253, 1978.

76. **Cohen, P., Burchell, A., Foulkes, J. G., and Cohen, P. T. W.,** Identification of the Ca^{2+}-dependent modulator protein as the fourth subunit of rabbit skeletal muscle phosphorylase kinase, *FEBS Lett.,* 92, 287, 1978.

77. **Srivasta, A. K., Waisman, D. M., Brostrom, C. O., and Soderling, T. R.,** Stimulation of glycogen synthase phosphorylation by calcium-dependent regulator protein, *J. Biol. Chem.,* 254, 583, 1979.

78. **Waisman, D. M., Singh, T. J., and Wang, J. H.,** The modulator-dependent protein kinase. A multifunctional protein kinase activatable by the Ca^{2+}-dependent modulator protein of the cyclic nucleotide system, *J. Biol. Chem.,* 253, 3387, 1978.

79. **Grand, R. J. A. and Perry, S. V.,** The binding of calmodulin to myelin basic protein and histone H2B, *Biochem. J.,* 189, 227, 1980.

80. **Itano, T., Itano, R., and Penniston, J. T.,** Interactions of basic polypeptides and proteins with calmodulin, *Biochem. J.,* 189, 455, 1980.

81. **Corbin, J. D., Keely, S. L., and Park, C. R.,** The distribution and dissociation of cyclic adenosine 3',5'-monophosphate-dependent protein kinases in adipose, cardiac and other tissues, *J. Biol. Chem.,* 250, 218, 1975.

82. **Uno, I., Ueda, T., and Greengard, P.,** Differences in properties of cytosol and membrane derived protein kinases, *J. Biol. Chem.,* 251, 2192, 1976.

83. **Rannels, S. R. and Corbin, J. D.,** Characterization of small cAMP-binding fragments of cAMP-dependent protein kinases, *J. Biol. Chem.,* 254, 8605, 1979.

84. **Kinzel, V. and Konig, N.,** Interaction of protease inhibitors with the catalytic subunit of cAMP-dependent protein kinase, *Biochem. Biophys. Res. Commun.,* 93, 349, 1980.

85. **Corbin, J. D., Soderling, T. R., and Park, C. R.,** Regulation of adenosine 3',5'-monophosphate-dependent protein kinase. I. Preliminary characterization of the adipose tissue enzyme in crude extracts, *J. Biol. Chem.,* 248, 1813, 1973.

86. **Keely, S. L., Corbin, J. D., and Park, C. R.,** Regulation of adenosine 3',5'-monophosphate-dependent protein kinase: regulation of the heart enzyme by epinephrine, glucagon, insulin and 1-methyl-3-isobutylxanthine, *J. Biol. Chem.,* 250, 4832, 1975.

87. **Palmer, W. K., McPherson, J. M., and Walsh, D. A.,** Critical controls in the evaluation of cAMP-dependent protein kinase activity ratios as indices of hormonal activation, *J. Biol. Chem.,* 255, 2663, 1980.

88. **Liang, W. Y. and Marsh, J. M.**, Reevaluation of the role of cyclic adenosine 3′,5′-monophosphate and protein kinase in the stimulation of steroidogenesis by luteinizing hormone in bovine corpus lu-team, *Endocrinology*, 100, 1571, 1977.

89. **Podesta, E. J., Dufau, M. L., and Catt, K. J.**, Adenosine 3′,5′-monophosphate dependent protein kinase of Leydig cells: in vitro activation and relationship to gonadotropin action upon cyclic AMP and steroidogenesis, *FEBS Lett.*, 70, 212, 1976.

90. **Dufau, M. L., Horner, K. A., Hayashi, K., Tsuruhara, T., Conn, P. M., and Catt, K. J.**, Action of cholerogen and gonadotropin in isolated Leydig cells. Functional compartmentalization of the hormone-activated cyclic AMP response, *J. Biol. Chem.*, 253, 3721, 1979.

91. **Keely, S. L.**, Prostaglandin E_1 activation of heart cAMP-dependent protein kinase: apparent disso-ciation of protein kinase activation from increases in phosphorylase activity and contractile force, *Mol. Pharmacol.*, 15, 235, 1979.

92. **Swillens, S., van Cauter, E., and Dumont, J. E.**, Protein kinase and cyclic 3′,5′-AMP. Significance of binding and activation constants, *Biochim. Biophys. Acta*, 364, 250, 1974.

93. **Cha, S.**, Kinetic behavior at high enzyme concentrations, *J. Biol. Chem.*, 245, 4814, 1970.

94. **Beavo, J. A., Bechtel, P. J., and Krebs, E. G.**, Activation of protein kinase by physiological concentrations of cyclic AMP, *Proc. Natl. Acad. Sci. U.S.A.*, 71, 3580, 1974.

95. **Gill, G. N. and McCune, R. W.**, Guanosine 3′,5′-monophosphate-dependent protein kinase, *Curr. Top. Cell. Reg.*, 15, 1, 1979.

96. **Lincoln, T. M. and Keely, S. L.**, Effects of acetylcholine and nitroprusside on cGMP-dependent protein kinase activity in the perfused rat heart, *Fed. Proc. Fed. Am. Soc. Exp. Biol.*, 39, 742, 1980.

97. **Szmigielski, A., Guidotti, A., and Costa, E.**, Endogenous protein kinase inhibitors. Purification, characterization and distribution in different tissues, *J. Biol. Chem.*, 252, 3848, 1977.

98. **Kuo, J. F.**, Changes in activities of modulators of cyclic AMP-dependent and cyclic-GMP dependent protein kinases in pancreas and adipose tissue of alloxan-induced diabetic rats, *Biochem. Biophys. Res. Commun.*, 65, 1214, 1975.

99. **Weber, H. and Rosen, O. M.**, Inhibition of adenosine 3′:5′-monophosphate-dependent protein ki-nase: comparison of a protein inhibitor with polyanions and substrate analogs, *J. Cyclic Nucleotide Res.*, 3, 425, 1977.

100. **Khandeleval, R. L., Vandenheede, J. R., and Krebs, E. G.**, Purification properties and substrate specificities of phosphoprotein phosphatase(s) from rabbit liver, *J. Biol. Chem.*, 251, 4850, 1976.

101. **Kato, K. and Bishop, J. S.**, Glycogen synthetase-D phosphatase. I. Some new properties of the partially purified enzyme from rabbit muscle, *J. Biol. Chem.*, 247, 7420, 1972.

102. **Antoniw, J. F. and Cohen, P.**, Separation of two phosphorylase kinase phosphatases from rabbit skeletal muscle, *Eur. J. Biochem.*, 68, 45, 1976.

103. **Tamara, S., Kikuchi, K., Hiraga, A., Kikuchi, H., Hosokawa, M., and Tsuiki, S.**, Character-ization of multiple forms of histone phosphatase in rat liver, *Biochim. Biophys. Acta*, 524, 349, 1978.

104. **Mellgren, R. L., Aylward, J. H., Killilea, S. D., and Lee, E. Y. C.**, The activation and dissociation of a nature high molecular weight form of rabbit skeletal muscle phosphorylase phosphatase by en-dogenous Ca^{2+}-dependent proteases, *J. Biol. Chem.*, 254, 648, 1979.

105. **Cohen, P., Nimmo, G. A., Burchell, A., and Antoniw, J. F.**, The substrate specificity and reg-ulation of the protein phosphatases involved in the control of glycogen metabolism, *Adv. Eng. Reg.*, 16, 97, 1978.

106. **Knight, B. L. and Teal, T. K.**, A comparison between heat-stable phosphatase inhibitors and ac-tivators from rabbit skeletal muscle and liver and their effects upon different preparations of phos-phoprotein phosphatase, *Eur. J. Biochem.*, 104, 521, 1980.

107. **Huang, F. L. and Glinsman, W. H.**, Inactivation of rabbit muscle phosphorylase phosphatase by cyclic AMP-dependent protein kinase, *Proc. Natl. Acad. Sci. U.S.A.*, 72, 3004, 1975.

108. **Rudolph, S. A. and Krueger, B.K.**, Endogenous protein phosphorylation and dephosphorylation, *Adv. Cyclic Nucleotide Res.*, 10, 107, 1979.

109. **Garrels, J. I.**, Two-dimensional gel electrophoresis and computer analysis of proteins synthesized by clonal cell lines, *J. Biol. Chem.*, 254, 7961, 1979.

110. **Gratecos, D. and Fischer, E. M.**, Adenosine 5′-0(3-thiotriphosphate) in the control of phosphorylase activity, *Biochem. Biophys. Res. Commun.*, 58, 960, 1974.

111. **Cassidy, P., Hoar, P. E., and Kerrick, W. G. L.**, Irreversible thiophosphorylation and activation of tension in functionally skinned rabbit ileum strips by [^{35}S]ATP-γ-S, *J. Biol. Chem.*, 250, 11148, 1979.

112. **Kerrick, W. G. L., Hoar, P. E., and Cassidy, P. S.**, Calcium-activated tension: the role of myosin light chain phosphorylation, *Fed. Proc. Fed. Am. Soc. Exp.*, 39, 1558, 1980.

113. **Berridge, M. J.**, The interaction of cyclic nucleotides and calcium in the control of cellular activity, *Adv. Cyclic Nucleotide Res.*, 6, 1, 1975.

114. **Rasmussen, H. and Goodman, D. B. P.,** Relationships between calcium and cyclic nucleotides in cell activation, *Physiol. Rev.,* 57, 421, 1977.

115. **Wolff, D. J. and Brostrom, C. O.,** Properties and functions of the calcium-dependent regulator protein, *Adv. Cyclic Nucleotide Res.,* 11, 27, 1979.

116. **Klee, C. B., Crouch, T. H., and Richman, P. G.,** Calmodulin, *Annu. Rev. Biochem.,* 49, 489, 1980.

117. **Wang, J. H. and Waisman, D. M.,** Calmodulin and its role in the second-messenger system, *Curr. Top. Cell. Reg.,* 15, 47, 1979.

118. **Conti, M. A. and Adelstein, R. S.,** Phosphorylation by cyclic adenosine 3':5'-monophosphate-dependent protein kinase regulates myosin light chain kinase, *Fed. Proc. Fed. Am. Soc. Exp. Biol.,* 39, 1569, 1980.

119. **LePeuch, C. J., Harech, J., and Demaille, J. G.,** Concerted regulation of cardiac sarcoplasmic reticulum calcium transport by cyclic adenosine monophosphate dependent and calcium-calmodulin-dependent phosphorylation, *Biochemistry,* 18, 5150, 1979.

120. **Huttner, W. B. and Greengard, P.,** Multiple phosphorylation sites in protein I and their differential regulation by cyclic AMP and calcium, *Proc. Natl. Acad. Sci. U.S.A.,* 76, 5402, 1979.

121. **Wallace, R. W. and Cheung, W. Y.,** Calmodulin. Production of an antibody in rabbit and development of a radioimmunoassay, *J. Biol. Chem.,* 254, 6564, 1979.

122. **Chafouleas, J. G., Dedman, J. R., Munjaal, R. P., and Means, A. R.,** Calmodulin. Development and application of a sensitive radioimmunoassay, *J. Biol. Chem.,* 254, 10262, 1979.

123. **Walker, J. D. and Walker, J. B.,** Properties of adenylate cyclase from senescent rat brain, *Brain Res.,* 54, 391, 1973.

124. **Govoni, S., Loddo, P., Spano, P. F., and Trabucchi, M.,** Dopamine receptor sensitivity in brain and retina of rats during aging, *Brain Res.,* 138, 565, 1977.

125. **Puri, S. K. and Volicer, L.,** Effect of aging on cyclic AMP levels and adenylate cyclase and phosphodiesterase activities in the corpus striatum, *Mech. Ageing Dev.,* 6, 53, 1977.

126. **Schmidt, M. J. and Thornberry, J. F.,** Cyclic AMP and cyclic GMP accumulation in vitro in brain regions of young, old, and aged rats, *Brain Res.,* 139, 169, 1978.

127. **Makman, M. H., Ahn, H. S., Thal, L. J., Sharpless, N. S., Dvorkin, B., Horowitz, S. G., and Rosenfeld, M.,** Evidence for selective loss of brain dopamine- and histamine-stimulated adenylate cyclase activities in rabbits with aging, *Brain Res.,* 192, 177, 1980.

128. **Cooper, B. and Gregerman, R. I.,** Hormone-sensitive fat cell adenylate cyclase in the rat. Influences of growth, cell size, and aging, *J. Clin. Invest.,* 57, 161, 1976.

129. **Kalish, M. J., Katz, M. S., Pineyro, M. A., and Gregerman, R. I.,** Epinephrine- and glucagon-sensitive adenylate cyclases in rat liver during aging. Evidence for membrane instability associated with increased enzymatic activity, *Biochim. Biophys. Acta,* 483, 452, 1977.

130. **Katz, M. S., Kalish, M. I., Pineyro, M. A., and Gregerman, R. I.,** Quantitation of epinephrine- and glucagon-sensitive adenylate cyclases of rat liver. Implications of alterations of enzymatic activities during preparation of particulate fractions and membranes, *Biochim. Biophys. Acta,* 540, 205, 1978.

131. **Katz, M. S., Kelly, T. M., Pineyro, M. A., and Gregerman, R. I.,** Activation of epinephrine and glucagon-sensitive adenylate cyclases of rat liver by cytosol protein factors. Role in loss of enzyme activities during preparation of particulate fractions, quantitation, and partial characterization, *J. Cyclic Nucleotide Res.,* 5, 389, 1978.

132. **Premont, J., Perey, M., and Bocksert, J.,** Adenosine-sensitive adenylate cyclase in rat striatal homogenates and its relationship to dopamine- and Ca^{2+}-sensitive adenylate cyclases, *Mol. Pharmacol.,* 13, 662, 1977.

133. **Gnegy, M. R., Vzunov, P., and Costa, E.,** Regulation of the dopamine stimulation of striatal adenylate cyclase by an endogenous Ca^{2+}-binding protein, *Proc. Natl. Acad. Sci., U.S.A.,* 73, 2887, 1976.

134. **Gnegy, M. E., Lucchelli, A., and Costa, E.,** Correlation between drug-induced supersensitivity of dopamine dependent striatal mechanism and the increase in striatal content of the Ca^{2+} regulated protein activator of cAMP phosphodiesterase, *Naunyn-Schmiedebergs Arch. Pharmacol.,* 301, 121, 1977.

135. **Roufogalis, B. D., Thornton, M., and Wade, D. N.,** Nucleotide requirement of dopamine sensitive adenylate cyclase in synaptosomal membranes from the striatum of the rat brain, *J. Neurochem.,* 27, 1533, 1976.

136. **Chen, T. C., Cote, T. E., and Kebabian, J. W.,** Endogenous components of the striatum confer dopamine sensitivity upon adenylate cyclase activity: the role of endogenous guanyl nucleotides, *Brain Res.,* 181, 139, 1980.

137. **Guidicelli, Y. and Pecquery, R.,** β-adrenergic receptors and catecholamine-sensitive adenylate cyclase in rat fat-cell membranes: influence of growth, cell size, and aging, *Eur. J. Biochem.,* 90, 413, 1978.

138. **Dax, E. M., Partilla, J. S., and Gregerman, R. I.,** Epinephrine stimulated lipolysis, β-adrenergic binding, adenylate cyclase, and intracellular cyclic AMP in rat adipocytes during maturation and aging, *J. Lipid Res.,* 22, 934, 1981.

139. **Jolly, S. R., Lombardo, Y. B., Lech, J. J. and Menahan, L. A.,** Effect of aging and cellularity on lipolysis in isolated mouse fat cells, *J. Lipid Res.,* 21, 44, 1980.

140. **Soderling, T. R., Corbin, J. D., and Park, C. R.,** Regulation of adenosine 3',5'-monophosphate-dependent protein kinase. II. Hormonal regulation of the adipose tissue enzyme, *J. Biol. Chem.,* 248, 1822, 1973.

141. **Cooper, B., Weinblatt, F., and Gregerman, R. J.,** Enhanced activity of hormone-sensitive adenylate cyclase during dietary restriction in the rat. Dependence on age and relation to cell size, *J. Clin. Invest.,* 59, 467, 1977.

142. **Masoro, E. J., Bertrand, H., Liepa, G., and Yu, B. P.,** Analysis of age-related changes in mammalian structure and function, *Fed. Proc. Fed. Am. Soc. Exp. Biol.,* 38, 1956, 1979.

143. **Yu, B. P., Bertrand, H. A., Masoro, E. J.,** Nutrition-aging influence of catecholamine-promoted lipolysis, *Metabolism,* 29, 438, 1980.

144. **Schmidt, M. J., Truex, L. L., Conway, R. G., and Routtenberg, A.,** Cyclic AMP-dependent protein kinase activity and synaptosomal protein phosphorylation in the brains of aged rats, *J. Neurochem.,* 32, 335, 1979.

145. **Schmidt, M. J., Truex, L. L., Ghetti, B., and Routtenberg, A.,** Cyclic AMP-dependent protein kinase activity in human brain across age, *J. Neurochem.,* 35, 261, 1980.

146. **Tsitouras, P. D., Kowatch, M. A., and Harman, S. M.,** Age-related alterations of isolated rat Leydig-cell function-gonadotropin receptors, adenosine 3',5'-monophosphate response, and testosterone secretion, *Endocrinology,* 105, 1400, 1979.

147. **Tsitouras, P. D., Kowatch, M. A., and Harman, S. M.,** HCG reverses secretory defect in Leydig cells from old rats, presented at *62nd Annu. Meet. of the Endocr. Soc.,* Program and Abstracts, Washington, D.C., June 18-20, 1980, 81.

148. **Lakatta, E. G.,** Age-related alterations in the cardiovascular response to adrenergic mediated stress, *Fed. Proc. Fed. Am. Soc. Exp. Biol.,* 39, 3173, 1980.

149. **Guarnieri, T., Filburn, C. R., Zitnik, G., Roth, G. S., and Lakatta, E. G.,** Contractile and biochemical correlates of β-adrenergic stimulation of the aged heart, *Am. J. Physiol.,* 239, H501, 1980.

150. **Froehlich, J. P., Lakatta, E. G., Beard, E., Spurgeon, H. A., Weisfeldt, M. L., and Gerstenblith, G.,** Studies of sarcoplasmic reticulum function and contraction duration in young adult and aged rat myocardium, *J. Mol. Cell. Cardiol.,* 10, 427, 1978.

151. **Kadoma, M., Sacktor, B., and Froehlich, J. P.,** Stimulation by cAMP and protein kinase of calcium transport in sarcoplasmic reticulum from senescent rat myocardium, *Fed. Proc. Fed. Am. Soc. Exp. Biol.,* 39, 2040, 1980.

Chapter 4

AGE-RELATED CHANGES IN HORMONE ACTION: THE ROLE OF HORMONE RECEPTORS

George S. Roth

TABLE OF CONTENTS

I. INTRODUCTION AND BACKGROUND

During the past decade there has been considerable interest in elucidating the molecular mechanisms by which hormones act on target cells to produce their various physiological effects. Although a great many questions still remain unanswered, substantial knowledge has been accumulated in this area. Figure 1 illustrates some of the better documented molecular steps in the actions of some representative hormones. Of course not all hormones affect all cells, nor do different cells always respond to given hormones in the same ways. Nevertheless, some relatively common features of these complex processes can be readily discerned.

The initial step in the actions of essentially all hormones is attachment to specific cellular proteins known as "receptors."[1-3] Operationally these may be divided into two general types: those located on the surface membrane and those located inside the cell. For most hormones which work through the former receptor class, entrance into the cell does not appear necessary. In some cases, however, controversy may exist on this point. Obviously, though, hormones must pass through the plasma membrane in order to bind to the intracellular receptor types. Many of the hormones interacting with membrane receptors exert their effects at least partially through the activation of "adenylate cyclase." This enzyme catalyzes the conversion of ATP to cyclic AMP, the so-called "second messenger," and inorganic pyrophosphate. Glucagon, catecholamines, ACTH, and dopamine are all hormones which work through elevation of intracellular cyclic AMP levels. These levels can be reduced by phosphodie-sterase enzymes which convert cyclic AMP to AMP. In some cases, phosphodiesterase activity has also been shown to be under hormonal control. Cyclic AMP levels determine the degree of activation of protein kinase enzymes which in turn phosphorylate various other proteins. This latter phosphorylation leads ultimately to specific biological effects. Among these are increased rates of lipolysis, muscle contraction and relaxation, glycogenolysis, regulation of microtubule function, and various enzyme inductions.[4] All of these are vitally important to normal physiological function and homeostatic balance.

Certain hormones which attach to cell membrane receptors do not appear to activate adenylate cyclase. Insulin is a prime example. It has been suggested that insulin may stimulate guanylate cyclase to elevate cellular cyclic GMP levels. However, this hypothesis is still rather tenuous. Indeed, it is still not certain what the "second messenger" for insulin actually is, or whether, in fact, such a mediator exists at all. It is certain, however, that insulin exerts a myriad of effects, depending on the cells with which it interacts. Some of these are stimulation of glucose transport and metabolism in adipocytes, stimulation of proteins synthesis in many cells types, specific enzyme inductions and enhancement of glycogen formation in liver.

Various other hormones have been shown to act through attachment to cell surface receptors, but the above examples will suffice for present purposes. On the other side of the coin, the intracellular (sometimes called "gene-active") hormones are found. Steroids probably comprise the largest group of hormones in this category. They appear to diffuse passively through the plasma membrane in most cases and then bind to receptors located in the cytoplasm.[2] After this initial attachment the receptor-hormone

HORMONE RESPONSIVE CELL

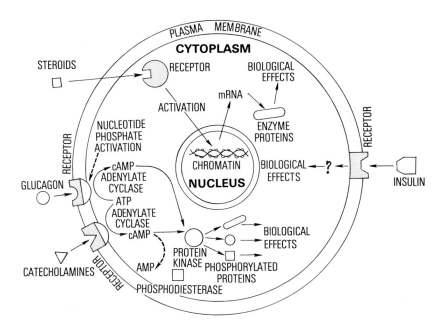

FIGURE 1. Hormone responsive cell. Different hormones exert their cellular effects in various ways. Initial interaction occurs at the level of specific receptors. Subsequent biochemical events may include activation of cellular enzymes, movement of hormone receptor complexes into the nucleus, and derepression of chromatin. Ultimately, diverse biological effects take place.

complex becomes "activated" in some way, allowing it to enter the nucleus. In the nucleus the complex binds to chromatin at specific sites. The nature of these sites, and the properties of certain steroid receptors which allow such recognition, have recently been the subject of several elegant investigations.[3] Equally impressive studies have demonstrated that certain messenger RNA templates are transcribed subsequent to the binding of receptor-hormone complexes to the chromatin. These in turn are translated into specific enzyme proteins which are implicated in various biological effects. Such responses include enzyme inductions, control of nutrient transport and metabolism, and inhibition of cell proliferation among others.[2,3] Additional intracellularly active hormones include thyroxin, triiodothyronine, and several other compounds. In the case of the thyroid hormones, binding may occur to cytoplasmic proteins or directly to chromosomal proteins.[5] It is the latter that appear to be the true receptors in some tissues based on ability to mediate thyroid hormone specific responses.

Having given some consideration to both the molecular biology involved in effecting hormone actions as well as the physiological actions themselves, it is important to realize that such processes are exquisitely sensitive to alteration by any number of factors. It is thence that the primary topic of this review is arrived at, namely the aging process and its relationship to the mechanisms of hormone action. Since aging is characterized by a decreased ability to adapt to many different conditions, it is not surprising that gerontologists have focused their attention on hormone actions as key examples of adaptive responsiveness which may be altered with age.[6–10] Representative examples of these studies and their implications will be discussed here. More than this, however, an attempt will be made to survey and evaluate the methodology and design of such investigations, with particular emphasis on those inherent technical and theoretical factors which must be considered in any legitimate study of the aging process.

II. EFFECTS OF AGING ON RESPONSIVENESS
TO HORMONES IN VIVO

A great number of responses to hormones in whole organisms have been shown to change during aging (for reviews see References 6 to 10). Generally in such situations, hormones are injected into animals and allowed sufficient time to reach target tissues where they produce biological effects. Measurements of particular responses may be made in the living organism or animals may be sacrificed and certain tissues removed, then examined physically and/or chemically. Such in vivo responses are quite complex and many factors must be considered in interpreting data even apart from age considerations. In the case of aging studies one must be aware of possible age differences in metabolism and distribution of hormones subsequent to their administration. In some situations a particular hormone may elicit many different responses, some of which may help to control others. Age changes in such regulatory responses might serve to alter any other effects that are directly under observation. If a particular response is to be measured in a tissue removed at some time after hormone is administered in vivo, what are the effects of age on the stability of the tissue, its physical integrity, and chemical composition? With such caveats in mind, let some representative examples of age studies on hormonal responsiveness in vivo be surveyed.

A. Isoproterenol Stimulation of Rat Salivary Gland DNA Synthesis and Cell Division

Numerous studies have examined the ability of the synthetic catecholamine, isoproterenol, to stimulate rat salivary gland DNA synthesis and cell division during aging.[11–15] Large numbers of rats are injected with the hormone, then ^{3}H-thymidine is administered to individual groups of five or six animals at various times. After 30 to 60 min these individual groups are sacrificed, their salivary glands removed, and the DNA extracted for specific radioactivity determinations. The time required to elicit stimulated DNA synthesis is progressively increased while the magnitude of this response is progressively decreased as rats age from 2 to at least 24 months (Figures 2 and 3). In addition, the induction of certain enzymes, as well as postulated RNA species required for DNA synthesis, are also delayed with increasing age. It would appear that the injected isporoterenol reaches the salivary glands at the same time in rats of all ages since stimulation of amylase secretion is not age dependent.[11] Consequently, several studies attempted to localize the initial biochemical event affected by age within the gland itself.[12–15] Unfortunately, however, the situation is more complicated than is first apparent since certain regulatory agents, in particular glucocorticoid hormones, seem to control the DNA synthesis; cell division response and the sensitivity to this control may be altered with increasing age.[13] Thus, in attempting to elucidate the causes of age related changes in ability of isoproterenol to stimulate DNA synthesis in vivo, glucocorticoid levels and sensitivity need to be examined as well.

B. ACTH Stimulation of Adrenal Androgen Excretion in Humans

The ability of ACTH to increase plasma levels of dehydroepiandrosterone sulfate (DS) was studied in humans aged 3 to 80 years.[16] Hormone was injected twice daily for 2 consecutive days and plasma DS was assayed on the 2nd and 3rd days. Basal levels of DS increased with age until approximately 20 years, then decreased progressively thereafter. After ACTH stimulation the percent increase in plasma DS was found

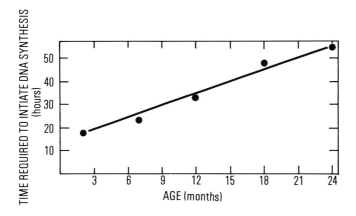

FIGURE 2. Effect of age on time required to initiate DNA synthesis in rat salivary glands following isoproterenol injection. Rats of various ages were injected with isoproterenol as described in the text and References 11 to 15. ^{3}H-thymidine was administered 30 min. prior to sacrifice at various times and DNA extracted for specific radioactivity determination as previously indicated in References 11 to 15. The time of onset of DNA synthesis was then determined for each age group.

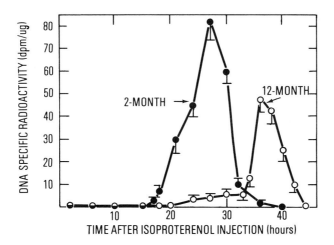

FIGURE 3. Effect of age on isoproterenol-stimulated DNA synthesis in rat salivary glands. Experimental procedures were as for Figure 2. Data from individual experiments on groups of 2- and 12-month-old rats are shown. Values represent means ± standard errors for three to six rats of each time point.

to be comparable in both young adult and sensecent subjects. However, because of much lower basal levels in the aged group, the absolute stimulation was five- to sixfold greater in the younger people. This type of phenomenon, which will also be discussed with respect to in vitro responses, is frequently observed in aging studies. It is therefore important to delineate the relationship between basal and stimulated levels, and to determine which is the more accurate measure of functional responsiveness.

Another consideration involves the time course of the response. Although many of the older subjects did not increase plasma (DS) levels substantially between days 2 and

3, levels in most younger subjects were still rising rapidly on day 3. Thus, an even greater age difference might be apparent if the study were conducted over a longer period of time. It is therefore important to determine time courses of responsiveness thoroughly for each age group in question, since as with the salivary gland stimulation by isoproterenol cited previously, age changes can occur both in magnitude and timing of hormone dependent processes. Without proper measurement of both, age-related differences may be missed.

Finally, ACTH was administered only at a single dose of 40 IU per injection. Such a regimen was undoubtedly necessitated by the limitations of human studies. The possibility exists, however, that different dose-response relationships may be observed in different age groups. Whether these are due to differential sensitivity at the target tissue level, or altered transport and metabolism of hormone, apparent differences in the response in question may ultimately be observed. It is therefore important to check dose-response relationship as well as time courses in such studies to avoid misinterpretation of the apparent presence or absence of age differences.

C. Thyroxine Stimulation of Cardiac Hypertrophy in Mice

Florini and co-workers measured the effects of thyroxine administration on induction of cardiac hypertrophy in adult (8 months) and senescent (26 months) euthyroid mice.[17] Ultimately, heart to body weight ratios reached the same values in both groups. However the response in the old mice lagged several days behind that of the young. In this respect, the data are somewhat similar to those obtained in the studies of isoproterenol stimulated salivary gland DNA synthesis previously cited. In the heart investigation it appeared that rates of cardiac protein synthesis took longer to become elevated following thyroxine stimulation of the old mice, and this delay seemed to account for the lag in hypertrophy. Protein synthesis was measured utilizing a 30 min ^{3}H-leucine perfusion in vitro. It is important to point out in comparing rates of protein synthesis in tissues of different aged animals that intergroup differences in specific radioactivities of amino acid pools can substantially prejudice results. To the credit of these workers, all values were calculated on the basis of individually determined ^{3}H-leucine-pool specific radioactivities for each heart. However, it was later determined by the same group that an even more exact procedure requires calculation of ^{3}H-leucyl t-RNA-pool specific radioactivities since it is this latter species which is the direct precursor of cellular proteins.

D. Thyroxine Stimulation of Basal Metabolic Rate and Oxygen Consumption in Thyroidectomized Rats

An older study of thyroid responsiveness in rodents contrasts the Florini study in that stimulation of basal metabolic rate and oxygen consumption are actually greater in the older age group.[18] These responses, however, are considerably more complex than the direct cardiac stimulation by thyroxine. In an effort to achieve comparable circulating hormone levels in both young and old rats, animals were thyroidectomized and thyroxine was administered in proportion to the 3/4 power of body weight. This figure is assumed to represent the metabolic mass of the test animals based on previous studies. After thyroidectomy, basal oxygen consumption fell by about one third for both age groups although intact levels were slightly higher in senescent rats. However, under the influence of the assumed identical circulating thyroxine levels, old animals were found to be significantly more responsive in terms of basal metabolic rate. Whether this apparent age difference represents a true increase in sensitivity or rather is simply a reflection of a reduced thyroxine clearance rate or some consequence of thyroidectomy has not been determined.

E. Estradiol Induction of Acetylcholinesterase in Rat Brain

Moudgil and Kanungo reported a progressive decrease with age in the ability of estradiol to induce the enzyme acetylcholinesterase in rat brain in vivo.[19] Age differences were observed in both intact and ovariectomized female animals. In addition, basal levels of acetylcholinesterase were progressively reduced with increasing age. Nevertheless, percent as well as absolute stimulation was reduced, since by 65 weeks of age no enzyme induction at all was detected.

It should be pointed out that enzyme activity was measured only at a single time point 4 hr after estradiol administration and only one dose of hormone was employed. Thus, the possibility that acetylcholinesterase might actually be inducible in the oldest rats, either at a later time or by a higher dose of estradiol, cannot be eliminated.

F. Androgen Stimulation of α-2-u Globulin Production in Rat Liver

Roy and his group observed that the livers of sexually mature rats produce α-2-u globulin in response to androgenic stimulation.[20] This protein has a molecular weight of 26,400 and is the principal urinary protein in adult moles. α-2-u Globulin appears to be synthesized in the hepatic parenchymal cells and requires the synergistic influence of various hormones including glucocorticoids, insulin, thyroid hormones, and growth hormone.

When senescent, 26-month-old animals were examined, it was observed that no α-2-u globulin was found in the urine following 25 days of testosterone administration.[20] This was in marked contrast to 5-month-old controls whose urine contained about 33 μg of this protein per day. It is surprising that a possible age related impairment in the entry of this hepatic protein into the urine was not considered in this study, as this might be an obvious explanation. Further supportive data for the androgenic insensitivity were obtained, however, and will be discussed. Nevertheless, this system, like all the other in vivo responsiveness situations discussed thus far, possesses an inherent complexity (e.g., regulation by many other hormones) and possible age effects on any of these control steps would certainly tend to contribute to apparent differences in responsiveness between mature and senescent animals.

III. EFFECTS OF AGING ON RESPONSIVENESS TO HORMONES IN VITRO

Having surveyed some representative examples of age related changes in responsiveness to hormones in vivo it is now appropriate to consider similar types of studies performed in vitro. Here, the overwhelming complexity of the whole organism has been minimized by removing particular cell or tissue types to isolated baths or cultures prior to administration of hormones. Thus the influence of intricate feedback and secondary regulatory mechanisms can be circumvented and the intrinsic responsiveness of given cells or tissues may be measured. Needless to say, such an approach is extremely valuable for aging studies. Nevertheless, new and different problems in interpreting the results of in vitro aging experiments soon become apparent. For example, what are the effects of age on the ability of particular tissues to survive sometimes harsh isolation procedures? Once isolated, do different nutritional requirements and culture conditions exist for tissues of different ages? What are the consequences of separating tissues from their customary innervation and micro environment? In isolating particular cell types, are recoveries comparable at different ages? All of these factors and many more must be considered in planning and evaluating any in vitro age studies, not to mention the possible differential age effects of isolation and culture conditions on the cellular components involved in mediating specific hormone dependent processes. This section will therefore deal with some representative changes in responsiveness to hormones in vitro with particular emphasis on such problematic considerations.

A. Isoproterenol Stimulation of Aortic Relaxation in Rats and Rabbits

Fleisch and his co-workers have carried out most of the work in this area.[21,22] Their basic finding is that with increased age, the ability of isporoterenol to elicit relaxation of rat and rabbit aortic strips is progressively decreased. The greatest reduction in this response occurs during the first 50% of the life span, although a slight reduction continues into later life.

The experimental protocol requires that helically cut thoracic aortic strips be placed in a tissue bath and made to contract with histamine or seratonin following alpha adrenergic receptor blockade by phentolamine. Isoproterenol is then administered at various concentrations and contraction measured. An important control is the use of $NaNO_2$ as a nonspecific relaxant. When aortic strips were exposed to this agent no age difference in contraction was observed. Thus, whatever problems might be inherent in the isolation and/or culturing conditions employed, the innate ability of tissues of all ages to contract did not appear to be disturbed. Instead, age differences seem to occur at the level of the specific β-adrenergic mechanism by which contraction is elicited. This is further demonstrated by the fact that this response is blocked by propranolol, by definition a β-adrenergic antagonist. As mentioned above, it is still possible that the specific adrenergic mechanism involved in this response in old animals is more disturbed by the isolation procedure than in young, or that the effects of denervation are differentially age-altered. These possibilities are very difficult to prove, however. Moreover, the fact that responsiveness to isoproterenol has also been found to be reduced in vivo in the case of stimulated salivary gland DNA synthesis[11-15] lends further support to the validity of Fleisch's conclusions.

B. Epinephrine Stimulation of Hepatic Adenylate Cyclase in Rats

Another β-adrenergic response, the ability of epinephrine to stimulate rat hepatic adenylate cyclase, was examined in vitro by Gregerman's group.[23] In contrasted to the adrenergic studies mentioned thus far, this response actually increases with increasing age. Again, the age difference appears to be specific to the β-adrenergic mechanism since glucagon and fluoride stimulation are increased only slightly in aged females and not at all in aged males (24 to 26 months). Glucagon works through a separate receptor from that of epinephrine and NaF in some cases is believed to reveal most of the total adenylate cyclase enzyme activity present.

Although the interpretation of these findings in mechanistic terms is not yet clear, these workers have raised several important theoretical and methodological points to be considered in performing such studies. First, stimulated enzyme activity should be expressed in absolute units rather than merely as fold increase of basal levels. It is not yet understood as to what factors contribute to basal adenylate cyclase activity, let alone how they might change during aging. Moreover, the relationship between basal and hormone stimulated levels also needs to be elucidated both in aging and nonaging studies.

Second, the nature of the tissue preparations in which adenylate cyclase is measured in vitro is extremely important in evaluating experimental results. Generally radioactively labeled ATP is added either to tissue whole homogenates or to particulate fractions obtained by various centrifugation and washing conditions. After incubation at various temperatures for various times, the cyclic AMP product is separated by ion exchange chromatography and quantitated. Kalish et al.[23] found that if their experiments were performed with particulates rather than homogenates, hormone stimulated values were substantially lowered and age differences were negligible. Thus it is extremely important to consider the possible differential age effects of in vitro preparation and environmental conditions not only on tissues and cells, but also on subcellular fractions in broken cell preparations.

Along these same lines, several tissues appear to possess supernatant factors which are required for full expression of adenylate cyclase activity. These factors are removed in the preparation of particulate fractions. Again, this level of control represents a possible age affected area to be included in any evaluation of such experiments.

Finally, the overall condition of the plasma membrane must be taken into account in studies of adenylate cyclase during aging. Differential stability of hormone, fluoride, and basal activities is apparent in rat liver with increasing age. The possible contribution of membrane lipid alterations to stability differences cannot be excluded. Such stability differences may be particularly important in some reports of altered adenylate cyclase activity during aging.

C. Norepinephrine Stimulation of Lipolysis in Human Adipocytes

Still another adrenergic response studied during aging is the norepinephrine stimulation of lipolysis in human adipocytes.[24] Biopsied subcutaneous adipose tissue was digested with collogenase to liberate adipocyte suspensions. Cells were then exposed to norepinephrine and lipolytic rates determined by measurement of free fatty acid and glycerol release.

In designing and interpreting their experiments, these investigators raised a most important consideration for aging studies on adipose, or for that matter, any tissue. Namely, to what extent are apparent age changes or lack of them simply due to changes in body weight or cell size? To distinguish between these two possibilities, Berger et al.[24] divided their subjects (aged 18 to 72 years) into an overweight and a normal weight group. Basal levels of adipocyte lipolysis were not seen to change with age in either group. However, when norepinephrine stimulated lipolysis was measured, progressive age related reduction in responsiveness was observed in the normal weight, but not the overweight group. In fact, the overweight subjects responded similarly to the oldest normal weight subjects. Thus, fat cell size as well as age may contribute to the degree of hormonal responsiveness in certain situations.

D. Insulin Stimulation of Glucose Oxidation and Lipid Synthesis in Human and Rat Adipocytes

Human as well as rat adipocyte and adipose tissue responsiveness to insulin in vitro was also studied during aging.[25] As in the norepinephrine study just mentioned, decreased responsiveness with increasing age was observed. Reductions were seen in rats and human cells and tissue segments for the stimulation of both CO_2 production and lipid synthesis. Somewhat reminiscent of the isoproternol stimulation of aortic relaxation,[21,22] the bulk of these reductions occur in the first half of the life span although some decline continues on into later life.

One problem with this relatively early study was that both glucose oxidation and lipid synthesis were expressed per gram of esterified fatty acid. No consideration of age differences in cell size or heterogeneity of cell sizes at a given age was made for either rat or human experiments, however. In light of the differences between obese and non-obese human adipocyte responsiveness to norepinephrine raised by Berger et al. it is difficult to determine whether age differences in insulin responsiveness might be more or less pronounced if expressed per cell and possible differences in cell sizes taken into account.

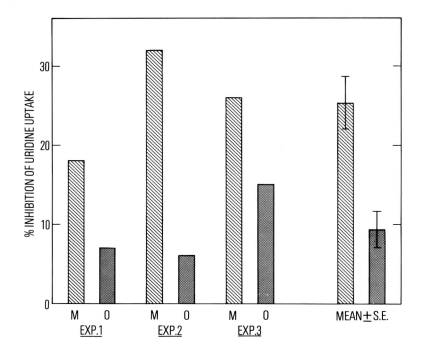

FIGURE 4. Effect of age on cortisol inhibition of uridine uptake in rat splenic leukocytes. Splenic leukocytes were prepared from 12- to 14-month-old, mature rats (M) hatched bars and 24- to 26-month-old senescent counterparts(0) filled bars. Assessment of cortisol inhibition of ^{3}H-uridine uptake was as described in the text and References 26 and 27. Values from three separate experiments using five pooled spleens of each age, along with means and standard errors are depicted.

E. Cortisol Inhibition of Uridine Uptake into Rat Splenic Leukocytes

The ability of the glucocorticoid hormone, cortisol, to inhibit uridine uptake into splenic leukocytes in vitro was shown to be reduced in 24- to 26-month-old rats when compared to 12- to 14-month-old counterparts (Figure 4).[26,27] Cells were incubated with or without 2×10^{-6} M hormone for 3 hr. ^{3}H-uridine was then added and cells were harvested, washed, and lysed after a 30 min exposure. Incorporation of ^{3}H was then assessed by scintillation counting of cellular lysates.

Cells were obtained by gently teasing apart spleens in the presence of culture medium. Erythrocytes were removed from the population by lysis in 0.83% ammonium chloride. Resultant leukocytes were found to be over 95% viable in both age groups. Moreover, morphological examination revealed that both populations consisted of over 95% lymphocytes. Thus, the cellular isolation procedure did not seem to alter differentially either age group. That fact that both groups also contained the same amount of cytoplasmic protein further supported their comparability for aging studies.

Another important point, also made in some of the studies previously cited, is that basal levels of responsiveness (in this case, uridine uptake) are essentially the same in cells for both mature and senescent rats. This observation suggests that preparation procedures have not damaged the metabolic integrity of the cells at least for the function in question. Thus, as with the studies by Fleisch et al. on aortic relaxation,[21,22] age changes occur in hormone specific responses rather than innate basal function.

F. Glucocorticoid Extension of Human Fibroblast Life Span In Vitro

Cristofalo and his co-workers have intensively studied the ability of glucocorticoid hormones to prolong the in vitro life span of WI-38 diploid human fibroblasts.[28] These cells have previously been shown to possess a limited proliferative capacity in culture, and can be serially passaged 50 to 60 times under normal conditions. If glucocorticoids are added to the culture medium, however, this life span can be extended 30 to 50%. The degree of extension is dependent upon the in vitro age at which hormone is first added to the culture.

Since in vitro fibroblast senescence appears to occur randomly (i.e., certain cells simply cease to undergo further divisions at various times), the effect of glucocorticoids seems to be one of encouraging particular cells to undergo more divisions than would normally be the case. This effect appears to be quite structurally specific for certain glucocorticoid molecules and other steroids are inactive in this regard. Thus, certain hormonal responses may be altered during in vitro as well as in vivo aging.

IV. THE ROLE OF HORMONE RECEPTORS IN REGULATING PHYSIOLOGICAL RESPONSIVENESS: STUDIES ON HORMONE RECEPTORS DURING AGING

Since so many responses to hormones (both in vivo and in vitro) are altered during aging, investigators have attempted to elucidate the mechanisms responsible for such changes. This has required a thorough knowledge of the basic molecular steps in the action of various hormones as discussed in the introductory section and depicted in Figure 1. For a number of reasons, the interaction of various hormones with their specific receptors has been the most intensely studied aspect of hormone action changes during aging.

First of all, attachment of hormones to receptors is the initial required step in the actions of essentially all hormones.[1-3] Thus, it is a logical place to begin examining age changes in these functions. Second, in many cases the degree of biological responsiveness is proportional to the amount of complexes which form between hormones and their receptors. This fact points out the importance of receptor binding in regulating some hormonal responses. Third, in many altered physiological states including development, disease, and certain biological cycles, changes occur in hormone receptor concentrations which appear to be closely, if not causally, related to similar alterations in physiological responsiveness.[8] Thus, gerontologists wondered whether similar changes in hormone receptor concentrations might be occuring during aging to account for some of the altered responsiveness characteristic of this period.

A. Intracellular Hormone Receptors

Initial studies focused on steroid hormone receptors since these are easily measured and they are present in almost all tissues. Steroid receptors are intracellular and in the absence of hormone in the environment are found in the cytoplasm.[2,3] For this reason adrenalectomized rats were employed for whole tissue measurements of glucocorticoid receptors. Homogenization, followed by ultracentrifugation yields cytoplasmic fractions. These are then incubated with radioactive hormone at 0 to 4° C. Duplicate samples containing, in addition, large excesses of unlabeled hormone are run in parallel to correct for nonsaturable, "nonspecific" binding. After binding equilibrium, which is approached in 1 to 2 hr, unbound radioactivity is quickly removed by adsorption to activated charcoal, and specific binding measured by scintillation counting of macromolecular-bound radioactivity. Using variations of this basic procedure, it was determined that the concentrations, but not the affinities of steroid receptors in a number of tissue types, including brain, adipose, liver, skeletal muscle, prostrate gland, etc., were reduced during aging (Table 1). Concentrations were generally expressed per unit protein although in essentially all cases, age related reductions were also apparent when data were expressed per cell or per unit DNA. Some of these receptors appear to be lost

Table 1
REDUCTIONS IN STEROID HORMONE RECEPTOR LEVELS DURING AGING

Hormone receptor	Tissue or cell	Ref.
Early Adulthood		
Glucocorticoid	Rat liver	29
	Rat thymus	29
Androgen	Rat cerebral cortex	30
Senescence		
Glucocorticoid	Rat splenic leukocyte	26, 27
	Rat cerebral cortex	31
	Rat cortical neuron	32
	Rat skeletal muscle	31
	Rat adipose tissue	31
	Rat adipocyte	33
	Human liver	34
	Human fibroblast (WI-38)	35
Androgen	Rat liver	20
	Rat ventral prostrate	36
	Rat lateral prostrate	37
	Rat hypothalamus	30
	Rat pituitary	30
	Rat testes	30
Estrogen	Rat uterus	38
	Mouse uterus	39
	Rat brain	40

most drastically in the early adult portion of the life span, while concentrations of others are reported not to change at all during aging. In addition, certain discrepancies or controversies may exist in the case of some of these investigations. First of all, studies in mice and rats have detected no change in hepatic glucocorticoid receptor levels.[31,41] This appears to be in contrast to the human situation where such a loss occurs when post-mortem livers of 30- to 40-year-old subjects are compared to those of 66- to 80-year-old counterparts,[34] and to a rat study showing receptor loss during early adulthood.[29] However, possible problems due to the use of post-mortem material cannot be excluded in the human work, nor can possible species differences. On closer examination, it would appear that the reported loss of rat hepatic corticosteroid receptors between 2 and 18 months of age is dependent on expression of concentration per wet tissue weight.[29] If the data are expressed per unit protein as in the two studies showing no age changes, receptor concentrations also appear to be static after about 9 months.

No significant differences in cerebral cortical corticosteroid receptor content between mice aged 8 to 12 months and 28 to 32 months were reported by Nelson et al.[42] In possible contrast, studies in the author's laboratory have shown an approximately 35% reduction in these receptor levels which occurs progressively from at least 3 to 25 or more months of age in rats.[31] Possibly again, species differences may account for this discrepancy. However, differences between the two studies may actually be insignificant if one considers that receptor losses between 13 and 25 months in the rat cortex are only 20 to 30%. The mouse data does show a 20% decrease, but numbers of animals are too small to allow statistical significance. It should be noted that when neuronal perikaryons are purified from cortices of mature and senescent rats, age reductions in corticosteroid receptor content are much more striking, about 65%.[32]

Androgen receptor concentrations in the prostrate gland also show differences with respect to age changes when prostate regions and different species are compared. For example, the rat ventral and lateral prostates show a loss of receptors during senescence[36,37] while the receptor content of the anterior and dorsal prostates remains constant with increasing age.[37] The prostate of dogs does not show an age-related change in androgen receptor levels.[43] Possibly, this difference from rat is due to the sixfold increase in cell content of the aged canine prostate as compared to young glands. This pronounced proliferation is not seen in the rat, and suggests that possibly receptor levels are somehow related to the ability of cells to divide. This hypothesis is supported by the work of Rosner and Cristofalo[35] on glucocorticoid receptors of WI-38 fibroblasts, where levels decrease with decreasing division potential in vitro. A study by Robinette and Mawhinney reported no change in rat seminal vesicle androgen receptor levels between 3 and 24 months of age.[37] More recently, however, the same investigators have actually reported a twofold increase in the concentration of this receptor if values are expressed per wet weight of tissue.[44] A similar increase was reported for seminal vesicle estrogen receptors. Whether such changes represent actual increases in receptor levels per cell is most crucial and still remains to be determined.

Despite these possible inconsistencies, it seems clear that many intracellular receptors are lost during aging. The functional significance of these findings will nevertheless be discussed.

B. Cell Surface Hormone Receptors

It was also desirable to perform aging studies on the hormone receptors located on the cell membrane in particular those for catecholamines since many responses mediated through these adrenergic systems were known to be altered during senescence. Unfortunately these studies lagged behind those on intracellular receptors due to theoretical and technical problems encountered in attempting such measurements. Although, investigators had been assessing the apparently "specific" displaceable binding of labeled catecholamines to membrane preparations for some time, it was pointed out by Cuatrecasas,[45] among others, in 1974 that such assays lacked several criteria necessary to the demonstration of true β-adrenergic receptors. First, the binding could not be blocked with specific antagonists such as propranalol, which inhibit biological responsiveness. Second, the time course of binding was much slower than for responsiveness. Third, the concentration curves for binding showed half maxima several order of magnitude higher than those for responsiveness, and fourth, the potency of various catecholamine stereoisomers in competing for binding was not in agreement with their biological effectiveness. Thus, numbers of catecholamine receptors determined by these early methods appeared to be much higher than those predicted by the kinetics of particular β-adrenergic responses.

Fortunately these problems were overcome within a year of the original published objections by the use of several potent labeled β-adrenergic antagonists which satisfy all the criteria laid down by Cuatrecasas. Among the most commonly employed were ^{3}H-propranalol,[46] ^{3}H-dihydroalprenolol,[47] and ^{125}I-hydroxybenzyl pindolol.[48] With the availability of these new ligands, a number of investigators made measurements of catecholamine-receptor concentrations in various tissues during aging. Although the results of these studies were less uniform in terms of progressive age-related reduction receptor concentrations, various cells and tissues have been shown to lose β-adrenergic catecholamine receptors during the aging process (Table 2).

Other types of cell membrane hormone receptors have now also been studied during

Table 2
REDUCTIONS IN MEMBRANE HORMONE RECEPTOR LEVELS DURING AGING

Hormone receptor	Tissue or cell	Ref.
Early Adulthood		
Catecholamine	Rat erythrocyte	49
	Rat pineal	50
Glucagon	Rat adipocyte	51
Insulin	Rat liver	52
	Rat adipocyte	53
Prolactin	Rat prostrate	54
Senescence		
Catecholamine	Human lymphocytes	55
	Rat adipocyte	56
	Rat cerebellum	50
	Rat corpus striatum	50
Gonadotropin	Rat testes	57
Dopamine	Rat corpus striatum	58
	Rabbit corpus striatum	59
	Rabbit frontal cortex	59
	Rabbit anterior limbic cortex	59
Insulin	Human fibroblast	60
Acetylcholine	Rat cerebral cortex	61
	Rat cerebellar cortex	61

the adult and senescence phase of the life span (Table 2). These include receptors for insulin, glucagon, acetylcholine, growth hormone, dopamine, prolactin, and gonado-tropins. Like the receptors for catecholamines and steroids, their time pattern of loss appears to vary depending on hormone and tissue, but many appear to be lost during the aging process.

As with the intracellular receptor situation, some possible discrepancies or contro-versies may exist in regard to these age studies. Such controversy over changes in human skin fibroblast insulin receptors will be discussed in the next section.

In related studies, rat hepatic insulin receptors were reported to decline in concen-tration by more than 50% between 2 and 12 months with only a slight decrease there-after.[52] However Sorrentino and Florini[62] reported that no significant changes in these receptors could be detected during the mouse life span. One problem in the latter study was extreme animal to animal variation. Another possible factor in the apparent dis-crepancy was that the mice were allowed food up until the time of the experiment. Since circulating insulin levels control insulin-receptor concentrations, the use of fasted animals, such as in the rat study, would probably have minimized the variation some-what and perhaps allowed detection of age changes.

As with steroid receptors, despite a few possibly controversial cases, a great number of membrane hormone receptors are lost during aging.

V. RELATIONSHIP OF RECEPTOR CHANGES TO ALTERED BIOLOGICAL RESPONSIVENESS DURING AGING

Having observed that many hormone-receptor concentrations are reduced during se-nescence, workers have more recently attempted to determine whether relationships exist between loss of receptors and responsiveness in particular tissues during aging. Some representative examples of these studies will be discussed here.

A. Androgen Receptors and Responsiveness

Testosterone receptors have been shown to be lost from both rat liver[20] and prostate[6,7] during aging. In liver, testosterone acts through its receptors to induce the synthesis of the protein α-2-u globulin. As mentioned above, the regulatory mechanisms, synthetic scheme, and physiochemical properties of this globulin have been well characterized. Roy and his co-workers showed that when androgen receptors were lost in old rats, the ability to induce α-2-u globulin concomittantly disappeared.[20]

The response to testosterone in the prostate gland has not been defined in such clear biochemical terms as that in the liver. It is known, however, that testosterone exerts a positive effect on prostatic protein and nucleic acid synthesis. In this context, it appears that testosterone is required for maintenance of prostatic size and cell content. Removal of testosterone in vivo by castration results in prostatic involution, reduction of cell number, and decreased wet weight. Shain's group found that the relative reductions in these parameters are inversely proportional to the ages of the orchiectomized rats up to at least 2 years.[63] Thus, they concluded that old animals are less sensitive to testosterone maintainance than young. They further suggested that such decreased androgen sensitivity in aged rats is related to a progressive reduction in androgen receptor concentration. Unfortunately, such a relationship cannot be conclusively proved in light of the indirect nature of the androgen response. Once again the innate complexity of measuring hormone action in vivo presents problems in interpreting experimental data. However, stronger support for the conclusion of these investigators might be mustered if similar reductions in testosterone stimulation of prostate protein synthesis could be observed in short-term explant or cell culture studies using prostates of different aged animals.

B. Estrogen Receptors and Responsiveness

Receptors for the female sex steroid, estradiol, are also lost with increasing age. A study by Kanungo's group demonstrated a progressive reduction in the specific binding of estrogen to these receptors as rats from 7 to 108 weeks.[40] This observation served as a possible explanation for a progressively reduced ability to induce the brain enzyme, acethylcholinesterase, with estradiol in vivo during aging.[19] In these receptor experiments, bound hormone was separated from free and less tedious measurements can be made by using charcoal or detran charcoal for this purpose. As stated previously, the latter procedure is currently preferred for such studies.

It has also been shown that estrogen receptors are lost from the uteri of aging rats[38] and mice.[9] Studies comparing estrogen responsiveness in the same groups of animals have not yet been reported. However, earlier studies by Singhal et al.[64] showed progressive reductions with age in the ability of estradiol to induce rat uterine phosphofructokinase and phosphohexase isomerase. A similar decrease was observed in estrogen stimulation of glycogen synthesis. However, time patterns of loss of response were not identical for the three parameters. Thus, as suggested in previous articles,[6,9] factors other than receptor changes may also contribute to altered hormonal responsiveness during aging.

C. Glucocorticoid Receptors and Responsiveness

Receptor concentrations and responsiveness to glucocorticoid hormones have been shown to be reduced in parallel during aging in at least three systems. One of the principal effects of glucocorticoid hormones on several cell types is an inhibition of nutrient transport and metabolism. As discussed in an earlier section, the ability of cortisol to inhibit uridine uptake is decreased in splenic leukocytes of senescent rats.[26,27] Such inhibition is believed to occur through a process initiated by binding of the steroid to cytoplasmic receptors and their translocation into the nucleus. There follows a period of postulated messenger RNA synthesis and translation into a "transport inhibitory protein."[65] A strong correlation exists between reduced glucocorticoid inhibition of uridine uptake and receptor concentration during aging.[26,27] Both processes exhibit similar dose-response curves and are reduced by 60% in 24-month-old rats as compared to 12-month-old control. Moreover, when binding of glucocorticoids to their receptors is blocked by steroids, which in themselves do not affect transport, no response to the former hormones occurs.

A similar biochemical scheme may be involved in the inhibition of glucose transport and metabolism by dexamethansone in adipocytes in vitro. Alternatively, Fain and Czech[66] have proposed that glucocorticoids may inhibit the synthesis of a labile protein, or proteins, involved in glucose transport by a process dependent on RNA synthesis. These two hypotheses need to be further resolved. In any case, however, the ability of dexamethasone to inhibit rat adipocyte glucose oxidation is progressively reduced about 70% from at least 2 to 26 months of age.[33] It is agreed that such inhibition is mediated initially by the binding of dexamethasone to cytoplasmic receptors. In fact, Olefsky has shown that progesterone, which prevents binding of dexamethasone to its receptor but has no affect on glucose transport, can block glucocorticoid action in fat cells.[67] A progressive reduction in glucocorticoid-receptor concentrations comparable in magnitude to the reduction in responsiveness is also seen between 2 and 26 months.[33]

Finally, the ability of cortisol to prolong diploid fibroblast life span and cell division in vitro is also reduced during aging.[35] The mechanisms involved in effecting this extension are still largely unresolved. However, dose-response curves for specific glucocorticoid uptake and binding to postulated receptors in WI-38 cells closely parallel those for prolongation of in vitro life span. Moreover, specificity studies have revealed that those glucocorticoid hormones with the highest affinity for the putative receptor also elicit the best responses.

D. Insulin Receptors and Responsiveness

Diploid fibroblasts have also been employed to compare age-related changes in insulin responsiveness to changes in insulin-receptor concentrations. In these cases, however, skin biopsies were obtained from human donors of different ages as opposed to the in vitro aging of the WI-38 system.[60] Fibroblasts were grown out from these explants and the ability of insulin to stimulate glucose uptake into the cells was assessed. A 90% reduction in this capacity was observed in exponentially growing fibroblasts from aged donors when compared to those of young adult counterparts. A 70% reduction in insulin-receptor concentrations was also detected in the senescent group. Thus, loss of these receptors may play a large role in the observed reduction in responsiveness.

It must be pointed out that age differences were only detected when exponentially growing, as opposed to confluent, cell cultures were employed. In fact Rosenbloom et al.[68] actually reported increased insulin-receptor levels in confluent skin fibroblasts of aged donors. These findings are similar to those of Rosner and Cristofalo[35] who found that in vitro age-related reductions in glucocorticoid receptors and response were most pronounced in exponentially growing cells, while at confluency older cultures appeared to possess more receptors than young.

E. Dopamine Receptors and Responsiveness

A number of investigators have observed that the ability of dopamine to stimulate adenylate cyclase in various rat brain regions is progressively altered with aging.[69-72]

Until recently, however, it was not possible to accurately measure actual dopamine receptors in these areas. Fortunately several investigators have pioneered the use of highly specific, radioactively labeled dopamine agonists and antagonists which allow receptor detection in membrane preparations with relative ease. Among these are haloperidol, apomorphine, and more recently, spiroperidol.[73,74] The latter appears to be the most specific dopamine-receptor antagonist yet discovered and it binds minimally to nonreceptor sites, a problem frequently encountered in early studies.

With the use of such agents, several groups have now reported that dopamine receptors are also lost from the brain during aging.[58,59,75] Various regions have been studied (primarily corpus striatum), and rats, mice, and rabbits have been utilized.

VI. HORMONE RECEPTOR CHANGES DURING AGING: MECHANISMS AND POSSIBLE CONTROL

Altered hormone-receptor concentrations seem to be closely related to changes in biological responsiveness during aging in a number of systems. It is therefore important to investigate the mechanisms by which receptor concentration change. Such mechanisms may be operative at least three levels, arbitrarily classified as ''cellular,'' ''molecular,'' and ''neuroendocrine-systemic.''

A. Cellular Mechanisms

Cellular mechanisms refer to those processes by which certain cell populations within complex tissues change in numbers and/or relative proportions during aging. Many of the initial studies on receptors and aging employed complex tissues such as liver and brain. Working with such heterogeneous systems, therefore, investigators could not determine whether receptors were lost from individual hormone target cells or whether target cells were merely lost from whole tissues. An early attempt to separate the glucocorticoid-responsive lymphocytes from other cells in rat spleens was carried out in the author's laboratory. Since thymic-derived lymphocytes seem to be exquisitely sensitive to the effects in steroids, Roth and colleagues prepared antisera against these cells of the thymus in hopes of distinguishing thymic or ''T'' lymphocytes from bone-marrow derived ''B'' lymphocytes and other splenic cell types. Thymic lymphocytes were prepared by teasing apart thymuses and injecting cell suspensions into rabbits. Booster injections were given at weekly intervals for several weeks. Following these injections, rabbits were bled by cardiac puncture and serum prepared. The serum was then sequentially absorbed with various nonthymic antigens including kidney, fetal liver, and bone marrow, according to the method of Balch and Feldman.[76] Specificity was determined by incubating thymic and bone-marrow derived lymphocytes with the resulting serum and lysing antisera reactive cells with complement.

Roth and colleagues then attempted to remove selectively the thymic lymphocyte population from the rest of the splenic cells so that glucocorticoid responsiveness might be assessed in complete and T-cell depleted splenic populations. Figure 5 shows the results of this experiment. About one third of the splenic leukocytes were removed by this manipulation and assumed to be thymic in origin. Unfortunately, the ability of cortisol to inhibit uptake of ^{3}H-uridine was not significantly different in the total and thymic lymphocyte-depleted populations. Thus glucocorticoid target cells seem to be randomly distributed throughout the thymic and nonthymic lymphocyte populations of the spleen. It was not possible, therefore, to isolate the desired hormone responsive cell population for analysis by this method.

For Roth and colleagues' next attempts at distinguishing between target-cell and hormone-receptor loss during senescence, they decided to employ defined populations of

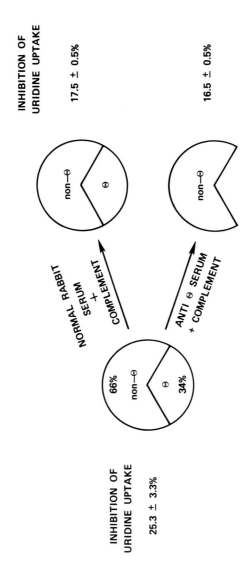

FIGURE 5. Effect of antithymocyte serum on cortisol inhibition of uridine uptake in rat splenic leukocytes. Antithymocyte serum was prepared as described in the text. Splenic leukocytes from mature, 12-month-old rats were split into two portions. One was treated with antithymocyte serum and complement, the other received normal rabbit serum and complement. Both were treated with cortisol and the degree of inhibition of ^{3}H-uridine uptake determined as for Figure 4. Values represent the means ± standard errors from triplicate determinations.

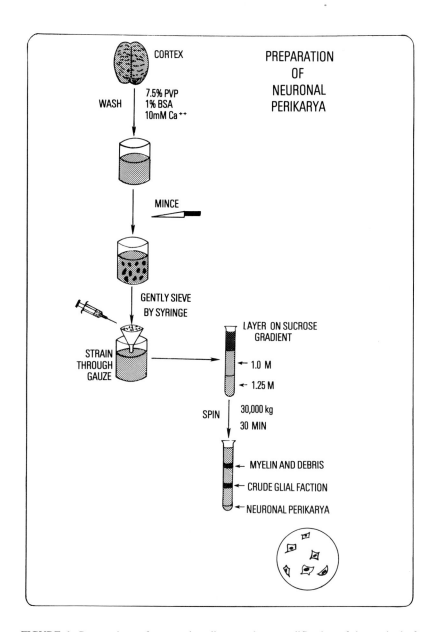

FIGURE 6. Preparations of neuronal perikaryons by a modification of the method of Sellinger et al.[79] Rat cerebral certices were washed and minced as described in the text and figure. After viewing and straining, cell suspensions were layered on discontinuous sucrose density gradients and sedimented to yield fractions greatly enriched for myelin and debris, glial cells, and neuronal perikarya, respectively.

static postmitotic cells. Two such populations were chosen for this purpose, rat cerebral cortical neurons and epididymal fat pad adipocytes. As mentioned in previous reports[32,33] the concentrations of glucocorticoid receptors in rat cerebral cortex and epididymal fat pad are progressively reduced from at least 2 to more than 26 months of age. Although both tissues are heterogeneous, they do contain populations of postmitotic cells (neurons and adipocytes) whose numbers remain constant throughout most of the life span.[77,78]

Neuronal perikarya were prepared by a modification of the mechanical disruption-

Table 3
PURITY, INTEGRITY, AND YIELD OF NEURONAL PERIKARYA FROM CORTICES OF MATURE AND SENESCENT RATS

Assessment	12–13 months	24–26 months
Cortex weights (g)	1.25 ± 0.05	1.20 ± 0.04
Neuron yield × 10^{-4} per cortex	350 ± 56	373 ± 17
Nanograms pellet protein per isolated neuron	1.39 ± 0.14	1.35 ± 0.22
Carbonic anhydrase (units/mg protein)		
Total cortex suspension	2.24 ± 0.12	2.01 ± 0.09
Neuronal fraction	1.88 ± 0.02	1.72 ± 0.04
Soluble glycine (nmol/mg protein)		
Total cortex suspension	1.44 ± 0.18	1.33 ± 0.17
Neuronal fraction	1.80 ± 0.03	1.87 ± 0.06

Note: Cerebral cortices were obtained from mature (12- to 13-month-old) and senescent (24- to 26-month-old) rats and cortical cell suspensions and neronal perikarya prepared as described in Figure 6. To ensure comparability of osmotic and centrifugal treatment, cortical suspensions were layered on gradients identical to those for neuronal preparation. However, the former were gently but completely resuspended in the gradient solutions and centrifuged at 20,000 r/min identically to the neuronal preparations. The entire cortical suspension was pelleted and was used for comparison with purified neuronal preparations. Assessment of protein, glycine, carbonic anhydrase, and neuronal yield were also as described in methods. Values represent the means ±SE for duplicate determinations from four to six individual rats of each age.

density gradient procedure of Sellinger et al.[79] (Figure 6). Cortices are minced in a viscous solution of 7.5% polyvinyl-pyrollidone; 1% bovine serum albumin and 10 mM calcium chloride suspensions are then sieved and filtered through gauge, layered on discontinuous sucrose gradients and sedimated. Neutronal perikaryons, being more dense than glia and debris, can be recovered in over 90% purity in the pellets of such gradients. Preparations from mature (12- to 13-month-old) and senescent (24- to 26-month-old) rats were found to be comparable with respect to yield, purity, protein content, and physiochemical integrity (Table 3). Carbonic anhydrase and soluble glucine are rough glial and neuronal markers, respectively. A 65% reduction in the concentration of glucocorticoid receptors was observed in the senescent cell population, however,[32] since cell numbers do not change during senescence and neurons do not proliferate, receptors do indeed appear to be lost from individual cells.

A similar experiment was performed on adipocytes isolated from rat epididymal fat pads. These cells were obtained by the method of Rodbell[80] which utilizes collagenase to digest away connective tissue and allows the buoyant fat cells to float free and be easily separated by fibroblasts, endothelial, cells etc. Like neurons, the adipocyte population is essentially static over most of the adult life span. A progressive reduction in the concentration of glucocorticoid receptors per cell and per unit protein was observed from at least 2 to 26 months.[33] As previously mentioned, this loss correlates well with a progressive reduction in the ability of steroids to inhibit glucose metabolism with increasing age. Loss of glucocorticoid receptors from adipocytes during aging, therefore, appears closely related to reduced responsiveness to these hormones.

B. Molecular Mechanisms

In at least the two systems previously listed, receptors actually appear to be lost from target cells rather than mere loss of target cells from target tissues. Thus, emphasis can

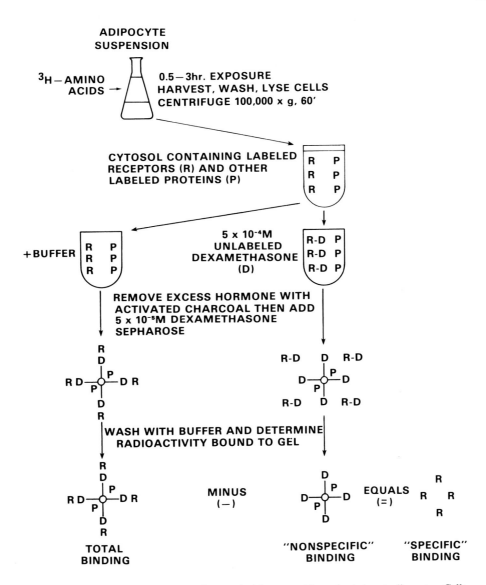

FIGURE 7. Measurement of putative glucocorticoid receptor biosynthesis in rat adipocytes. Cells are labeled with radioactive amino acids for varying time periods, lysed and receptor-containing cytosols are prepared. These are divided into two parts, one of which is treated with excess unlabeled dexamethasone to complex with putative receptors. Activated charcoal is then used to remove excess hormone and dexamethasone Sepharose® is added to specifically bind receptors. The gel is then washed and radioactivity determined by scintillation counting. "Specific" binding is determined operationally by subtracting "non-specific," nonsaturable binding from total binding.

be placed on molecular mechanisms which occur within target cells. Causes of decreased receptor levels may include reduced rates of receptor synthesis, increased rates of degradation, and the possible presence of nonfunctional receptors in aged cells.

The use of affinity chromatography to purify hormone receptors from crude cell and tissue extracts should prove to be a highly useful technique in examining the above possibilities. Selective removal of receptors from the other 99+% of the cellular proteins will allow labeling with radioactive amino acids for various time periods to determine synthetic and degradative kinetics. Figure 7 illustrates the method currently used in the author's laboratory to make such measurements. Purification will also allow preparation of specific antisera against receptors. These will be important tools by which receptors can be detected immunochemically as well as functionally. Since current assays depend upon the ability of receptors to specifically bind radioactive hormones, nonfunctional, blocked or masked receptors cannot be measured. Many nonfunctional enzyme populations have already been reported to appear during aging.[81,82] Thus, immunochemical measurement of receptors will allow determination of whether apparently reduced levels during senescence are due to loss of functionality.

C. Neuroendocrine-Systemic Mechanisms

Even if molecular mechanisms are found to be involved in apparent loss of hormone receptors during aging, another level of modulation may be interposed. Many receptors have recently been found to be under the control of hormones and other chemical agents (for reviews see References 7 and 83). Thus, molecular properties such as functional integrity, synthetic and degradative schemes, etc., may actually be under physiological control. During aging such control may become altered (like so many other regulatory systems) to result in altered receptor levels.

Age-related changes in the internal environment of organisms as opposed to changes actually intrinsic to particular cells have become a classical distinction in gerontology. Thus it will also be necessary to determine which or both of these alternatives is true in the case of hormone receptors and responsiveness. An answer may be possible through the use of parabiosis or transplant experiments. Such techniques have been applied with limited success in vivo. Perhaps it may also be possible in the case of responsive cell populations to perfuse cultures from different aged hormones with sera or fluids of different aged animals, in a sense an in vitro parabiosis.

VII. SUMMARY AND CONCLUSIONS

Changes in certain hormone-receptor concentrations may provide explanations for many cases of altered responsiveness to hormones during aging. Generally responsiveness changes are reductions with increasing age, but in some cases no change or even increases have been reported. Since hormonal responsiveness may be measured either in vivo or in vitro, different factors must be considered in evaluating data obtained by these two different approaches. For in vivo studies, these include possible age differences in metabolism and distribution of hormones as well as in secondary regulatory responses. For in vitro studies, one must be aware of possible age differences in the sensitivity of cells and tissues to isolation and cultures procedures as well as differential nutritional requirements.

In attempting to explain altered hormone responsiveness in biochemical terms, it must be remembered that many events are candidates for age-related modification. Since hormone binding to receptors is the initial and in many cases a regulatory step in hormone actions, receptor changes during aging have been studied extensively. Close, if not causal, relationships have been established between receptor and responsiveness loss in numerous cases. Efforts are now underway to elucidate those mechanisms by which receptor levels are altered with age. In this regard, hormone-receptor systems offer interesting models in which to study the molecular control of gene expression and regulation of many physiological processes during aging.

REFERENCES

1. **Cuatrecasas, P.,** Membrane receptors, *Annu. Rev. Biochem.,* 43, 169, 1974.
2. **King, R. J. B. and Mainwaring, W. I. P.,** *Steroid-Cell Interactions,* University Park Press, Baltimore, 1974.
3. **O'Malley, B. W. and Means, A. R.,** Eds., *Receptors for Reproductive Hormones,* Plenum Press, New York, 1973.
4. **Greengard, P.,** Phosphorylated proteins as physiological effectors, *Science,* 199, 146, 1978.
5. **Latham, K. R., Ring, J. C., and Baxter, J. D.,** Solubilized nuclear receptors for thyroid hormones, *J. Biol. Chem.,* 251, 7388, 1976.
6. **Roth, G. S. and Adelman, R. C.,** Age related changes in hormone binding by target cells and tissues: possible role in altered adaptive responsiveness, *Exp. Gerontol.,* 10, 1, 1975.
7. **Roth, G. S.,** Changes in hormone binding and responsiveness target cells and tissues during aging, in *Explorations in Aging,* Cristofalo, V. J., Roberts, J., and Adelman, R. C., Eds., Plenum Press, New York, 1975, 195.
8. **Roth, G. S.,** Hormone action during aging: alterations and mechanisms, *Mech. Ageing Dev.,* 9, 497, 1979.
9. **Roth, G. S.,** Hormonal receptor and responsiveness changes during aging: genetic modulation, in *Genetic Effects on Aging,* Bergsma, D. and Harrison, D. H., Eds., Liss, New York, 1978, 365.
10. **Roth, G. S.,** Hormone receptor changes during adulthood and senescence: significance for aging research, *Fed. Proc. Fed. Am. Soc. Exp. Biol.,* 38, 1910, 1979.
11. **Adelman, R. C., Stein, G. S., Roth, G. S., and Englander, D.,** Age-dependent regulation of mammalian DNA synthesis and cell proliferation in vivo, *Mech. Ageing Dev.,* 1, 49, 1972.
12. **Roth, G. S., Karoly, K., Britton, V. J., and Adelman, R. C.,** Age-dependent regulation of isoproterenol stimulated DNA synthesis in rat salivary gland in vivo, *Exp. Gerontol.,* 9, 1, 1974.
13. **Roth, G. S., Karoly, K., Adelman, A., and Adelman, R. C.,** Regulation of isoproterenol stimulated DNA synthesis in rat salivary gland in vivo by adrenal glucocorticoids, *Exp. Gerontol.,* 9, 13, 1974.
14. **Roth, G. S. and Adelman, R. C.,** Age-dependent regulation of mammalian DNA synthesis and cell division in vivo by glucocorticoids, *Exp. Gerontol.,* 9, 27, 1974.
15. **Roth, G. S. and Adelman, R. C.,** Possible changes in tissue sensitivity in the age-dependent stimulation of DNA synthesis in vivo, *J. Gerontol.,* 28, 298, 1973.
16. **Yamaji, T. and Ibayashi, H.,** Plasma dehydroepiandrosterone sulfate in normal and pathological conditions, *J. Clin. Endocrinol. Metab.,* 29, 273, 1969.
17. **Florini, J. R., Saito, Y., and Manowitz, E. J.,** Effect of age on thyroxine induced cardiac hypertrophy in mice, *J. Gerontol.,* 28, 293, 1973.
18. **Grad, B.,** The metabolic responsiveness of young and old female rats to thyroxine, *J. Gerontol.,* 24, 5, 1969.
19. **Moudgil, V. K. and Kanungo, M. S.,** Effect of age of the rat on induction of acetylcholinesterase of the brain by 17β-estradiol, *Biochim. Biophys. Acta,* 329, 211, 1973.
20. **Roy, A. K., Milin, B. S., and McMinn, D. M.,** Androgen receptors in rat liver: hormonal and developmental regulation of the cytoplasmic receptor and its correlation with the androgen dependent synthesis of α2μ-globulin, *Biochim. Biophys. Acta,* 354, 213, 1974.
21. **Fleisch, J. H., Maling, H. M., and Brodie, B. B.,** Beta-receptor activity in the aorta, *Circ. Res.,* 26, 151, 1970.
22. **Fleisch, J. H. and Hooker, C. S.,** The relationship between age and relaxation of vascular smooth muscle in the rabbit and rat, *Circ. Res.,* 38, 243, 1976.
23. **Kalish, M. I., Katz, M. S., Piñeyro, M. A., and Gregerman, R. I.,** Epinephrine- and glucagon-sensitive adenylate cyclases of rat liver during aging, *Biochim. Biophys. Acta,* 483, 452, 1977.
24. **Berger, M., Preiss, H., Hesse-Wortmann, C., and Gries, F. A.,** Altersabhangigkeit der Fettzellgrosse und der Lipotytischen Aktivitat im menschlichen Fettgewebe, *Gerontologia,* 17, 312, 1971.
25. **Gries, F. A., and Steinke, J.,** Comparative effects of insulin on adipose tissue segments and isolated fat cells of rats and man, *J. Clin. Invest.,* 46, 1413, 1967.
26. **Roth, G. S.,** Age related changes in glucocorticoid binding by rat splenic leukocytes: possible cause of altered adaptive responsiveness, *Fed. Proc. Fed. Am. Soc. Exp. Biol.,* 34, 183, 1975.
27. **Roth, G. S.,** Reduced glucocorticoid responsiveness and receptor concentration in splenic leukocytes of senescent rats, *Biochim. Biophys. Acta,* 399, 145, 1975.
28. **Cristofalo, V. J.,** Metabolic aspects of aging in human diploid cells, Holeckova, E. and Cristofalo, V. J., Eds., *Aging in Cell and Tissue Culture,* Plenum Press, New York, 1970, 83.
29. **Petrovic, J. S. and Markovic, R. Z.,** Changes in cortisol binding to soluble receptor proteins in rat liver and thymus during development and ageing, *Dev. Biol.,* 45, 176, 1975.

30. **Chouknyiska, R. and Vassileva-Popova, J. G.,** Effect of age on the binding of ^{3}H testosterone with receptor protein from rat brain and testes, *C. R. Acad. Bulg. Sci.,* 30, 133, 1977.

31. **Roth, G. S.,** Age-related changes in specific glucocorticoid binding by steroid responsive tissues of rats, *Endocrinology,* 94, 82, 1974.

32. **Roth, G. S.,** Reduced glucocorticoid binding site concentration in cortical neuronal perikarya from senescent rats, *Brain Res.,* 107, 345, 1976.

33. **Roth, G. S. and Livingston, J. N.,** Reductions in glucocorticoid inhibition of glucose oxidation and presumptive glucocorticoid receptor content in rat adipocytes during aging, *Endocrinology,* 99, 831, 1976.

34. **Singer, S., Ito, H., and Litwack, G.,** ^{3}H-cortisol binding by young and old human liver cytosol proteins in vitro, *Int. J. Biochem.,* 4, 569, 1973.

35. **Rosner, B. A. and Cristofalo, V. J.,** Specific binding of ^{3}H-dexamethasone in WI-38 monolayers: changes with increased in vitro age, *Fed. Proc. Fed. Am. Soc. Exp. Biol.,* 37, 888, 1978.

36. **Shain, S. A., Boesel, R. W., and Axelrod, L. R.,** Aging in the rat prostate, reduction in detectable ventral prostate androgen receptor content, *Arch. Biochem. Biophys.,* 167, 247, 1973.

37. **Robinette, C. L. and Mawhinney, M. G.,** Cytosol binding of dihydrotestosterone in young and senile rats, *Fed. Proc. Fed. Am. Soc. Exp. Biol.,* 36, 344, 1977.

38. **Holinka, C. F., Nelson, J. F., and Finch, C. E.,** Effect of estrogen treatment on estradiol binding capacity in uteri of aged rats, *Gerontologist,* 15, 30, 1975.

39. **Nelson, J. F., Holinka, C. F., and Finch, C. E.,** Age-related changes in estradiol binding capacity of mouse uterine cytosol, in Abstr. of the 29th Annu. Meet. of the Gerontol. Soc., New York, October 1976, 34.

40. **Kanungo, M. S., Patnaik, S. W., and Koul, O.,** Decrease in 17-β estradiol receptor in brain of aging rats, *Nature (London),* 353, 366, 1975.

41. **Latham, K. R. and Finch, C. E.,** Hepatic glucocorticoid binders in mature and senescent C57B1/6J male mice, *Endocrinology,* 98, 1480, 1976.

42. **Nelson, J. F., Holinka, C. F., Latham, K. R., Allen, J. K., and Finch, C. E.,** Corticosterone binding in cytosols from brain regions of mature and senescent male C57B1/6J mice, *Brain Res.,* 115, 345, 1976.

43. **Shain, S. A. and Boesel, R. W.,** Androgen receptors of the aging canine prostate, in Proc. of the 59th Annu. Meet. of the Endocrine Soc., Toronto, October 1977, 332.

44. **Robinette, C. L. and Mawhinney, M. G.,** Effects of aging on the estrogen receptor in rat seminal vesicles, *Fed. Proc. Fed. Am. Soc. Exp. Biol.,* 37, 283, 1978.

45. **Cuatrecasas, P.,** Problems in receptor identification: catecholamines, *N. Eng. J. Med.,* 291, 206, 1974.

46. **Atlas, D., Steer, M. L., and Levitzki, A.,** Stereospecific binding of propranolol and catecholamines to the β-adrenergic receptor, *Proc. Natl. Acad. Sci. U.S.A.,* 71, 4246, 1974.

47. **Lefkowitz, R. J., Mukherjee, C., Coverstone, M., and Caron, M. G.,** Stereospecific ^{3}H(−)alprenolol binding sites, β-adrenergic receptors and adenylate cyclase, *Biochem. Biophys. Res. Commun.,* 60, 703, 1974.

48. **Aurbach, G. D., Fedak, S. A., Woodward, C. J., Palmer, J. S., Hauser, D., and Troxler, F.,** β-adrenergic receptor: stereospecific interaction of iodinated β-blocking agent with high affinity site, *Science,* 186, 1223, 1974.

49. **Bylund, D. B., Tellez-Inon, M. T., and Hollenberg, M. D.,** Age-related parallel decline in beta-adrenergic receptors, adenylate cyclase and phosphodiesterase activity in rat erythrocyte membranes, *Life Sci.,* 21, 403, 1977.

50. **Greenberg, L. H., Dix, R. K., and Weiss, B.,** Age-related changes in ^{3}H-dihydroalprenolol binding in rat brain, *Science,* 201, 61, 1978.

51. **Livingston, J. N., Cuatrecasas, P., and Lockwood, D. H.,** Studies of glucagon resistance in large rat adipocytes: ^{125}I-labeled glucagon binding and lipolytic capacity, *J. Lipid Res.,* 15, 26, 1974.

52. **Freeman, C., Karoly, K., and Adelman, R. C.,** Impairments in availability of insulin to liver in vivo and in binding of insulin to purified hepatic plasma membranes during aging, *Biochem. Biophys. Res. Commun.,* 54, 1573, 1973.

53. **Olefsky, J. M. and Reaven, G. M.,** Effects of age and obesity on insulin binding to isolated adipocytes, *Endocrinology,* 96, 1486, 1975.

54. **Barkey, R. J., Shani, J., and Barzilai, D.,** Specific binding of prolactin to seminal vesicle, prostate and testicular homogenates of immature, mature and aged rats, *J. Endocrinol.,* 74, 163, 1977.

55. **Schocken, D. D. and Roth, G. S.,** Reduced beta adrenergic receptor concentrations in aging man, *Nature (London),* 267, 856, 1977.

56. **Guidicelli, Y. and Pecquery, R.,** β-adrenergic receptors and catecholamine sensitive adenylate cyclase in rat fat cell membranes: influence of growth, cell size and aging, *Eur. J. Biochem.,* 90, 413, 1978.

57. **Vassileva-Popova, J.,** Developmental changes in gonadal binding of gonadotropins, *Proc. 5th Asia Oceania Congr. Endocrinol.,* 1, 242, 1974.

58. **Joseph, J. A., Berger, R. E., Engel, B. T., and Roth, G. S.,** Age related changes in the nigrostriatum: a behavorial and biochemical analysis, *J. Gerontol.,* 33, 643, 1978.

59. **Makman, M. H., Ahn, H. S., Thal, L., Dvorkin, B., Horowitz, S. G., Sharpless, N., and Rosenfeld, M.,** Decreased brain biogenic amine-stimulated adenylate cyclase and spiroperidol binding sites with aging, *Fed. Proc. Fed. Am. Soc. Exp. Biol.,* 37, 548, 1978.

60. **Ito, H., Orimo, H., and Shimada, H.,** Reduced insulin action in vitro and the binding of ^{125}I-insulin to the cultured human skin fibroblasts with aging, in Abstr. of the 5th Int. Congr. of Endocrinol., Hamburg, July 18 to 24, 1976, 261.

61. **James, T. C. and Kanungo, M. S.,** Alterations in atropine sites of the brain of rats as a function of age, *Biochem. Biophys. Res. Commun.,* 72, 170, 1976.

62. **Sorrentino, R. M. and Florini, J. R.,** Variations among individual mice in binding of growth hormone and insulin to membranes from animals of different ages, *Exp. Aging Res.,* 2, 191, 1976.

63. **Shain, S. A. and Boesel, R. W.,** Aging-associated diminished rat prostate androgen receptor content concurrent with decreased androgen dependence, *Mech. Ageing Dev.,* 6, 219, 1977.

64. **Singhal, R. L., Valadares, H. R. E., and Ling, G. M.,** Estrogenic regulation of uterine carbohydrate metabolism during senescence, *Am. J. Physiol.,* 217, 793, 1969.

65. **Makman, M. H., Nakagawa, S., and White, A.,** Studies on the mode of action of adrenal steroids on lymphocytes, *Recent Progress Hormone Res.,* 23, 195, 1967.

66. **Fain, J. N. and Czech, M. P.,** Glucocorticoid effects on lipid modilization and adipose tissue metabolism, in *Handbook of Physiology; Section 7: Endocrinology,* Vol. 6, Greep, R. and Astwood, E., Eds., Williams & Wilkens, Baltimore, 1974, 169.

67. **Olefsky, J.,** Effect of dexamethasone on insulin binding, glucose transport, and glucose oxidation of isolated rat adipocytes, *J. Clin. Invest.,* 56, 1499, 1975.

68. **Rosenbloom, A. L., Goldstein, S., and Yip, C. C.,** Insulin binding to cultured human fibroblasts increases with normal and precocious aging, *Science,* 193, 412, 1976.

69. **Walker, J. B. and Walker, J. P.,** Properties of adenylate cyclase from senescent rat brain, *Brain Res.,* 54, 391, 1973.

70. **Puri, S. and Volicer, L.,** Effect of aging on cyclic AMP levels and adenylate cyclase and phosphodiesterase activities in the rat corpus striatum, *Mech. Aging Dev.,* 6, 53, 1977.

71. **Govoni, S., Loddo, P., Spano, P. F., and Trabucchi, M.,** Dopamine receptor sensitivity in and retina of rats during aging, *Brain Res.,* 138, 565, 1977.

72. **Schmidt, M. J. and Thornberry, J. F.,** Cyclic AMP and cyclic GMP accumulation in vitro in brain regions of young, old and aged rats, *Brain Res.,* 139, 169, 1978.

73. **Burt, D. R., Creese, I., and Snyder, S. H.,** Properties of ^{3}H-haloperidol and ^{3}H-dopamine binding associated with dopamine receptors in calf brain membranes, *Mol. Pharmacol.,* 12, 800, 1976.

74. **Creese, I., Schneider, R., and Snyder, S. H.,** ^{3}H-spiroperidol labels dopamine receptors in pituitary and brain, *Eur. J. Pharmacol.,* 46, 377, 1977.

75. **Finch, C. E.,** personal communication, 1978.

76. **Balch, C. M. and Feldman, J. D.,** Thymus-dependent (T) lymphocytes in the rat, *J. Immunol.,* 112, 79, 1974.

77. **Brizzee, D. R., Sherwood, N., and Timiras, P.,** A comparison of cell populations at various depth levels in cerebral cortex of young adult and aged Long-Evans rats, *J. Gerontol.,* 23, 289, 1968.

78. **Stiles, J. W., Francendese, A. A., and Masoro, E. J.,** Influence of age on the size and number of fat cells in the epididymal depot, *Am. J. Physiol.,* 229, 1561, 1975.

79. **Sellinger, O. Z., Azcurra, J. M., Johnson, D. E., Ohlsson, W. G., and Lodin, Z.,** Independence of protein synthesis and drug uptake in nerve cell bodies and glial cells isolated by a new technique, *Nature (London), New Biol.,* 230, 253, 1971.

80. **Rodbell, M.,** Metabolism of isolated fat cells, I. Effects of hormones on glucose metabolism and lipolysis, *J. Biol. Chem.,* 250, 8353, 1975.

81. **Reiss, V. and Rothstein, M.,** Age-related changes in isocitrate lyase from the free living nematode, *Turbatrix aceti, J. Biol. Chem.,* 250, 826, 1975.

82. **Gershon, H. and Gershon, D.,** Inactive enzyme molecules in aging mice: liver aldolase, *Proc. Natl. Acad. Sci. U.S.A.,* 70, 909, 1973.

83. **Roth, G. S., Chang, W. C., and Gesell, M. S.,** Changes in hormone receptors during aging, role in altered hormonal responsiveness, in *Physical and Chemical Bases of Biological Information Transfer,* Vol. 2, Vassileva-Popova, J., Ed., Plenum Press, New York, 1978, 123.

Chapter 5

FEMALE REPRODUCTIVE SENESCENCE

Richard W. Steger, William E. Sonntag, and Joseph Meites*

TABLE OF CONTENTS

*Aided by National Institutes of Health research grants AG00416 from the National Institute on Aging, and AM04784 from the National Institute for Arthritis, Metabolism, and Digestive Diseases.

I. INTRODUCTION

Innumerable techniques have been used to study female reproductive physiology and these basically should all be useful in a comparative study of reproductive processes in old and young subjects. In the following chapter, the authors attempt to review much of the published information on age-related changes of the structure and function of the female reproductive axis. In many instances the techniques used in the cited study are pointed out to the reader. In some instances special precautions in analyzing data are discussed, but space limitations prevent discussion of techniques in detail. In general, the reader should gain some understanding of what already is in the literature, the areas that are still awaiting investigation, and techniques that might be used for studying the reproductive decline.

One precaution that underlies most of the information in this chapter is a careful evaluation of the experimental model. It is essential to separate gross pathological changes from ''normal'' or ''physiological'' changes associated with age. The reader should be aware of definitions or criteria of aging such as those discussed by Strehler[1] in his recent book in order to judge the relevance of his or her study to the aging phenomena. Finally, care must be taken in comparing results among species or even strains of the same species since markedly different events are associated with aging. For example, women and CBA mice show a marked or even complete depletion of oocytes while many other species and mouse strains still have a relatively large population of oocytes near the end of their natural life span.[2-4] Likewise, postmenopausal women have markedly elevated gonadotropin levels, while old rodents generally have low gonadotropin levels.

II. CHANGES IN THE REPRODUCTIVE TRACT

A. Age-Related Changes in the Vagina

Gross and microscopic evaluations of the postmenopausal vagina have shown a decreased depth and caliber with age, together with decreased elasticity and expansive ability.[5,6] The vagina rugae regress and the color often changes due to loss of vascularity and/or chronic inflammation.[5,7] The vagina exfolative cytology reflects the decreased steroid production of the older women, and the vaginal epithelium becomes markedly thin.[8] In the postmenopausal vagina collagen replaces many of the elastic fibers in the lamina propria, lipofuscin granules accumulate in muscle cells, and glycogen is very low or absent.[8] The vaginal microflora and fauna are also changes with age due to biochemical and secretory changes in the vaginal wall.[8]

B. Age-Related Changes in the Cervix

Gross inspection of the postmenopausal cervix reveals a decrease in size, a reduction in width of the cervical canal, and a reduction in quantity, but thickening of cervical mucus.[9,10] Microscopic examination of the aging cervix reveals a progressive atrophy of the cervical crypts and stenosis of the ducts, sometimes leading to retention cysts.[9] The height of endocervical columnar epithelium is reduced and the ectocervical squamous epithelium becomes thinner.[11,12] There is some replacement of columner epithelium with squamous epithelium, and the junctional zone moves into the endocervical canal after the menopause.[5,12,13] Progressive hyalinization of the stroma also is seen with aging.[12]

C. Uterine Changes with Age

A variety of techniques have been used to study the effects of advancing age on the uterus. Gross observations of the postmenopausal human uterus show atrophy and an approximate weight loss of 50% if hypertrophy and hyperplasia are not present, a shrinkage of fibroids, and a reduced vascularity.[5,14–17] In the rat, uterine atrophy is seen in old anestrous, but not in constant estrous or repeat-pseudopregnant old rats, emphasizing the importance of defining the reproductive state of the animal under study.[80,83] The dry weight fraction of the rabbit uterus does not change between 34 to 204 weeks of age, but uterine blood flow decreases and there is an increasing frequency of spontaneous uterine tumors.[33a,33b,152–153]

D. Uterine Histology and Age

The postmenopausal endometrium exhibits several histological profiles:[4,5,12,17–19] (1) most commonly, a thin and atrophic mucosa; (2) mucosa of varying thickness with "Swiss cheese-type" hyperplasia without proliferation; or (3) active hyperplasia, either diffused or in scattered patches, sometimes polyploid. Cystic atrophy is characterized by a low functionalis not clearly demarcated from the basalis. The endometrial glands become narrow and are lined with cuboidal as opposed to columner cells. There is often moderate to severe cystic dialation of some glands. There is a dramatic decrease in the number of cilia and microvilli and secretory material.[20] The uterus of old rats and mice shows similar decreases in microvilli and secretory material.[20–21]

In the postmenopausal myometrium, fibrous replacement of smooth muscle cells is common.[12] Also seen is a severe muscular hypertrophy of myometrial vessels with thickening of the subendothelial layers and occasional calcification of the media.[5] Similar changes are seen in the guinea pig.[22] Lipofusion and "lipoidal-hemosiderin" deposits have been described in the myometrium of the old rat, mouse, and pig.[23–25]

E. Changes with Age in Uterine Collagen and Elastin

In the rat, mouse, and hamster a progressive deposition of uterine collagen was seen with age, while the opposite was true in the rabbit.[26–36] In the mouse, both total collagen content and collagen concentration increased with age, but there were no differences between horns which had contained or not contained fetuses as a result of unilateral ovariectomy.[37] Collagen in the rat becomes less theromolabile and more resistant to collagenase with age.[36] Despite the increase in collagen content, the old rat uterus was demonstrated to have less capacity for collagen synthesis.[30]

F. Physiological Responses of the Aging Uterus

Stromal and endometrial cells in the uterus of old mice retained their capacity to proliferate in response to estrogen and progesterone, but lumen closure was not seen.[29,38] A decrease in the decidualization reaction was one of the most prominent aging effects in the mouse as was the increased incidence of fetal resorbtions.[24,28,29,38–46] Similar changes have been described in the uterus of the old hamster.[47–53]

G. Biochemical Response of the Aging Uterus

There is a decreased uterine RNA and DNA content in 15-month-old, as compared to 4-, 7-, and 11-month-old mice, and although estrogen stimulates *de novo* RNA synthesis, the response is decreased with age.[43,54,55] Protein concentration in the mouse uterus is unchanged with age when expressed on a wet-weight basis, but decreased by 15 months when expressed on a dry-weight basis.[55] Results such as these explain some of the apparent contradictions in gerontologic research, since various investigators use protein content, wet-weight, or dry-weight, as a basis to compare other biochemical parameters such as nucleic acid content, enzyme activity, and hormone binding.

Glycogen content has been described in the uterus of both the old mouse and hamster.[43,56] More significantly the decrease in the old hamster uterus was measured during preimplantation stages, a time when the embryo is still dependent upon uterine glycogen. A decreased uterine alkaline phosphatase activity in the mouse and a decreased uterine phosphofructokinase and phosphohexose isomerase in the rat have been demonstrated with advancing age.[42,43,57,58]

Old rabbits, mice, constant estrous and anestrous rats, but not old pseudopregnant rats, show a decreased uterine estradiol uptake with age.[59-61] In a recent study, it was shown that the absolute amount of uterine estrogen receptors in old rats was less than half the amount found in young animals, although progesterone receptor levels were similar in both groups.[62] Administration of progesterone failed to decrease estrogen receptor levels in old rats. Finally the sedimentation values of young and old rats were found to differ, but it was not determined if these changes could account for differences in physiological responses of the uterus. A lack of age changes in the uterine progesterone receptor in the old hamster also has been reported.[63]

H. Effect of Advancing Age on Implantation Rate and Timing

In the mouse and hamster there was a progressive decrease in implantation rate despite a constant ovulation rate.[47,64,65] In the hamster it has been shown that implantation failure is the major cause of embryonic mortality in old animals.[49,52] When implantation takes place in old hamsters, the timing is often delayed.[51] Much of the implantation failure in old animals has been attributed to the lack of lumen closure and other uterine factors as opposed to hormonal defects.[27,28,38,39]

I. Age-Related Changes in the Oviduct (Fallopian Tube)

Relatively few studies have been undertaken to describe the effects of age on oviductal structure and function, and some of the observations described in the literature are contradictory. Soriero[54] states that there are few histological changes except for the loss of cyclic changes for up to 15 years after menopause. Several authors claim that cilia are rarely found in the postmenopausal oviduct,[66,67] but others find that ciliated cells still are present in the infundibulum and ampulla at 20 to 30 years postmenopause.[68] An increased collagen content and a decrease of smooth muscle together with a flattening of the tubal mucosa was also seen with advancing age.[69] A recent study has shown age-related changes in the human fallopian tube ultrastructure.[70]

Numerous studies in the old uterus have localized collagen and elastin histochemically, quantitated it biochemically, and characterized it using various physiochemical procedures. In the human uterus, collagen increased from age 15 to 30 years, remained constant from ages 30 to 49, and then decreased 60% during postmenopausal involution.[14-15] The same studies showed that collagen from old uterus had increased resistance to collagenase digestion, decreased thermal shrinkage temperature, and increased fluorescent properties. The postmenopausal uterus demonstrated a 43% loss in elastin as compared to the uterus from young women.[15] The remaining elastin had an increased hydroxyproline content.

A primary block in ova transport at the ampullary-isthmic junction and a retention of oocytes and blastocytes in the oviduct is seen in the old mouse and hamster, respectively, but no tubal locking of oocytes was observed in the old rat.[71]

III. EFFECT OF ADVANCING AGE ON THE OVARY

The ovary has a dual role in reproductive processes, and both the gametogenic and steroidogenic functions decline in the aging female. Several excellent reviews have described in detail the aging events in ovaries of both women and laboratory species.[3,72,73] In general, women show a marked depletion in oocyte number at the time of the menopause, an almost complete lack of developing follicles,[74] and a very large reduction in estrogen and progesterone synthesis.[72] The ovaries of other mammals also show functional changes with age, but not nearly to the degree as seen in postmenopausal women.[75,76]

A. Studies on Ovarian Morphological Changes With Age

Morphological changes in the aging ovary have been described at the gross, light-microscopic and electron-microscopic level in numerous papers and gynecological texts. In women, the ovary becomes progressively smaller and more fibrotic with age and the surface becomes grayish-yellow and relatively smooth.[10,12,72] There is a diminution of primordial and Graafian follicles,[74] although a recent ultrastructural study has demonstrated that apparently normal primordial follicles are present in postmenopausal ovaries.[77] In this study, most differentiating or advanced follicles were undergoing atretic changes. Other postmenopausal changes include a high incidence of stromal hyperplasia,[10,12,72] hylanization of collagen elements,[78] thickening of the tunica albuginea,[12] arteriosclerotic changes in the vessels of the hilus and medulla,[78] the occasional presence of hilar cell hyperplasia,[10,72] and stromal calcification and/or hemorrhage.[12] Finally, there are numerous corpora albicantia composed of collagen fibers and derived from both regressing corpora lutea and relatively recent atretic follicles.[72]

The rat, by contrast, although showing a decrease in oocyte number, has numerous oocytes present at the end of the reproductive period and continuing to the end of the life span.[79] The aging female rat progresses from regular to irregular estrous cycles, then to a constant estrus (CE) or a pseudopregnant-like (PP) condition, and finally to an anestrous (AN) state, each characterized by a different ovarian morphology.[80] Irregularly cycling rats show a reduced number of follicles, both atretic and nonatretic, luteinized follicles with entrapped oocytes, follicular cysts composed of elongated thecal cells, and other cysts presumably of rete ovarii origin.[81,82] The ovary of the CE rat is characterized by numerous 1 to 3 mm fluid filled cysts, no corpura lutea, and many small preantral and medium sized antral follicles.[80,83–84] The old PP rat has a hyperluteinized ovary with numerous small preantral and medium antral follicles, whereas the AN rat has only small atrophic ovaries which lack antral follicular development.[80,83–84] Changes in the ovarian interstitial tissue with age has also been demonstrated using light and electron microscopy.[85]

Mice also have oocytes persisting throughout their life span, with the interesting exception of the CBA strain which show an almost complete depletion of oocytes before the end of their life span.[73,75,86] With age, pigmentation of the interstitum, luteinization of follicles without ovulation, generalized amyloydosis, rete hyperplasia, and cyst accumulation are seen in the mouse.[87,88] A recent series of reports by Quattropani[89,90] described the aging guinea pig ovary by using light, scanning, and electron microscopy. The principle emphasis of these studies was the age-related accumulation of serious cysts arising from the rete ovarii. A few morphological studies of the aged ovary in other species, such as the dog,[91] hamster,[92] rabbit,[93] and cow[94] have been published.

B. Oocyte Number and Reproductive Decline

As mentioned previously, the most evident change in the ovary with advancing age is the depletion in number of oocytes and developing follicles. Most mammalian ovaries have obtained their full complement of oocytes by the time of birth and oocyte numbers then decrease progressively.[95] With the exception of women and CBA mice,[73–75,96] most animals retain a considerable, although reduced, number of oocytes throughout their life span.

Oocyte depletion has been cited as a cause of reproductive failure, but several sets of experiments have argued against this hypothesis. In the rat, it has been shown that with advancing age, follicular numbers decline, but the ovulation rate does not.[82] Furthermore, unilateral ovariectomy does not cause a premature cessation of reproduction.[93] Likewise, in the rabbit there is no decrease in maternal age at the last litter after unilateral ovariectomy.[93] Finally, ovaries transplanted from old to young ovariectomized rats can ovulate and maintain cyclic reproductive function.[83]

More extensive studies have been done in the mouse, where it was demonstrated that irradiated young mice with ovaries retaining only 1000 to 2000 oocytes are still fertile while old mice with 2000 to 3000 oocytes were not.[97-99] As seen in the rat, follicular numbers decrease with age, but ovulation rate does not,[64] and unilateral ovariectomy does not prevent the maintenance of ovulation and pregnancy.[27,73,100]

The evaluation of ovarian response to gonadotropic stimulation has been studied with a variety of procedures. Administration of exogenous gonadotropins has been used to study ovarian responses in postmenopausal women and a variety of laboratory animals. Despite high endogenous gonadotropin levels in postmenopausal women, 5,000 to 50,000 IU of HCG has been shown to increase urinary estrogen levels[101] and ovarian venous androstenedione and testosterone, but not estradiol levels,[102-103] and to alter vaginal cytology in postmenopausal, but not in ovariectomized women.[104] LH, HCG, or crude pituitary extracts can induce ovulation in noncycling old rats,[105-110] and stimulate Δ^5-3β-hydroxysteroid dehydrogenase activity in the old mouse.[111] The ovulatory response to HCG is reduced in the old rabbit.[93]

Transplants of ovaries from old donor rats to young ovariectomized recipients has shown conclusively that the old rat ovary is capable of near normal function when provided with the proper hormonal milieu.[106,112] Unilateral ovariectomy, which induces compensatory hypertrophy in the remaining ovary, has also been used to study ovarian responsiveness. The data on the effects of unilateral ovariectomy are somewhat contradictory, but indicate equal ovarian response. Ingram[109] demonstrated compensatory ovarian hypertrophy in 14-month-old rats, but Labhsetwer[113] did not see compensatory hypertrophy in 9- to 10-month-old rats. In the latter study, young and old rats responded equally to PMSG, suggesting a hypothalamic or pituitary defect. Howland and Preiss[114] also demonstrated compensatory hypertrophy in old rats and furthermore observed that hemiovariectomy sometimes induced ovulation in the remaining previously inactive ovary.

Ovarian response in old rats also has been demonstrated by stimulation of pituitary LH and FSH release by gonadotropin releasing hormone (LHRH) or through hypothalamic stimulation by using stress, central acting drugs, or electrical stimulation of the hypothalamus (see Section V). It is important to note that in some of these studies vaginal smears were used to monitor the resumption of cycles and ovulation. In fact, changes in vaginal smear patterns in old rats are not always accompanied by ovulation as assessed by laparotomy or ovarian histology.

C. Gonadotropin Binding by the Old Ovary

In order for gonadotropins to stimulate ovarian function they must first bind to membrane receptors.[115] Several methods to study ovarian gonadotropin binding have been used. Radioautography with ^{125}I-labeled LH and FSH was used to demonstrate the binding of these hormones to the postmenopausal ovarian cortical stroma and the hilus.[116] Although only semiquantitative in nature, radioautography shows that growing follicles and corpora lutea in the aged rat ovary retain their capacity to bind LH and FSH in a manner qualitatively similar to that of ovaries from young cyclic rats.[84] A quantitative study of ^{125}HCG binding to granulosa cells isolated from old and young ovarian follicles showed similar numbers of HCG-binding sites.[117] The dissociation constant (kd) of the high affinity HCG receptor, as determined by Scatchard plot analysis, also was unchanged with age.

D. Steroidogenic Capacity of the Old Ovary

Serum steroid levels provide an estimate of ovarian steroidogenesis, but many other factors besides steroid synthesis influence this parameter. First of all, the adrenal produces androgens, estrogens, and progestrones in addition to glucocorticoids and mineralocorticoids, and it has been documented that the adrenal contributes significantly to serum steroid levels in postmenopausal women.[102,103,118–120] Ovariectomy in postmenopausal patients in some, but not all instances, results in a further reduction of already low serum estrogen levels.[121,122] The rate of steroid metabolism can also affect serum values and the metabolic clearance rate for estrogen decreases approximately 25% in postmenopausal, as compared to young women,[123] although it appears to remain unchanged in the female rat.[124] Finally, ovarian venous blood may be a better indicator of ovarian steroidogenesis than peripheral blood, since the postmenopausal ovary produces chiefly androgens which are converted in the periphery to androgens.[125–129] Reported values for serum steroid levels vary markedly as shown in Table 1. Whether these differences are due to the manner of selecting patients for the study and/or variations in radioimmunoassay procedures must be considered.

The urinary excretion of steroids, usually expressed as $\mu g/24$ hr has also been used to estimate postmenopausal ovarian steroidogenesis.[122] Although subject to the same limitations of analysis as discussed for serum steroid measurements, the collection procedure is noninvasive and should tend to negate any short-term fluctuations in serum steroid levels.

Localization and quantitation of enzymes involved in ovarian steroidogenesis have also been used to study aging effects. Histochemical studies, although not usually quantitative, have shown the presence of several enzymes necessary for steroid synthesis, such as glucose-6-PO_4-dehydrogenase and 3β-hydroxysteroid dehydrogenase (3β-HSD)[130] in the postmenopausal ovarian cortical stroma. Similarly, histochemical procedures have been used to show similar 3β-HSD distribution in young and old rats,[84] but aged estrous and diestrous C57BL mice exhibited lower histochemically demonstratable 3β-HSD in thecal, luteal, and interstitial cells than young estrous mice.[131] PMS and HCG restored luteal and interstitial 3β-HSD in old mice.

When rat ovarian 3β-HSD activity was measured histochemically, using several different substrates, it was demonstrated that aging was associated with changes in the use of steroid substrate and distribution of 3β-HDS.[132] This study emphasizes the precautions that must be taken in evaluating an assay for enzyme activity since changes in the substrate gave markedly different results.

Biochemical determination of enzyme activity provides a better quantitative estimate of activity than histochemical procedures, but does not indicate where changes occur, unless elaborate microdissection or other separatory procedures are used. Using biochemical procedures, total ovarian 3β-HSD activity per milligram protein was less in old than in young rats.[133] Similar results were seen in the C57BL/6J mouse and, in addition, total activity was restored by PMSG and/or HCG administration.[111] 3β-HSD was not different in old (12 to 14 month) and young (3 month) pregnant C57BL mice, despite a higher incidence of fetal death and resorbtion in the older mice.[134] In an elaborate series of experiments, Erickson et al.[117] using Lineweaver-Burke plot analysis of saturation curves, showed similar Km and Vmax for ovarian granulosa cell aromatase enzymes in old and young rats.

An exciting new procedure, using duterium-labeled steroids to study estrogen pro-

Table 1
SERUM STEROID LEVELS IN AGING FEMALES

Women (Postmenopausal)

Steroid	Level[a]	Ref.
Estradiol	1–10 pg/mℓ	123
	11–15 pg/mℓ	118, 125, 136–138
	16–20 pg/mℓ	102, 103
	>20 pg/mℓ	137, 138
Estrone	0–30 pg/mℓ	123, 126
	>30 pg/mℓ	136, 139, 140
Progesterone	0–0.25 ng/mℓ	123, 139
	>0.25 ng/mℓ	102, 103, 125
Adrostenedione	0–1.0 ng/mℓ	123, 125
	>1.0 ng/mℓ	102, 103

Rats

	Estradiol (pg/mℓ)	Progesterone (ng/mℓ)	Testosterone (pg/mℓ)	Ref.
Young				
Estrus	19.2 ± 1.9	14.0 ± 2.2	77 ± 2	141, 142
Proestrus				
a.m.	53.7 ± 5.4	11.7 ± 2.4	209 ± 16	
p.m.	72.1 ± 6.4	31.0 ± 3.9	436 ± 55	
Diestrus	29.0 ± 2.0	16.7 ± 2.6	142 ± 21	
Old				
Constant estrus	33.6 ± 3.3	15.5 ± 2.8	150 ± 29	
Pseudopregnant-like	28.7 ± 4.8	25.2 ± 6.5	106 ± 16	
Anestrus	19.8 ± 2.5	6.5 ± 0.88	83 ± 15	

[a]Levels average 150 pg/mℓ in young women.

duction rates, has recently been developed by Pinkus et al.[135] This technique uses stable isotope-labeled compounds and gas chromatography-mass spectrometry to carry out experiments usually disallowed with radiotracer methodology. Preliminary data show low production rates of estradiol in postmenopausal women. The results from Pinkus[135] are comparable to studies using radiotracer techniques where H^3-estrone was administered to postmenopausal patients and H^3-estradiol production was followed.[119]

E. Effects of Age on Corpora Lutea Function

Corpora lutea (CL) formation and function may also be adversely affected by aging, but its relationship to decline in reproductive processes has been debated. In the postmenopausal ovary, only corpora atretica or corpora albicantia remain,[72,116] but decreased luteal function in the perimenopausal period has been described by several different techniques. Morphological studies, the presence of decreased levels of serum progesterone accompanied by dysfunctional uterine bleeding, increased incidences of miscarriages, and changes in the cyclic pattern of basal body temperature, all suggest altered CL function.[72,76,137,138,143]

In the old rat, luteal cells are morphologically altered but still show normal LH binding and normal to increased 3β-HSD activity.[84,99] Interestingly, the substrate specificity for 3β-HSD is altered in old rat CL.[132] Although the number of CL decrease in old rats, this decrease does not occur until a decrease in litter size has taken place.[144]

The CL in old mice are also altered morphologically,[32,64,73,145–147] and 3β-HSD activity has been reported to decline.[75,131] Alterations in serum progesterone in old C57/BL/6J mice are associated with prolonged gestational lengths and increased frequencies of fetal resorbtions.[78,79] Despite a change in CL function, many investigators do not always see this as the overall cause for decreased litter size.[27,47,146,148,149] For example, progesterone administration to aged mice or rabbits increases the implantation rate, but not subsequent embryonic survival.[145,146,150]

Hamsters likewise show reduced CL growth and progesterone production with age.[52,151]

IV. PITUITARY AND AGING

The pituitary gland has been the subject of numerous gerontological studies. In postmenopausal women, the pituitary shows decreased weight[154,155] which differs from the rabbit,[34] mouse,[156] and rat[61,157,158] in whom an increased pituitary weight with age has been reported. However, in other reports, no changes in relative pituitary weights were shown from age 40 to 80 in men.[159,160] It was pointed out that such data must be interpreted cautiously since diverse terminal diseases may grossly affect pituitary morphology. In the rat, increased pituitary weights were noted in old constant estrous, old pseudopregnant-like and old anestrous rats, as compared to young cycling females.[80] Vascularity of the human pituitary is decreased after the age of 40 or 50.[161]

Caution must be used in evaluating pituitary morphology since the pituitary is easily damaged during removal and autolytic changes affecting staining procedures occur rapidly after death.[162] Although pituitary pathologies were once thought to be relatively unimportant in the elderly, considerable data show important changes, such as microscopic tumors and disturbances in the blood supply,[162] indicating that data on the pituitary gland in aging animals must be viewed with caution in order to differentiate between physiological and pathological changes.

Histological examination of the pituitary of aging women reveals an increase of connective tissue.[163] This is also evident in rats,[164,165] mice,[156,166] and hamsters.[167] Women show an 8 to 10% increase in basophils and a 40 to 50% decrease in acidophils with age.[168] The basophils in postmenopausal women are often vacuolated.[169] Rats also show a vacuolation of basophils with age, but the relative proportion of cell types remains unchanged in nonvirgin rats.[165,170] Pituitary adenomas are especially common in the old rat.[170,171]

Electron microscopic identification of pituitary cell types provides a better means of cell identification than histology at the light microscope level, but few if any studies in old women or experimental animals have been undertaken. The relatively new and powerful immunocytochemical methods of pituitary cell identification[172] have recently been used to describe mammotropes[173,174] and thyrotropes[175] in young and old human pituitaries, but the authors are unaware of any descriptions of gonadotropin producing cells.

A. Pituitary Hormone Content

Pituitary hormone content varies with age as described by numerous investigators, but the data in the literature are sometimes contradictory. For example, a two- or three-fold increase in pituitary LH content after the menopause was reported by Ryan,[155] while Albert et al.[176] reported increased FSH, but unchanged LH levels. Pituitary LH and FSH levels vary in old rats, depending on the reproductive state.[157,158] In the rabbit the total LH content was reported to be unchanged with age, but the LH concentration is lower in old rabbits.[34]

Several precautions must be observed in analyzing pituitary hormone levels. First of all, data from bioassays and radioimmunoassays are not always in agreement,[177] and the possibility of the existence of altered forms of pituitary hormones with age cannot be discounted.[178] Many factors such as sex steroids dramatically affect pituitary hormone content and it is important to take these into consideration. Finally, it is important to realize that changes in pituitary hormone content cannot differentiate between changes in synthesis and secretory activities of the gland.

B. Effect of Age on Pituitary Responsiveness to LHRH

With the availability of synthetic LHRH decapeptide, it has been possible to test the effects of age on pituitary response to hypothalamic stimulation. Dose and method of administration of LHRH must be carefully evaluated since, for example, steady infusion of LHRH to monkeys does not effect LH release while pulsatile administration causes an LH surge.[179] Likewise, multiple small LHRH injections are more effective in inducing an LH surge in rats than one large dose.[83,180] Finally, steroids such as estradiol markedly increase the LH response to LHRH.[180,181]

Pituitary responsiveness to LHRH persists in women up to 100 years of age,[182–185] but there may be a different sensitivity to dose and a differential age effect on LH and FSH release. In old intact female rats, a reduced LH responsiveness to a single injection of LHRH has been reported,[186,187] but multiple injections cause equal LH release in old and young rats.[83,188] Old and young ovariectomized rats or intact rats injected with estrogen respond equally to LHRH.[187,189] A differential LH/FSH response to LHRH may occur in old as compared to young rats.[124,190]

C. Effects of Age on Serum Gonadotropin Levels and Prolactin

A better indication of pituitary secretion than pituitary content is serum hormone levels. However, certain precautions still must be observed. As discussed previously, immuno- and bioactivity of the hormones may change with age, as can metabolic clearance of the hormones. Metabolic clearance of LH and FSH were reported to be unchanged with age in women,[191,192] but data for other species are lacking. Disease states often suppress gonadotropin levels in postmenopausal women,[193] indicating that health status must also be closely monitored to avoid misinterpretation of data.

It is generally agreed that in postmenopausal women there is marked elevation of serum LH and FSH.[104,137,138,182–185,194,200] FSH levels may increase to a much greater extent than LH levels.[137,138,185] Urinary gonadotropins are also elevated in the menopausal and perimenopausal period.[154,201,202]

Parabiotic studies indirectly indicated increased gonadotropin levels in old mice,[203] but almost all studies in the rat showed normal or decreased basal LH levels in old female rats.[83,114,204,205] Depending on the reproductive state, old rats have either elevated or unchanged basal levels of FSH.[83,114,141] Numerous reports confirm the loss of cyclic gonadotropin and steroid release in old female rats.[80,83,110,114,141,204,206,207]

Serum prolactin levels decline with age in women.[199,208] This decrease parallels the fall in estrogens[199,209] and can be reversed by estrogen replacement.[210]

Serum and pituitary prolactin levels increase with age in the rat.[83,157,211,212] Ovariectomy lowers prolactin in old constant estrous and pseudopregnant rats, but not in old anestrous females.[205] Estrogen further increases prolactin levels in these three classes of old rats.[205,213]

D. Negative Feedback Relationships in Old Females

Ovarian steroids exert a strong influence on serum and pituitary gonadotropin levels. Ovariectomy results in large increases in serum LH and FSH, and estrogen replacement lowers both gonadotropins. The effects of age on the negative feedback control of LH and FSH have been tested in women and several laboratory species, often with contradictory results due to different procedures and differences in age or strain of animals.

As previously discussed, the postmenopausal endocrine profile is characterized by low sex steroid levels and high gonadotropin levels. It is generally agreed that sex steroid replacement in postmenopausal women lowers LH and FSH,[140,200,210,214–217] but it may take higher doses of lower gonadotropins in older women,[218] and it may not be possible to lower levels to those seen in the premenopausal period.[219] A differential LH and FSH response to low doses of estrogen also has been observed in older women.[219] Although a variety of steroid preparations and doses were used in the cited studies, in only a few of the studies were serum steroid levels monitored to see if equal levels were maintained in young and old patients.

Basal serum gonadotropin levels in old rats are either normal or slightly reduced.[141] After ovariectomy serum LH increases in old rats, but at a lesser rate and magnitude than in young rats.[83,186,189,205,212] FSH in old ovariectomized rats increases either to an equal or a reduced level as compared with young rats.[83,205] Estrogen suppresses gonadotropin levels in old female rats. After multiple estradiol injections, serum estradiol levels become similar,[124] suggesting that metabolism of this steroid does not differ between young and old female rats.

E. Positive Feedback Relationships in Old Females

A preovulatory surge of estradiol has been shown by many investigators to be the "trigger" for the ovulatory surge of LH and FSH. Ovulatory-like surges of LH and FSH in women, monkeys, and rats can be induced with a proper time course injection of estrogen or progesterone. An age-related change in positive feedback relationships may explain changes in cyclic activity, and several studies have been reported recently.

In women, studies have shown that estrogen and/or progesterone can induce LH and FSH surges in postmenopausal or castrate women.[198,200,218,220] Estrogen-primed ovariectomized old female rats show a reduced positive feedback release of LH in response to either estrogen or progesterone,[83,186,189,204,221] but FSH appears to be less affected by age.[83,124] In the latter study, a progressive loss of estrogen and progesterone positive feedback was seen as supporting an hypothesis on differential aging of different areas in the hypothalamus and limbic systems controlling gonadotropin release.

V. AGE-RELATED CHANGES IN THE HYPOTHALAMUS

Aging in female rats is characterized by the absence of cyclic variations in serum LH and FSH,[141,205] and estradiol and progesterone.[141] Furthermore, the large increase in serum LH and FSH in response to ovariectomy was attenuated in old female rats.[83,124,205] Although a decrease in pituitary responsiveness to LHRH may partly be responsible for these deficiencies, the degree of pituitary involvement in the decline in reproductive function is still controversial. The autonomic nervous system has been shown to have an important role in the control of anterior pituitary function[222–224] and these effects have been shown to be mediated by the secretion of hypothalamic peptide hormones.[225] The demonstration that catecholamine metabolism is decreased and serotonin metabolism increased in aging male and female rats[226] implies that changes in synthesis, metabolism, or release of hypothalamic hypophysiotropic hormones are responsible for some of the reproductive deficits in aging female rats. This conclusion is further substantiated by the finding that electrical stimulation of the preoptic area which has been shown to contain cell bodies for LHRH, or injection of central acting drugs can at least temporarily reinitiate estrous cycles in old constant estrous females.[107,227–232] There are few experiments as yet on the regulation of hypothalamic hormones in aged animals. This is partly attributable to the inherent difficulties in measuring peptide synthesis, the difficulties in measuring plasma concentrations of hypothalamic hormones, and the limited conclusions that can be drawn from assaying LHRH content. The present section will review studies on hypothalamic LHRH content in aged and young female rats and discuss LHRH distribution, synthesis, and release.

A. Hypothalamic LHRH Content in Young and Aged Rats

Studies of constant estrous or repetitive pseudopregnant rats generally reveal little alteration in LHRH content in comparison to young cycling females. In young female rats there are fluctuations in LHRH content that vary throughout the estrous cycle. Kalra[233] has shown that in the rostral hypothalamic area, including the MPOA and OVLT, temporal increases in LHRH are greatest on diestrus II, with smaller increases in proestrus. The cyclic fluctuations in LHRH content have been confirmed by Araki et al.[234] However, the greatest LHRH content in the latter study occurred primarily at 0800 hr on estrus with a smaller increase at 1700 hr on diestrus II. Although the differences between these two studies are probably the result of temporal sampling factors, the increases in rostral hypothalamic LHRH in each case were hypothesized to result from alterations in synthesis and transport of LHRH to areas responsible for the release of hormone into the portal vasculature. Although these variations occurred throughout the estrous cycle, basal content of LHRH in rostral areas was unaffected by castration[234,235] or estrogen replacement.[235]

Under certain specific instances, content of LHRH in the arcuate-median eminence region is directly related to the concentration of gonadal steroids.[236] LHRH content fluctuates throughout the estrous cycle, with a major decrease occurring on the day of proestrus.[234] In a more detailed study, Kalra and Kalra[237] found that MBH-LHRH decreased between 1400 and 1445 hr on proestrus. An LH surge occurred at 1605 hr. Although the decrease in LHRH content was highly correlated with increases in serum LH, changes in LHRH content during estrus or diestrus were not highly correlated with serum LH.[237,238] In castrated rats, LHRH content in MBH areas decreased up to 21 days after ovariectomy.[234,235] Studies from the authors' laboratory have confirmed the effect of circulating steroids on LHRH content.[236] Ovariectomy decreased LHRH content while estrogen reversed this effect. Progesterone acted synergistically with estrogen in increasing LHRH content. Thus, under certain specific circumstances, decreases in LHRH content are correlated with increases in serum LH, suggesting that LHRH was released into the portal vasculature and was responsible for the elevated concentration of LH in serum.

Increases in LHRH in portal blood, however, are not always consistant with increases in serum LH and FSH. Eskay et al.[239] failed to observe increased LHRH in portal blood immediately preceding the LH surge. These differences may reflect the nonphysiological nature of sampling portal blood, temporal sampling factors, and the potential of anesthetics in interfering with the release of LHRH.

In aged female rats, Pi et al.[158] reported no changes in stalk-median eminence LHRH and FSH-RH activity in constant estrous and anestrous animals compared to adult female rats in estrus or diestrus, respectively. In subsequent experiments designed to give greater sensitivity to the LHRH bioassay, Peng et al.[241] reported increased activity in constant estrous animals and no change in anestrous animals. Clemens and Meites[157] found increased FSH-RH activity in the stalk-median eminence extracts of constant estrous animals and inferred that LHRH activity was decreased because of low pituitary content of LH. Miller and Riegle[242] found no significant differences in LHRH activity of intact or ovariectomized aged females compared to young animals. Data from the authors' laboratory has extended much of the bioassay data on LHRH content using RIA.[142] In young cycling females, LHRH content was elevated on the morning of proestrus and fell that afternoon. Content was again elevated on the morning of estrus. Although content of LHRH in the MBH of repetitive pseudopregnant animals was not different from young animals, MBH-LHRH in constant estrous females was lower than in young estrous rats. Anestrous females, however, had lower LHRH content than any other group. Rostral hypothalamic LHRH in aged females was similar to young females. It was concluded that constant estrous and repetitive pseudopregnant animals have sufficient LHRH for cyclic release of gonadotropins, but lack the stimulus for cyclic LHRH release. Anestrous females may lack sufficient LHRH to stimulate basal release of LH. In each of the above studies, the endogenous levels of estrogen and progesterone varied between young and aged animals. The content of LHRH in ovariectomized estrogen primed animals remains to be determined.

B. Hypothalamic Distribution of LHRH

Many of the previous studies have determined total hypothalamic LHRH content to assess differences in LHRH synthesis or release between young and aged animals. LHRH is not uniformly distributed throughout the hypothalamus. In young animals, LHRH activity has been localized using bioassay techniques in the medial basal tuberal region of the hypothalamus as well as more rostral regions including the suprachiasmatic nucleus, ventral portions of the medial preoptic area, and anterior hypothalamus.[243] Similar studies using RIA combined with serial sectioning of the hypothalamus in different planes[244,245] and a punch technique for specific hypothalamic nuclei[246,247] have confirmed the bioassay data and further localized LHRH in the retrochiasmatic, arcuate- and median-eminence regions, the prechiasmatic region including the preoptic, anterior hypothalamic region, and in the organum vasculosum of the lamina terminalis (OVLT).

Localization of LHRH using bioassay and radioimmunoassay techniques have generally produced consistant results and are in agreement with immunocytochemical (ICC) evidence which finds LHRH immunoreactive processes in the median eminence and OVLT. However, ICC techniques employed to localize perikarya responsible for the synthesis of the decapeptide are not in complete agreement. At the present time, it is generally accepted that the majority of LHRH perikarya reside within the preoptic-septal area[248] and LHRH within the median eminence and OVLT are derived from these regions.[249-251] The difficulty in localizing LHRH perikarya may result not only from differences in ICC techniques, but also from the use of antisera that have different antigenic properties.[252-254] Hoffman et al.,[252] for example, used five different antisera against LHRH conjugated through different amino acids. These antisera subsequently bound to the decapeptide at different positions. LHRH perikarya were found in the medial preoptic, preoptic periventricular, and medial septal areas with fibers projecting to the OVLT, median eminence, and thalamic regions. These cell bodies were identified only with antisera against LHRH conjugated through the N or C terminal of the hormone.

King et al.[253] studied the differences in LHRH content in four hypothalamic areas using an antiserum against LHRH adsorbed on polyvinylpyrrolidone (PVP) that fails to bind LHRH with modified C or N terminals (Arimura #422) and an antiserum against glu-1-LHRH conjugated to human serum albumin through the 1-glutamyl position (Arimura #743). This latter antiserum was shown to bind LHRH in central portions of the decapeptide. Results indicated that the arculate and MPOA areas have higher concentrations of LHRH immunoreactivity as determined by antiserum #743 than by #422. Both the median eminence and OVLT regions exhibited similar levels of LHRH as determined by both antisera. These results would seem to indicate that immunoreactive LHRH in perikarya is bound at the C or N terminal, while that found in fiber regions is the mature decapeptide. This conclusion is further supported by data which demonstrate three different molecular weight species of immunoreactive LHRH after chromatography on Sephadex® G-25.[255,256] These presumptive prohormone species are more concentrated in areas presumed to be responsible for LHRH synthesis, while primarily the mature decapeptide is found in the median eminence and OVLT regions.[253] Furthermore, estradiol implants for 2 weeks into ovariectomized female rats increased both mature and high molecular weight forms of immunoreactive LHRH.[257] Together, these data provide strong evidence for the existence of an LHRH prohormone that may be enzymatically cleaved into the mature form of LHRH when it is transported down the axon terminal. Because areas of synthesis are discrete from areas of release, each must be assessed independently and the specific antiserum may be important in determining differences between these areas.

C. Plasma Concentrations of LHRH

The preferred methods for assessing changes in hypothalamic function with age are to observe alterations in LHRH synthesis, metabolism, or release. The difficulties and problems of sampling portal blood to assess LHRH release have previously been discussed and methods developed for determining LHRH release in vitro may not be indicative of release in vivo. These methods will not be reviewed in the present section. The difficulty in determining plasma concentrations of LHRH is due to the low plasma concentrations of LHRH,[258] the short half-life of the hormone, and interference in the RIA by lipids and plasma proteins.[259,260] When LHRH is incubated in unextracted serum, it loses both its biological[261] and immunological[260-263] activity. Furthermore, serum LHRH values are affected by method of iodination and purification of tracer, differences between antisera, and affinity of antiserum.[263] Extraction procedures used to purify plasma LHRH in young animals have been partially successful, but this may be more complex in aging animals. Plasma from young animals extracted with acetone and ether had low plasma LHRH concentrations and linear dose-response curves. Extracted plasma from aged animals had high concentrations of LHRH and nonlinear dose-response curves.[264] This suggests that extraction procedures that may be adequate for determining plasma LHRH in young animals may not be valid for aged animals. More recently adsorbtion of LHRH from plasma with florisil has proved useful in measuring plasma LHRH.[265,266] The capability of this method in determining plasma levels of LHRH in aged animals remains to be determined.

D. Metabolism of LHRH

Peptidases that are capable of metabolizing LHRH are present in the hypothalamus[267] and their activity and/or concentration is increased by estradiol,[268] LH,[269] and prostaglandins.[270] Enzyme activity was decreased by progesterone and gonadectomy.[268] Changes in enzymes that degrade LHRH have not been investigated as a function of age and their importance in alterations of reproductive function remain to be determined.

E. Synthesis of LHRH

Synthesis of LHRH has been studied in intact and sliced hypothalami,[271,272] and in cell-free homogenates,[273–275] using incorporation of tritiated amino acids into LHRH. The large number of hypothalami needed per incubation has made these techniques prohibitive to use with aging animals. Recently, Hall and Steinberger[276] have used a specific antiserum against LHRH to percipitate ^{3}H-LHRH generated in vitro. This method overcomes the problems with classical methods of purification by chromatography or bioassay. Sundberg and Knigge[277] have measured in vitro synthesis of LHRH by comparing incubated vs. nonincubated hypothalami and comparing changes in LHRH content. This is a valuable technique, but has restricted usefulness because of the inability to differentiate metabolism of a prohormone for LHRH from true *de novo* synthesis.

F. Role of Putative Neurotransmitters in the Decline of Reproductive Function

Administration of progesterone, epinephrine,[107] L-dopa, or iproniazid[227–231] to aged rats classified as constant estrus resulted in resumption of estrous cycles. Watkins et al.[232] suggested that the hypothalamo-hypophysial axis may be less responsive to the effects of L-dopa, while Clemens[278,279] proposed that changes in the MPOA may contribute to alterations in reproductive processes in aging females. Lesions of the MPOA in young females result in a repetitive pseudopregnant state and animals began to cycle again after injections of dopamine agonists. If lesions extend to anterior hypothalamic areas, animals go into constant estrus. Whether specific changes in MPOA and anterior hypothalamic areas contributes to the aging process remains to be determined. However, with advancing age there are decreases in the number of hypothalamic neurons[280] as well as decreases in uptake of ^{3}H-estrogen in the hypothalamus[281] and estrogen receptors in the cortex.[282] Other experimenters have hypothesized that the primary cause of senile deviations of the estrous cycle are the result of changes in the synthesis, turnover, or release of putative neurotransmitters.[231,283] In aged mice, Finch[284] has observed incorporation of ^{3}H-tyrosine into brain catecholamines in the hypothalamus, decreased turnover of ^{3}H-norepinephrine and ^{3}H-dopamine, reduction in strial dopamine, slowed catabolism of catecholamines, and reduced uptake of dopamine into synaptosomes. The action of central acting drugs in the reinitiation of estrous cycles suggests that similar changes in putative neurotransmitters may take place in aged rats. Studies by Simpkins et al.[226] show that dopamine and norepinephrine content and turnover are lower in aged male rats and there also is increased turnover of 5-HT. Similarly, in female rats, Huang[286] has reported decreases in norepinephrine and dopamine turnover. Although the specific regulation of LHRH, LH, FSH, and prolactin by catecholamines and indoleamines is still controversial,[287] there is strong evidence that changes in reproductive function with age are caused by neurotransmitter imbalances leading to changes in hypothalamic control of hypophysial functions. This has been termed the "cascading effect" of aging, implying that changes in catecholamines induce alterations in hypothalamic releasing/inhibiting hormones and, hence, gonadotropins.[231,283]

VI. CONCLUSIONS

It is clear from this review that there is a gradual decline in the reproductive system with aging in all mammalian species studied thus far, including man. However, there are some important differences as well as similarities in the causes that lead to reproductive senescence in man and animals. In women approaching the menopause, there is a gradual decline in number of ovulations for the 2- to 3-year period preceding the menopause. The ovaries are apt to develop cystic follicles and the number of ovulations decrease, resulting in shortening of the cycles. The number of ova remaining in the ovaries at the time of the menopause is reduced to about 10,000 from approximately 600,000 to 700,000 at the time of birth. The ovaries during the perimenopausal period secrete reduced amounts of estrogen and progesterone, resulting in increased secretion of FSH and LH by the anterior pituitary. In the postmenopausal period, the ovaries become fibrotic and atrophic, and most of the remaining follicles gradually disappear. The ovaries may continue to produce small amounts of estrone converted from androstenedione, although the major source of androstenedione appears to be from the adrenals. The atrophy of the reproductive tract is due mainly to loss of ovarian hormones. FSH and LH continue to rise and to be maintained at high levels during the postmenopausal period, indicating that there are no major deficiencies in hypothalamo-pituitary function during this period. Thus, the major reason for the decline and ultimate cessation of menstrual cycles in women lies in ovarian failure, and is not due to any disabilities in hypothalamo-pituitary function.

In aging female rats, the primary reason for the reproductive decline and cessation of estrous cycles does not lie in the ovaries, but rather in the hypothalamo-pituitary system. In aging female rats, the cycles first tend to become irregular and are usually lengthened rather than shortened as in women approaching the menopause. Instead of 4- or 5-day estrous cycles, the cycles may be prolonged to 6 to 9 days, and are usually characterized by lengthening of the estrous phase of the cycle and sometimes of the diestrous phase. From irregular cycles, the aging rat usually progresses to constant estrus, characterized by ovaries with well developed and often cystic follicles, but no corpora lutea due to failure to ovulate. This is usually followed by irregular and prolonged periods of pseudopregnancy, up to 30 days or more in length, characterized by ovaries with many corpora lutea that are actively secreting progesterone. The oldest female rats usually show an anestrous condition, characterized by shrunken ovaries with only small follicles, and little evidence of estrogen secretion as indicated by the atrophic, infantile-appearing uterus. Most of these old anestrous rats also have prolactin-secreting pituitary tumors. It is remarkable, however, that the ovaries from all of these categories of aging rats are capable of normal or near normal function when transplanted to young ovariectomized rats, where they increase in size and function. Administration of pituitary gonadotropins or LHRH also can reactivate the functions of these ovaries. Thus, the ovaries of female rats are potentially capable of activity for practically all of their entire life span, but do not function normally because of faults that develop in the hypothalamo-pituitary system with aging.

In the aging female rats, the authors have reported that there is a reduced capacity to secrete LH and FSH and an increased ability to secrete prolactin. LH and FSH show no cyclic changes in the old rats, and the total amount of these gonadotropins secreted are lower than during the estrous cycle. As a result, there also are no cyclic changes in estrogen or progesterone secretion by the ovaries, and the total amounts of these hormones secreted also are less than during the normal estrous cycle. The primary fault appears to lie in the hypothalamus, which the authors have found to be deficient in catecholamines, particularly norepinephrine which stimulates gonadotropin secretion via LHRH release, and the hypothalamus produces increased amounts of serotonin which mainly inhibits gonadotropin secretion. There also is evidence for a decrease in estrogen uptake by the hypothalamus of old rats. When the hypothalamo-pituitary system of old rats is challenged, as by ovariectomy or by ovariectomy followed by estrogen or estrogen-progesterone administration, the usual increases in LH and FSH release are greatly attenuated as compared with the much greater rises in serum LH and FSH seen in young or mature rats. Reinitiation of estrous cycles has been produced in old constant estrous rats by direct electrical stimulation of the preoptic area of the hypothalamus or by administration of drugs that increase catecholamines such as L-dopa or iproniazid. Progesterone and ACTH also are very effective in reestablishing estrous cycles in old constant estrous rats. In old pseudopregnant rats, estrous cycles have been reinitiated by administration of an ergot drug (lergotrile) or a prostaglandin, which apparently rid the ovaries of their numerous corpora lutea. Thus in aging female rats, the changes in hypothalamic rather than in the ovarian function appear to be mainly responsible for loss of reproductive functions.

REFERENCES

1. **Strehler, B. L.,** *Time Cells and Aging,* 2nd ed., Academic Press, New York, 1977, 5.
2. **Talbert, G. B.,** Aging of the reproductive system, in *Handbook of the Biology of Aging,* Finch, C. E. and Hayflick, L., Eds., D. Van Nostrand, New York, 1977, 318.
3. **Talbert, G. B.,** Effect of aging of the ovaries and female gametes on reproductive capacity, in *The Aging Reproductive System,* Schneider, E. L., Ed., Raven Press, New York, 1978, 59.
4. **Steger, R. W.,** Aging and the hypothalamo-hypophyseal-gonadal-axis, in *Aging and Reproductive Physiology,* Hafez, E. S. E., Ed., Ann Arbor Science, Ann Arbor, Mich., 1976, 51.
5. **Lang, W. R. and Aponte, G. E.,** Gross and microscopic anatomy of the aged female reproductive organs, *Clin. Obstet. Gynecol.,* 10, 454, 1967.
6. **Masters, W. H., and Johnson, V. E.,** *Human Sexual Response,* Little, Brown, Boston, 1966, 233.
7. **Schiff, I. and Wilson, E.,** Clinical aspects of aging of the female reproductive system, in *The Aging Reproductive System,* Schneider, E. L., Ed., Raven Press, New York, 1978, 9.
8. **Steger, R. W. and Hafez, E. S. E.,** Age associated changes in the human vagina, in *The Human Vagina,* Hafez, E. S. E. and Evans, T. N., Ed., Elsevier/North Holland, Amsterdam, 1977.
9. **Hammond, C. B.,** Menopause, an American way, in *The Management of the Menopause and Post-menopausal Years,* Campbell, S., Ed., University Park Press, Baltimore, 1976.
10. **Rakoff, A. E. and Nowrooz, K.,** The female climacteric, in *Geriatric Endocrinology,* Greenblatt, R. B., Ed., Raven Press, New York, 1978, 165.
11. **Crompton, A. E.,** Cervical colposcopic changes associated with the menopause, in *The Management of the Menopause and Postmenopausal Years,* Campbell, S., University Park Press, Baltimore, 1976.
12. **Kuppe, G., Metzger, H., and Ludwig, H.,** Aging and structural changes in the female reproductive tract, in *Aging and Reproductive Physiology,* Hafez, E. S. E., Ed., Ann Arbor Science, Ann Arbor, Mich., 1976, 21.
13. **Fluhman, C. F.,** *The Cervix Uteri and Its Diseases,* W. B. Saunders, Philadelphia, 1961.
14. **Woessner, J. F.,** Aging of human uterus connective tissue, *J. Gerontol.,* 17, 453, 1962.
15. **Woessner, J. F.,** Age-related changes of the human uterus and its connective tissue framework, *J. Gerontol.,* 18, 220, 1963.
16. **Lang, W. R.,** Cervical portio from menarche on: a colposcopic study, *Ann. N.Y. Acad. Sci.,* 97, 653, 1962.
17. **Speert, H.,** The endometrium in old age, *Surv. Gynecol. Obstet.,* 89, 551, 1949.
18. **McBride, J. M.,** The normal postmenopausal endometrium, *J. Obstet. Gynaec. Br. Emp.,* 61, 691, 1954.
19. **Bigelow, B.,** Comparison of ovarian and endometrial morphology spanning the menopause, *J. Obstet. Gynecol.,* 11, 487, 1958.
20. **Steger, R. W., Huang, H. H., Kuppe, G., Meites, J., Hafez, E. S. E., and Ludwig, H.,** Effect of age on uterine surface ultrastructure, in *Scanning Electron Microscopy/1976,* IIT Research Institute, Chicago, 1976, 359.
21. **Jones, E. C.,** The endometrium and effects of aging (mouse), in *Scanning Electron Microscopic Atlas of Mammalian Reproduction,* Hafez, E. S. E., Ed., Igaku Shoin, Tokyo, 1975, 190.
22. **Rogers, J. B. and Taylor, R. C.,** Age changes in the uterus and ovary of the guinea pig, *Anat. Rec.,* 121, 448, 1955.
23. **Warbrick, J. G.,** A pigment in the rat's uterus, *Q. J. Microsc. Sci.,* 97, 11, 1956.
24. **Biggers, J. D.,** Problems concerning the uterine causes of embryonic death, with special reference to the effects of ageing of the uterus, *J. Reprod. Fertil. Suppl.,* 8, 27, 1969.
25. **Bal, H. S. and Getty, R.,** Changes in the histomorphology of the uterus of the domestic pig with advancing age, *J. Gerontol.,* 28, 160, 1973.

26. **Burack, E., Wolfe, J. M., Lansing, W., and Wright, A. W.,** The effect of age upon the connective tissue of the uterus, cervix and vagina of the rat, *Cancer Res.,* 1, 227, 1941.
27. **Finn, C. A.,** Reproductive capacity and litter size in mice, effect of age and environment, *J. Reprod. Fertil.,* 6, 205, 1963.
28. **Finn, C. A.,** The ageing uterus and its influence on reproductive capacity, *J. Reprod. Fertil. Suppl.,* 12, 31, 1970.
29. **Finn, C. A.,** Uterine function in aged animals, in *The Uterus,* Finn, C. A. and Porter, D. G., Eds., Publishing Sciences Group, Acton, Mass., 1975, 100.
30. **Kao, K. T., Lu, S. C., Hitt, W., and McGarack, T. H.,** Connective tissue VI: synthesis of collagen by rat uterine slices, *Proc. Soc. Exp. Biol. Med.,* 109, 4, 1962.
31. **Kao, K. and McGarack, T.,** Connective tissue. I. Age and sex influence on protein composition of rat tissues, *Proc. Soc. Exp. Biol. Med.,* 101, 153, 1959.
32. **Loeb, L.,** Aging processes in the ovaries of mice belonging to strains differing in the incidence of mammary carcinoma, *Arch. Pathol.,* 46, 401, 1948.
33. **Maurer, R. R. and Foote, R. H.,** Uterine collagenase and collagen in young and ageing rabbits, *J. Reprod. Fertil.,* 30, 301, 1972.
34. **Maurer, R. R. and Foote, R. H.,** Maternal ageing and embryonic mortality in the rabbit. II. Hormonal changes in young and ageing females, *J. Reprod. Fertil.,* 31, 15, 1972.
35. **Rahima, A. and Soderwall, A. L.,** Uterine collagen content in young and senescent pregnant golden hamsters, *J. Reprod. Fertil.,* 49, 161, 1974.
36. **Schaub, M. C.,** Changes in the collagen in the aging and in the pregnant uterus of white rats, *Gerontologia,* 10, 137, 1964/1965.
37. **Wolfe, J. M., Buracke, E., Lansing, W., and Wright, A. W.,** The effects of advancing age on the connective tissue of the uterus, cervix and vagina of the rat, *Am. J. Anat.,* 70, 135, 1942.
38. **Loeb, L., Suntzeff, V., and Burns, E. L.,** Changes in the nature of the stroma in vagina, cervix and uterus of the mouse produced by long continuous injections of oestrogen and by advancing age, *Am. J. Cancer,* 35, 159, 1939.
38. **Finn, C. A. and Martin, L.,** The cellular response of the uterus of the aged mouse to oestrogen and progesterone, *J. Reprod. Fertil.,* 20, 545, 1969.
39. **Finn, C. A.,** Embryonic death in aged mice, *Nature (London),* 194, 499, 1962.
40. **Finn, C. A.,** The initiation of the decidual cell reaction in the uterus of the aged mouse, *J. Reprod. Fertil.,* 11, 423, 1966.
41. **Finn, C. A., Fitch, S. M., and Harkness, R. D.,** Collagen content of barren and previously pregnant uterine horns in old mice, *J. Reprod. Fertil.,* 6, 405, 1963.
42. **Holinka, C. H. and Finch, C. E.,** Age related changes in the decidual responses of the C57BL/6J mouse uterus, *Biol. Reprod.,* 16, 385, 1977.
43. **Holinka, C. F., Hetland, M. D., and Finch, C. E.,** The response to a single dose of estradiol in the uterus of ovariectomized C57BL/6J mice during aging, *Biol. Reprod.,* 17, 262, 1977.
44. **Hollander, W. F. and Strong, L. C.,** Intrauterine mortality and placental fusions in the mouse, *J. Exper. Zool.,* 115, 131, 1950.
45. **Shapiro, M. and Talbert, G. B.,** The effect of maternal age on decidualization in the mouse, *J. Gerontol.,* 29, 145, 1974.
46. **Talbert, G. B.,** Effect of maternal age on postimplantation reproduction failure in mice, *J. Reprod. Fertil.,* 24, 449, 1971.
47. **Blaha, G. C.,** Reproductive senescence in the female golden hamster, *Anat. Rec.,* 150, 405, 1964.
48. **Blaha, G. C.,** Effects of age, treatment and method of induction on deciduomata in the golden hamster, *Fertil. Steril.,* 18, 477, 1967.
49. **Connors, T. J., Thorpe, L. W., and Soderwall, A. L.,** An analysis of preimplantation embryonic death in senescent golden hamsters, *Biol. Reprod.,* 6, 131, 1972.
50. **Parkening, T. A.,** Apposition of uterine luminal epithelium during implantation in senescent golden hamsters, *J. Gerontol.,* 34, 335, 1979.
51. **Parkening, T. A. and Soderwell, A. J.,** Delayed embryonic development and implantation in senescent golden hamsters, *Biol. Reprod.,* 8, 427, 1973.
52. **Thorneycroft, I. H. and Soderwall, A. L.,** The nature of the litter size loss in senescent hamsters, *Anat. Rec.,* 165, 343, 1969.
53. **Thorpe, L. W., Connors, T. J., and Soderwall, A. L.,** Closure of the uterine lumen at implantation in senescent golden hamsters, *J. Reprod. Fertil.,* 39, 29, 1974.
54. **Soriero, A. A.,** The aging uterus and fallopian tubes, in *The Aging Reproductive System,* Schneider, E. L., Ed., Raven Press, New York, 1978.
55. **Soriero, A. A. and Talbert, G. B.,** The effect of estrogen on protein and RNA concentration and on *de novo* synthesis of RNA in the uterus of aging ovariectomized mice, *J. Gerontol.,* 30, 265 1976.

56. **Parkening, T. A. and Soderwall, A. L.,** Histochemical localization of glycogen in preimplantation and implantation stages of young and senescent golden hamsters, *J. Reprod. Fertil.,* 41, 285, 1974.
57. **Singhal, R. L. and Valadares, R. E.,** Influence of age on uterine enzyme induction, *Fed. Proc. Fed. Am. Soc. Exp. Biol.,* 26, 854, 1967.
58. **Singhal, R.. L., Valadares, H. R. E., and Ling, G. M.,** Estrogenic regulation of uterine carbohydrate metabolism during senescence, *Am. J. Physiol.,* 217, 793, 1969.
59. **Gosden, R. G.,** Uptake and metabolism in vivo of tritiated oestradiol-17β in tissues of ageing female mice, *J. Endocrinol.,* 68, 153, 1976.
60. **Larson, L. L., Spilman, C. H., and Foote, R. H.,** Uterine uptake of progesterone and estradiol in young and aged rabbits, *Proc. Soc. Exp. Biol. Med.,* 141, 463, 1972.
61. **Peng, M. T. and Peng, Y. M.,** Changes in the uptake of tritiated estradiol in the hypothalamus and adenohypophysis of old female rats, *Fertil. Steril.,* 24, 539, 1973.
62. **Saiduddin, S. and Zassenhaus, H. P.,** Estrous cycles, decidual cell response and uterine estrogen and progesterone receptor in Fischer 344 virgin aging rats, *Proc. Soc. Exp. Biol. Med.,* 161, 119, 1979.
63. **Blaha, G. C. and Leavitt, W. W.,** Uterine progesterone receptors in aged golden hamster, *J. Gerontol.,* 33, 810, 1978.
64. **Harman, S. M. and Talbert, G. B.,** The effect of maternal age on ovulation, corpora lutea of pregnancy and implantation failure in mice, *J. Reprod. Fertil.,* 23, 33, 1970.
65. **Soderwall, A. L., Kent, H. A., Turbyfill, C., and Britenbaker, A. L.,** Variation in gestation length and litter size of the golden hamster, mesocricetus auratus, *J. Gerontol.,* 15, 246, 1960.
66. **Ferenczy, A., Richard, R. M., Agale, F. J., Durkenson, M., and Dempsy, F. W.,** Scanning electron microscopy of the human fallopian tube, *Science,* 175, 783, 1972.
67. **Gaddum-Rosse, P., Rumery, R. E., Blandau, R. J., and Thiersch, J. B.,** Studies on the mucosa of postmenopausal oviducts: surface appearance, ciliary activity, and the effect of estrogen treatment, *Fertil. Steril.,* 26, 951, 1975.
68. **Patek, E., Nilsson, L., and Johannisson, E.,** Scanning electron microscopic study of the human fallopian tube, *Fertil. Steril.,* 23, 719, 1972.
69. **Novak, E. and Everett, H. S.,** Cyclical and other variations in the tubal epithelium, *Am. J. Obstet. Gynecol.,* 16, 499, 1928.
70. **Shimoyama, T.,** Electron microscopic studies of the mucous membrane of the human fallopial tube in the embryonal, pregnancy and senile period, *J. Jap. Obstet. Gynecol. Soc.,* 12, 132, 1965.
71. **Parkening, T. A.,** Retention of ova in oviducts of senescent mice and hamsters, *J. Exp. Zool.,* 196, 307, 1976.
72. **Asch, R. H. and Greenblatt, R. B.,** The aging ovary: morphological and endocrine correlations, in *Geriatric Endocrinology,* Greenblatt, R. B., Ed., Raven Press, New York, 1978, 141.
73. **Jones, E. C.,** The ageing ovary and its influence on reproductive capacity, *J. Reprod. Fertil. Suppl.,* 12, 17, 1970.
74. **Block, E.,** A quantitative morphological investigation of the follicular system in women: variations at different ages, *Acta Anat.,* 14, 108, 1953.
75. **Krohn, P. L.,** Ageing processes in the female reproductive tract, *Lect. Sci. Basis Med.,* 7, 285, 1958.
76. **Talbert, G. B.,** Effect of maternal age on reproductive capacity, *A. J. Obstet. Gynecol.,* 102, 451, 1968.
77. **Costoff, A. and Mahesh, V. B.,** Primordial follicles with normal oocytes in the ovaries of postmenopausal women, *J. Am. Geriatr. Soc.,* 23, 193, 1975.
78. **Thung, P. J.,** Ageing changes in the ovary, in *Structural Aspects of Aging,* Bourne, J., Ed., Hafner, New York, 1961, 109.
79. **Mandl, A. M. and Shelton, M.,** A quantitative study of oocytes in young and old nulliparous laboratory rats, *J. Endocrinol.,* 18, 444, 1959.
80. **Huang, H. H. and Meites, J.,** Reproductive capacity of aging female rats, *Neuroendocrinology,* 17, 289, 1975.
81. **Burack, E. and Wolfe, J. M.,** The effect of anterior hypophyseal administration on the ovaries of old rats, *Endocrinology,* 64, 676, 1959.
82. **Peluso, J. J., Steger, R. W., Huang, H. H., and Meites, J.,** Alterations in the pattern of follicular development and steroidogenesis in the ovary of aging cycling rats, *Exp. Age Res.,* 5, 319, 1979.
83. **Huang, H. H.,** *Relation of Neuroendocrine System to Loss of Reproductive Function in Aging Female Rats,* Ph.D. dissertation, Michigan State University, East Lansing, Mich., 1977.
84. **Steger, R. W., Peluso, J. J., Huang, H. H., Hafez, E. S. E., and Meites, J.,** Gonadotropin binding sites in the ovary of aged rats, *J. Reprod. Fertil.,* 48, 205, 1976.
85. **Crumeyrolle-Arias, M., Scheib, D., and Aschheim, P.,** Light and electron microscopy of the ovarian interstial tissue in the senile rat. Normal aspect and response to HCG of "deficiency cells" and "epithelial cords," *Gerontology,* 22, 185, 1976.

86. **Jones, E. C. and Krohn, P. L.,** The effect of hypophysectomy on the age changes in the ovaries of mice, *J. Endocrinol.,* 21, 497, 1961.

87. **Green, J. A.,** Some effects of advancing age on the histology and reactivity of the mouse ovary, *Anat. Rec.,* 129, 333, 1957.

88. **Thung, P. L., Boot, L. M. and Mühlbook, O.,** Senile changes in the oestrous cycle and in ovarian structures in some inbred strains of mice, *Acta Endocrinol.,* 23, 8, 1956.

89. **Quattropani, S. L.,** Serous cysts of the aging guinea pig ovary. I. Light microscopy and origins, *Anat. Rec.,* 188, 351, 1977.

90. **Quattropani, S. L.,** Serous cysts of the aging guinea pig ovary. II. Scanning and transmission electron microscopy, *Anat. Rec.,* 190, 285, 1978.

91. **Schottever, A.,** Veitrag zur Festellung der Eianzahl in vershiedenen Altersperioden bei der Hündin, *Anat. Anz.,* 65, 177, 1928.

92. **Rolle, G. K. and Charipper, H. A.,** The effect of advancing age upon the histology of the ovary, uterus and the vagina of female golden hamster *(Cricetus auratus),* *Anat. Rec.,* 105, 281, 1949.

93. **Adams, C. E.,** Ageing and reproduction in the female mammal with particular reference to the rabbit, *J. Reprod. Fertil. Suppl.,* 12, 1, 1970.

94. **Erickson, B. H.,** Development and senescence of the postnatal bovine ovary, *J. Anim. Sci.,* 25, 800, 1966.

95. **Franchi, L. L., Mandl, A. M., and Zuckerman, S.,** The development of the ovary and the process of oogenesis, in *The Ovary,* Zuckerman, S., Mandl, A. M., and Eckstein, P., Eds., Academic Press, New York, 1962.

96. **Novak, E. R.,** Ovulation after 50, *Obstet. Gynecol.,* 36, 903, 1970.

97. **Arai, H.,** On the postnatal development of the ovary (albino rat), with special reference to the number of ova, *Am. J. Anat.,* 27, 405, 1920.

98. **Ingram, D. L.,** Fertility and oocyte numbers after X-irradiation of the ovary, *J. Endocrinol.,* 17, 81, 1958.

99. **Mandl, A. M.,** Corpora luten in senile virgin laboratory rats, *J. Endocrinol.,* 18, 438, 1959.

100. **Biggers, J. D., Finn, C. A., and McLaren, A.,** Long-term reproductive performance of female mice. I. Effect of removing one ovary, *J. Reprod. Fertil.,* 3, 303, 1962.

101. **Poliak, A., Jones, G., Goldberg, B., Soloman, B., and Woodruff, J. D.,** Effect of human chorionic gonadotropin on postmenopausal women, *Am. J. Obstet. Gynecol.,* 101, 731, 1968.

102. **Greenblatt, R. B., Colle, M. L., and Mahesh, V. B.,** Ovarian and adrenal steroid production in the postmenopausal women, *Obstet. Gynecol.,* 47, 383, 1976.

103. **Greenblatt, R. B., Oettinger, M., and Bohler, C. S. S.,** Estrogen-androgen levels in aging men and women, *J. Am. Geriatr. Soc.,* 24, 173, 1976.

104. **Mills, T. M. and Mahesh, V. B.,** Gonadotropin secretion in the menopause, *Clin. Obstet. Gynecol.,* 4, 71, 1977.

105. **Aschheim, P.,** Contenu hypophysaire en hormone luteinisante (LH) et reaction histophysiologique á la LH circulante du tissue interstitial ovarian chez divers bypes de ratte seniles, *C.R. Acad. Sci.,* 267, 1397, 1968.

106. **Aschheim, P.,** Aging in the hypothalamic-hypophyseal ovarian axis in the rat, in *Hypothalamus, Pituitary and Aging,* Everitt, A. V. and Burgess, J. A., Eds., Charles C Thomas, Springfield, Ill., 1976, 376.

107. **Clemens, J. A., Amenomori, Y., Jenkins, T., and Meites, J.,** Effects of hypothalamic stimulation, hormones and drugs on ovarian function in old female rats, *Proc. Soc. Exp. Biol. Med.,* 132, 561, 1969.

108. **Everett, J. W.,** The restoration of ovulatory cycles and corpus luteum formation in persistant estrous rats, *Endocrinology,* 27, 681, 1940.

109. **Ingram, D. L.,** The vaginal smear of senile laboratory rats, *J. Endocrinol.,* 19, 182, 1959.

110. **Meites, J., Huang, H. H., and Simpkins, J. W.,** Recent studies on neuroendocrine control of reproductive senescence in rats, in *The Aging Reproductive System,* Schneider, E. L., Ed., Raven Press, New York, 1978, 213.

111. **Albrecht, E. D., Koos, R. D., and Gottlieb, S. F.,** Pregnant mare serum and human chorionic gonadotropin stimulate ovarian Δ^5-3β hydroxysteroid dehydrogenase in aged mice, *Fertil. Steril.,* 28, 762, 1977.

112. **Peng, M. T. and Huang, H. H.,** Aging of hypothalamic-pituitary-ovarian function in the rat, *Fertil. Steril.,* 23, 535, 1972.

113. **Labhsetwar, A. P.,** Age-dependent changes in the pituitary-gonadal relationship: a study of ovarian compensatory hypertrophy, *J. Endocrinol.,* 39, 387, 1967.

114. **Howland, B. E. and Preiss, C.,** Effect of aging on basal levels of serum gonadotropins, ovarian compensatory hypertrophy and hypersecretion of gonadotropins after ovariectomy in female rats, *Fertil. Steril.,* 26, 271, 1975.

115. **Richards, J. S. and Midgley, A. R.,** Protein hormone action: a key to understanding ovarian follicular and luteal cell development, *Biol. Reprod.,* 14, 82, 1976.
116. **Peluso, J. J., Steger, R. W., Jaszczak, S., and Hafez, E. S. E.,** Gonadotropin binding sites in the human postmenopausal ovary, *Fertil. Steril.,* 27, 789, 1976.
117. **Erickson, G. F., Hsueh, A. J. W., and Lu, K. H.,** Gonadotropin binding and aromatose activity in granulosa cells of young PE and old CE rats, *Biol. Reprod.,* 20, 182, 1979.
118. **Baird, D. T. and Guevara, A.,** Concentrations of unconjugated estrone and estradiol in peripheral plasma in nonpregnant women throughout the menstrual cycle, castrate and postmenopausal women and in men, *J. Clin. Endocrinol. Metab.,* 29, 879, 1969.
119. **Grodin, J. M., Siiteri, P. K., and MacDonald, P. C.,** Source of estrogen production in postmenopausal women, *J. Clin. Endocrinol. Metab.,* 36, 207, 1973.
120. **Vermeulen, A.,** The hormonal activity of the postmenopausal ovary, *J. Clin. Endocrinol. Metab.,* 42, 247, 1976.
121. **Paulsen, C. A., Leach, R. B., Sandberg, H., Sheinfield, S., and Maddock, W. O.,** Function of the postmenopausal ovary. Comparison of urinary estrogen and gonadotropin excretion and response to administration of FSH in postmenopausal and ovariectomized women, *J. Am. Geriatr. Soc.,* 6, 803, 1958.
122. **Procope, B. J.,** Studies on urinary excretion, biological effects and origin of oestrogens in postmenopausal women, *Acta Endocrinol. (Copenhagen), Suppl.,* p. 135, 1968.
123. **Longcope, C.,** Metabolic clearance and blood production of estrogens in postmenopausal women, *Am. J. Obstet. Gynecol.,* 111, 778, 1971.
124. **Steger, R. W., Huang, H. H., Chamberlain, D., and Meites, J.,** Changes in the control of gonadotropin secretion in the transition period between regular cycles and constant estrus in the old female rat, *Biol. Reprod.,* 22, 595, 1980.
125. **Abraham, G. E., Lobotsky, J., and Lloyd, C. W.,** Metabolism of testosterone and androstenedione in normal and ovariectomized women, *J. Clin. Invest.,* 48, 696, 1969.
126. **Judd, H. L., Judd, G. E., Lucas, W. E., and Yen, S. S. C.,** Endocrine function of the postmenopausal ovary: concentration of androgens and estrogens in ovarian and peripheral vein blood, *J. Clin. Endocrinol. Metab.,* 39, 1020, 1974.
127. **Longcope, C., Kate, T. and Horton, R.,** Conversion of blood androgens to estrogens in normal adult men and women, *J. Clin. Invest.,* 48, 2191, 1969.
128. **Mattingly, R. F. and Huang, W. Y.,** Steroidogenesis of the menopausal and postmenopausal ovary, *Am. J. Obstet. Gynecol.,* 103, 679, 1969.
129. **Pourtman, J., Thijssen, J. H., and Schwartz, F.,** Androgen production and conversion to estrogens in normal postmenopausal women and in selected breast cancer patients, *J. Clin. Endocrinol. Metab.,* 37, 101, 1973.
130. **Novaks, E. R., Goldberg, B., Jones, G. S., and O'Toole, R. V.,** Enzyme histochemistry of the postmenopausal ovary associated with normal and abnormal endometrium, *Am. J. Obstet. Gynecol.,* 93, 669, 1965.
131. **Albrecht, E. O., Koos, R. D., and Wehrenberg, W. B.,** Ovarian Δ^5-3β-hydroxysteroid dehydrogenase and cholesterol in the aged mouse during pregnancy, *Biol. Reprod.,* 13, 158, 1975.
132. **Leathem, J. H. and Murono, E. P.,** Ovarian Δ^5-3β-hydroxysteroid dehydrogenase in aging rats, *Fertil. Steril.,* 26, 996, 1975.
133. **Leathem, J. H. and Shapiro, B. H.,** Aging and ovarian Δ^5-3β-hydroxysteroid dehydrogenase in rats, *Proc. Soc. Exp. Biol. Med.,* 148, 793, 1975.
134. **Wehrenberg, W. B., Gottlieb, S. F., Levinet, D., and Ramsay, L.,** Ageing and ovarian Δ^5-3β-hydrosteroid dehydrogenase in the pregnant mouse, *J. Endocrinol.,* 70, 183, 1976.
135. **Pinkus, J. L., Chalres, D., and Chattoraj, S. C.,** Deuterium-labeled steroids for study in humans. II. Preliminary studies on estrogen production rates in pre and post-menopausal women, *Hormone Res.,* 10, 44, 1979.
136. **Rader, M. D., Flickiner, G. L., and deVilla, G. O.,** Plasma estrogens in postmenopausal women, *Am. J. Obstet. Gynecol.,* 116, 1069, 1973.
137. **Sherman, B. M. and Korenman, S. G.,** Hormonal characteristics of the human menstrual cycle throughout reproductive life, *J. Clin. Invest.,* 55, 699, 1975.
138. **Sherman, B. M., West, J. H., and Korenman, S. G.,** The menopausal transition: analysis of LH, FSH, estradiol and progesterone concentrations during menstrual cycles of older women, *J. Clin. Endocrinol. Metab.,* 42, 629, 1976.
139. **Judd, H. L., Lucas, W. E., and Yen, S. S. C.,** Serum 17β-estradiol and estrone levels in postmenopausal women with and without endometrial cancer, *J. Clin. Endocrinol. Metab.,* 43, 272, 1976.
140. **Yen, S. S. C., Tsai, C. C., Naftolin, F., Vandenberg, G., and Judd, H.,** Circulating estradiol, estrone and gonadotropin levels following the administration of orally active 17β-estradiol in postmenopausal women, *J. Clin. Endocrinol. Metab.,* 34, 671, 1972.

141. **Huang, H. H., Steger, R. W., Bruni, J., and Meites, J.,** Changes in patterns of sex steroid and gonadotropin secretion in aging female rats, *Endocrinology,* 103, 1855, 1978.

142. **Steger, R. W., Huang, H. H., and Meites, J.,** Relation of aging to hypothalamic LHRH content and serum gonadal steroids in female rats, *Proc. Soc. Exp. Biol. Med.,* 161, 251, 1979.

143. **Collett, M. E., Wertenberger, G. E., and Fiske, V. M.,** The effect of age upon the pattern of the menstrual cycle, *Fertil. Steril.,* 5, 437, 1954.

144. **Labhsetwar, A. P.,** Ageing changes in pituitary-ovarian relationships, *J. Reprod. Fertil. Suppl.,* 12, 99, 1970.

145. **Gosden, R. G.,** Corpus luteum adequacy in the aging pregnant mouse, *Eur. J. Obstet. Gynec. Reprod. Biol.,* (Suppl.), S109, 1974.

146. **Gosden, R. G.,** Ovarian support of pregnancy in ageing inbred mice, *J. Reprod. Fertil.,* 42, 423, 1975.

147. **Harman, S. M. and Talbert, G. B.,** Structural changes in corpora lutea and decline of reproductive function in aging female mice, *Am. Zool.,* 74, 757, 1967.

148. **Parkening, T. A., Lau, I., Saksana, S. K., and Chang, M. C.,** Circulating plasma levels of pregnenolene, progesterone, estrogen, LH and FSH in young and aged C57BL/6 mice during various stages of pregnancy, *J. Gerontol.,* 33, 191, 1978.

149. **Parkening, T. A., Saksena, S. K., and Lau, I. F.,** Postovulatory levels of progestogens, oestrogens, LH and FSH in the plasma of aged golden hamsters exhibiting a delay in fertilization, *J. Endocrinol.,* 78, 147, 1978.

150. **Larson, L., Spilman, C. H., Dunn, H. O., and Foote, R. H.,** Reproductive efficiency in aged female rabbits given supplemental progesterone and estradiol, *J. Reprod. Fertil.,* 33, 31, 1973.

151. **Blaha, G. C. and Leavitt, W. W.,** Ovarian steroid dehydrogenase histochemistry and circulating progesterone in aged golden hamsters during the estrous cycle and pregnancy, *Biol. Reprod.,* 11, 156, 1974.

152. **Larson, L. L. and Foote, R. H.,** Uterine blood flow in young and aged rabbits, *Proc. Soc. Exp. Biol. Med.,* 141, 67, 1972.

153. **Greene, H. S. N.,** Uterine adenomata in the rabbit, *J. Exp. Med.,* 73, 273, 1941.

154. **Albert, A.,** Human urinary gonadotropins, *Recent Prog. Horm. Res.,* 12, 266, 1956.

155. **Ryan, R. J.,** The luteinizing hormone content of human pituitaries. I. Variations with sex and age, *J. Clin. Endocrinol.,* 22, 300, 1965.

156. **Blumenthal, H. T.,** Aging processes in the endocrine glands of various strains of normal mice: relationship of hypophyseal activity to aging changes in other endocrine glands, *J. Gerontol.,* 10, 253, 1955.

157. **Clemens, J. A. and Meites, J.,** Neuroendocrine status of old constant-estrous rats, *Neuroendocrinology,* 7, 249, 1971.

158. **Pi, W. P., Huang, H. H., and Peng, M. T.,** Pituitary luteinizing hormone and follicle stimulating hormone concentrations and stalk median eminence LH-releasing factor and FSHRF levels of old female rats, *J. Formosan Med. Assoc.,* 72, 485, 1974.

159. **Bakke, J. L., Lawrence, N., Knudtson, K. P., Roy, S., and Needman, G. H.,** A correlative study of the content of TSH and cell morphology of the human adenohypophysis, *Am. J. Clin. Pathol.,* 41, 576, 1964.

160. **Calloway, N. O., Foley, C. F., and Lagerbloom, P.,** Uncertainties in geriatric data. II. Organ size. *J. Am. Geriatr. Soc.,* 13, 20, 1965.

161. **Bourne, G. H.,** Aging changes in the endocrines, in *Endocrines and Aging,* Gitman, L., Ed., Charles C Thomas, Springfield, Ill., 1967, 66.

162. **Duchen, L. W. and Schurr, P. H.,** The pathology of the pituitary gland in old age, in *Hypothalamus, Pituitary and Aging,* Everitt, A. V. and Burgess, J. A., Eds., Charles C Thomas, Springfield, Ill., 1976, 137.

163. **Verzar, F.,** Anterior pituitary function in age, in *The Pituitary Gland,* Vol. 2, Harris, G. W. and Donovan, B. T., Eds., University of California Press, Berkeley, Calif., 1966, 444.

164. **Lansing, W. and Wolfe, J. M.,** Changes in the fibrillar tissue of the anterior pituitary of the rat associated with advancing age, *Anat. Rec.,* 83, 355, 1942.

165. **Wolfe, J. M.,** The effects of advancing age on the structure of the anterior hypophyses and ovaries of female rats, *Am. J. Anat.,* 72, 361, 1943.

166. **Weiss, J. and Lansing, A. I.,** Age changes in the fine structure of anterior pituitary of the mouse, *Proc. Soc. Exp. Biol.,* 82, 460, 1953.

167. **Spagnoli, H. H. and Charipper, H. A.,** The effects of aging on the histology and cytology of the pituitary gland of the golden hamster (*Cricetus auratus*) with brief reference to simultaneous changes in the thyroid and testes, *Anat. Rec.,* 121, 117, 1955.

168. **Baggart, J. H.,** *Edinburgh Med. J.,* 42, 113, 1935.

169. **Timiras, P. S.,** *Developmental Physiology and Aging,* Macmillan, New York, 1972.
170. **Wolfe, J. M., Bryan, R. and Wright, A. W.,** Histological observation on the anterior pituitary of old rats with particular reference to the spontaneous apparition of pituitary adenomata, *Am. J. Cancer,* 34, 352, 1938.
171. **Saxton, J. A.,** The relation of age to the occurance of adenomalike lesions in the rat hypophysis and to their growth after transplantation, *Cancer Res.,* 1, 227, 1941.
172. **Nakane, P. K.,** Simultaneous localization of multiple tissue antigens using the peroxidase-labeled antibody method: a study on pituitary glands of the rat. *J. Histochem. Cytochem.,* 16, 557, 1969.
173. **Baker, B. L. and Ya-Yen, Y.,** An immunocytochemical study of human pituitary mammatropes from fetal life to old age, *Am. J. Anat.,* 148, 217, 1977.
174. **Kovacs, K., Ryan, N., Horvath, E., Pane, G., and Ezrin, C.,** Prolactin cells of the human pituitary gland in old age, *J. Gerontol.,* 32, 534, 1977.
175. **Ryan, N., Kovacs, K., and Ezrin, C.,** Thyrotrops in old age, a immunocytological study of human pituitary glands, *Endokrinologie,* 73(2), 191, 1979.
176. **Albert, A., Randall, R. V., Smith, R. A., and Johnson, C. E.,** Urinary excretion of gonadotropins as a function of age, in *Hormones and the Aging Process,* Engle, E. T. and Pincus, G., Eds., Academic Press, New York, 1956, 49.
177. **Leung, F. C.,** Studies on the Relationship Among Bioassay and Radioligand Assays for Prolactin, Ph.D. dissertation, University of California, Berkeley, Calif., 1978.
178. **Prentice, L. G. and Ryan, R. J.,** LH and its subunits in human pituitary, serum and urine, *J. Clin. Endocrinol. Metab.,* 40, 303, 1975.
179. **Wildt, L., Marshall, G., Hausler, A., Plant, T. M., Belchet, P. F., and Knobil, E.,** Amplitude of pulsatile GnRH input and pituitary gonadotropin secretion, *Fed. Proc. Fed. Am. Soc. Exp. Biol.,* 38, 978, 1979.
180. **Aiyer, M. S., Chiappa, S. A., and Fink, G.,** A priming effect of luteinizing hormone releasing factor on the anterior pituitary gland in the female rat, *J. Endocrinol.,* 62, 573, 1974.
181. **Aiyer, M. S. and Fink, G.,** The role of sex steroid hormones in modulating the responsiveness of the anterior pituitary gland to luteinizing hormone releasing factor in the female rat, *J. Endocrinol.,* 62, 553, 1974.
182. **Dekretser, D. M., Burger, H. G., and Dumpys, R.,** Patterns of serum LH and FSH in response to 4 hour infusions of LHRH in normal women during menstrual cycle, on oral contraceptives, and in postmenopausal state, *J. Clin. Endocrinol. Metab.,* 46, 227, 1978.
183. **Hashimato, T., Miyai, K., Izumi, K., and Kumahara, Y.,** Gonadotropin response to synthetic LHRH in normal subjects, correlation between LH and FSH, *J. Clin. Endocrinol. Metab.,* 37, 910, 1973.
184. **Kuhahara, Y., Miyai, K., Hashimato, T., and Onishi, T.,** Aging and anterior pituitary function—responses of PRL, TSH and gonadotropins and TRH and LH-RH in normal subjects, *J. Geriat.,* 12, 363, 1975.
185. **Scaglia, H., Medina, M., Pinto-Ferrerra, A. L., Vazques, G., Gaul, C., and Perez-Palacies, G.,** Pituitary LH and FSH secretion and responsiveness in women of old age, *Acta Endocrinol., (Copenhagen),* 81, 673, 1976.
186. **Howland, B. E.,** Reduced gonadotropin release in response to progesterone or gonadotropin releasing hormone (GnRH) in old female rats, *Life Sci.,* 19, 219, 1976.
187. **Watkins, B. E., Meites, J., and Riegle, G. D.,** Age-related changes in pituitary responsiveness to LHRH in the female rat, *Endocrinol.,* 97, 543, 1975.
188. **Miller, A. E. and Riegle, G. D.,** Serum LH levels following multiple LHRH injections in aging rats, *Proc. Soc. Exp. Biol. Med.,* 157, 484, 1978.
189. **Peluso, J. J., Steger, R. W., and Hafez, E. S. E.,** Regulation of LH secretion in aged female rats, *Biol. Reprod.,* 16, 212, 1977.
190. **Steger, R. W. and Peluso, J. J.,** Hypothalamic-pituitary function in the old irregularly cycling rat, *Exp. Age. Res.,* 5, 303, 1979.
191. **Coble, Y. D., Jr., Kohler, P. O., Cargille, C. M., and Ross, G. T.,** Production rates and metabolic clearance rates of human FSH in pre-menopausal and post-menopausal women, *J. Clin. Invest.,* 48, 359, 1969.
192. **Kohler, P. O., Ross, G. T., and Odell, W. D.,** Metabolic clearance and production rates of human luteinizing hormone in pre- and post-menopausal women, *J. Clin. Invest.,* 47, 38, 1968.
193. **Warren, M. P., Siris, E. S., and Petrovich, C.,** The influence of severe illness on gonadotropin secretion in the postmenopausal female, *J. Clin. Endocrinol. Metab.,* 45, 99, 1977.
194. **Hashimato, T., Miyai, K. and Izumi, K.,** Effect of clomiphene on basal and LRH-induced gonadotropin secretion in postmenopausal women, *J. Clin. Endocrinol.,* 42, 593, 1976.
195. **Lauritzen, C.,** The hypothalamic anterior pituitary system in the climacteric age period, *Front. Hormone Res.,* 3, 20, 1975.

196. **Mills, T. M. and Mahesh, V. B.,** Pituitary function in the aged, in *Geriatric Endocrinology,* Greenblatt, R. B., Ed., Raven Press, New York, 1978, 1.

197. **Monroe, S. E. and Menon, K. M.,** Changes in reproductive hormone secretion during the climacteric and postmenopausal periods, *Clin. Obstet. Gynecol.,* 20, 113, 1977.

198. **Odell, W. D. and Swerdloff, R. S.,** Progesterone-induced luteinizing and follicle stimulating hormone surge in post-menopausal women: a simulated ovulatory peak, *Proc. Nat. Acad. Sci. U.S.A.,* 61, 529, 1968.

199. **Reyes, F. I., Winter, J. S. D., and Faiman, C.,** Pituitary-ovarian relationships preceding menopause. I. Cross-sectional study of serum follicle stimulating hormone, luteinizing hormone, prolactin, estradiol and progesterone levels, *Am. J. Obstet. Gynecol.,* 129(5), 557, 1977.

200. **Wise, A. J., Gross, M. A., and Schlach, D. S.,** Quantitative relationships of the pituitary-gonadal axis in postmenopausal women, *J. Lab. Clin. Med.,* 81, 28, 1973.

201. **Adamopoulos, D. A., Loraine, J. A., and Dore, G. A.,** Endocrinological studies in women approaching the menopause, *J. Obstet. Gynaecol. Br. Commonw.,* 78, 62, 1971.

202. **Papanicolaou, A. D., Loraine, J. A., and Dore, G. A.,** Endocrine function in postmenopausal women, *J. Obstet, Gynaecol. Br. Commonw.,* 76, 317, 1969.

203. **Tagasugi, N.,** Gonadotropic activity of the anterior hypophysis of old female mice as demonstrated by parabiosis with young partners, *J. Fac. Sci. Tokyo Univ. Sect. 9,* 10, 193, 1963.

204. **Gosden, R. G. and Bancroft, L.,** Pituitary function in reproductively senescent female rats, *Exp. Gerontol.,* 11, 157, 1976.

205. **Huang, H. H., Marshall, S., and Meites, J.,** Capacity of old versus young female rats to secrete LH, FSH and prolactin, *Biol. Reprod.,* 14, 538, 1976.

206. **Finch, C. E., Jonec, V., Wisner, J. R., Jr., Sinha, Y. N., DeVellis, J. S., and Swerdloff, R. S.,** Hormone production by the pituitary and testes of male C57BL/6J mice during aging, *Endocrinology,* 101, 1310, 1977.

207. **Meites, J., Huang, H. H., and Riegle, G. D.,** Relation of the hypothalamo-pituitary-gonadal system to decline of reproductive function in aging female rats, in *Hypothalamus and Endocrine Function,* Labrie, F., Meites, J., and Pelletier, G., Eds., Plenum Press, New York, 1976.

208. **Yamaji, T., Shimamato, K., Ishibashi, M., Kosaka, K. and Orimo, H.,** Effect of age and sex on circulation and pituitary prolactin levels in human, *Acta Endocrinol. (Copenhagen),* 83, 711, 1976.

209. **Vekemens, M. and Robyn, C.,** Influence of age on serum prolactin levels in women and men, *Br. Med. J.,* 4, 738, 1975.

210. **Robyn, C. and Vekemans, M.,** Influence of low dose oestrogen on circulating prolactin, LH and FSH levels in post-menopausal women, *Acta Endocrinol. (Copenhagen),* 83, 9, 1976.

211. **Kawashima, S., Asai, I., and Wakabayashi, K.,** Prolactin secretion in normal and neonatally estrogenized persistent-diestrous rats at advanced ages, *Psychoneuroendocrinology,* Workshop Conf. Int. Soc. Psychoneuroendocrinol., Karger, Basel, 1974, 128.

212. **Shaar, C. J., Euker, J. S., Riegle, G. D., and Meites, J.,** Effects of castration and gonadal steroids on serum LH and prolactin in old and young rats, *J. Endocrinol.,* 66, 45, 1975.

213. **Ratner, A. and Peake, G. T.,** Maintenance of hyperprolactinemia by gonadal steroids in androgen-sterilized and spontaneously constant estrous rats, *Proc. Soc. Exp. Biol. Reprod.,* 146, 680, 1974.

214. **Larson-Cohn, V. and Wallentin, L.,** Metabolic and hormonal effects of post-menopausal oestrogen replacement treatment, *Acta Endocrinol. (Copenhagen),* 86(3), 583, 1977.

215. **Nillius, S. J. and Wide, L.,** Effects of oestrogen on serum levels of LH and FSH, *Acta Endocrinol. (Copenhagen),* 65, 583, 1970.

216. **Ricciard, I., Bruni, G., Imparato, E., Marino, L., and Pesando, P.,** Effect of quinestral on plasma and urinary gonadotropins of post-menopausal women, *Horm. Metab. Res.,* 7, 323, 1975.

217. **Wallantin, L. and Larsson-Cohn, U.,** Metabolic and hormonal effects of post-menopausal oestrogen replacement treatment, *Acta Endocrinol. (Copenhagen),* 86(3), 597, 1977.

218. **Tasi, C. C. and Yen, S. S. C.,** Acute effects of intraveneous infusion of 17β-estradiol on gonadotropin release in pre- and post-menopausal women, *J. Clin. Endocrinol. Metab.,* 32, 766, 1971.

219. **Franchimont, P., Legros, J. J., and Meurice, J.,** Effects of several estrogens on serum gonadotropin levels in post-menopausal women, *Horm. Metab. Res.,* 4, 288, 1972.

220. **Kempers, R. B. and Ryan, R. J.,** Acute effects of intravenous infulsion of 17β-hydroxyprogesterone on gonadotropin release, *Fertil. Steril.,* 28, 631, 1977.

221. **Lu, K. H., Huang, H. H., Chen, H. T., Kurcz, M., Mioduszewski, R., and Meites, J.,** Positive feedback by estrogen and progesterone on LH release in old and young rats, *Proc. Soc. Exp. Biol. Med.,* 154, 82, 1977.

222. **Wurtman, R. J.,** Brain monoamines and endocrine function, in *Neurosciences Research Symposium Summaries,* Vol. 6, LeBlanc, C. M., Ed., MIT Press, Cambridge, Mass., 1972, 171.

223. **Meites, J. and Clemens, J. A.,** Hypothalamic Control of Prolactin Secretion, in *Vitamins and Hormones,* Vol. 20, Academic Press, New York, 1972, 165.

224. **McCann, S. M., Kalra, P. S., Donoso, A. O., Bishop, W., Schneider, H. P. G., Fawcett, C. P., and Krulich, L.,** The role of monoamines in the control of gonadotropin and prolactin secretion, in *Brain Endocrine Interaction,* Knigge, K. M., Scott, D. E., and Weindl, A., Eds., Karger, Basel, 1972, 224.

225. **Schally, A. V., Arimura, A., Baba, Y., Wair, R., Matsuo, H., Redding, T., Debeljuk, L., and White, W.,** Isolation and properties of the FSH and LH-releasing hormone, *Biochem. Biophys. Res. Commun.,* 43, 393, 1971.

226. **Simpkins, J. W., Mueller, G. P., Huang, H. H., and Meites, J.,** Evidence for depressed catecholamine and enhanced serotonin metabolism in aging male rats; possible relation to gonadotropin secretion, *Endocrinology,* 100, 1672, 1977.

227. **Cooper, R. L., Brandt, S. J., Linnoila, M., and Walker, R. F.,** Induced ovulation in aged female rats by L-dopa implants into the medial preoptic area, *Neuroendocrinology,* 28, 234, 1979.

228. **Huang, H. H., Marshall, S., and Meites, J.,** Induction of estrous cycles in old non-cyclic rats by progesterone, ACTH, ether stress or L-dopa, *Neuroendocrinology,* 20, 21, 1976.

229. **Lehman, J. R., McArthur, D. A., and Hendricks, S. E.,** Pharmacological induction of ovulation in old and neonatally androgenized rats, *Exp. Gerontol.,* 13, 107, 1978.

230. **Linnoila, M. and Cooper, R. L.,** Reinstatement of vaginal cycles in aged female rats, *J. Pharmacol.,* 199, 477, 1976.

231. **Quadri, S. K., Kledzik, G. S., and Meites, J.,** Reinitiation of estrous cycles in old constant-estrous rats by central-acting drugs, *Neuroendocrinology,* 11, 248, 1973.

232. **Watkins, B. E., McKay, D. W., Meites, J., and Riegle, G. D.,** L-dopa effects on serum LH and prolactin in old and young female rats, *Neuroendocrinology,* 19, 331, 1975.

233. **Kalra, S. P.,** Circadian rhythm in luteinizing hormone-releasing hormone (LH-RH) content of preoptic area during the rat estrous cycle, *Brain Res.,* 104, 354, 1976.

234. **Araki, S., Ferin, M., Zimmerman, E. A., and Van deWiele, R. L.,** Ovarian modulation of immunoreactive gonadotropin-releasing hormone (GN-RH) in the rat brain: evidence for a differential effect of anterior and mid-hypothalamus, *Endocrinology,* 96, 644, 1975.

235. **Kobayashi, R. M., Lu, K. H., Moore, R. Y., and Yen, S. C.,** Regional distribution of hypothalamic luteinizing hormone-releasing hormone in proestrous rats: effects of ovariectomy and estrogen replacement, *Endocrinology,* 102, 98, 1978.

236. **Chen, H. T., Geneau, J., and Meites, J.,** Effects of castration, steroid replacement and hypophysectomy on hypothalamic LHRH and serum LH, *Proc. Soc. Exp. Biol. Med.,* 156, 127, 1977.

237. **Kalra, S. P. and Kalra, P. S.,** Temporal changes in the hypothalamic and serum luteinizing hormone-releasing hormone (LH-RH) levels and circulating ovarian steroids during the rat oestrous cycle, *Acta Endocrinol.,* 85, 449, 1977.

238. **Barr, G. D. and Barraclough, C. A.,** Temporal changes in medial basal hypothalamic LH-RH correlated with plasma LH during the rat estrous cycle and following electrochemical stimulation of the preoptic area in pentobarbital-treated proestrous rats, *Brain Res.,* 148, 413, 1978.

239. **Eskay, R. .L., Mical, R. S., and Porter, J. C.,** Relationship between luteinizing hormone releasing hormone concentration in hypophysical portal blood and luteinizing hormone release in intact, castrated, and electrochemically-stimulated rats, *Endocrinology,* 100, 263, 1977.

240. **Sarkar, D. K., Chiappa, S. A., Fink, G., and Sherwood, N. M.,** Gonadotropin-releasing hormone surge in pro-oestrous rats, *Nature (London),* 264, 461, 1976.

241. **Peng, Y., Tsai, Y., and Peng, M.,** A further study on the luteinizing of old rats by an in vitro method, *J. Formosan Med. Assoc.,* 77, 16, 1975.

242. **Miller, A. E. and Riegle, G. D.,** Hypothalamic LH-releasing activity in young and aged intact and gonadectomized rats, *Exp. Age. Res.,* 4, 145, 1978.

243. **Crighton, D., Schneider, H., and McCann, S.,** Localization of LH-releasing factor in the hypothalamus and neurohypophysis as determined by an in vitro method, *Endocrinology,* 87, 323, 1970.

244. **King, J. C., Williams, T. H., and Arimura, A. A.,** Localization of luteinizing hormone-releasing hormone in rat hypothalamus using radioimmunoassay, *J. Anat.,* 120, 275, 1975.

245. **Wheaton, J. E., Krulich, L., and McCann, S. M.,** Localization of luteinizing hormone-releasing hormone in the preoptic area and hypothalamus of the rat using RIA, *Endocrinology,* 97, 30, 1975.

246. **Kizer, J. S., Palkovits, M., Brownstein, M. J.,** Releasing factors in the circumventricular organs in the rat brain, *Endocrinology,* 98, 311, 1976.

247. **Palkovits, M., Arimura, A., Brownstein, M., and Saavedra, J. M.,** Luteinizing hormone releasing hormone (LHRH) content of the hypothalamic nuclei in the rat, *Endocrinology,* 95, 554, 1974.

248. **Ibata, Y., Watanabe, K., Kinoshita, H., Kubo, S., and Sano, Y.,** The localization of LHRH neurons in the rat hypothalamus and their pathway to the median eminence, *Cell Tissue Res.,* 198, 381, 1979.

249. **Barry, J., Dubois, M. P. and Poulain, P.,** LRF producing cells of the mammalian hypothalamus, *Z. Zellforsch. Mikrosk, Anat.,* 146, 351, 1973.

250. **Sétáló, G., Vigh, S., Schally, A. V., Arimura, A., and Flerkó, B.,** Immunohistological study of the origin of LH-RH containing nerve fibers of the rat hypothalamus, *Brain Res.,* 103, 597, 1976.

251. **Alpert, L. C., Brawer, J. R., Jackson, I. M. D., and Reichlin, S.,** Localization of LHRH in neurons of frog brains, *Endocrinology,* 98, 910, 1976.

252. **Hoffman, G. E., Knigge, K. M., Moynihan, J. A., Melnyk, U., and Arimura, A.,** Neuronal fields containing luteinizing hormone releasing hormone (LHRH) in mouse brain, *Neuroscience,* 3, 219, 1978.

253. **King, J. C., Elkind, K. E., Gerall, A. A., and Millar, R. P.,** Investigation of the LHRH system in the normal and neonatally steroid-treated male and female rat, in *Brain Endocrine Interaction. III: Neural Hormones and Reproduction,* Scott, D. E., Kozlowski, G. P., and Weindl, A., Eds., Karger, Basal, 1978, 97.

254. **Sternberger, L. A. and Hoffman, G. E.,** Immunocytology of luteinizing hormone releasing hormone, *Neuroendocrinology,* 25, 111, 1978.

255. **Millar, R. P., Aehnelt, C., Rossier, G., and Hendricks, S.,** Evidence for the existence of higher molecular-weight precursor of luteinizing hormone-releasing hormone (LH-RH), *IRCS J. of Med. Sci.,* 3, 603, 1976.

256. **Millar, R. P., Aehnelt, C., and Rossier, G.,** Higher molecular weight immunoreactive species of luteinizing hormone releasing hormone: possible precursors of the hormones, *Biochem. Biophys. Res. Commun.,* 74, 720, 1977.

257. **Millar, R. P., Denniss, P., Tobler, C., King, J. C., Schally, A. V., and Arimura, A.,** Presumptive prohormonal forms of hypothalamic peptide hormones, in *Cell Biology of Hypothalamic Neurosecretion,* Vincent, J. and Kordon, C., Eds., Centre National de la Recherche Scientifique, Paris, 1977, Chapter 30.

258. **Nett, T. M., Akbar, A. M., and Niswender, G. D.,** Serum levels of luteinizing hormone and gonadotropin-releasing hormone in cycling, castrated and anestrous ewes, *Endocrinology,* 94, 713, 1974.

259. **de la Cruz, K. G., and Arimura, A.,** Evidence for the presence of immunoreactive plasma LH-RH which is unrelated to LH-RH decapeptide, in *Prog. 57th Annu. Meet. Am. Endocrinol. Soc. Abstr.,* 1975, 103.

260. **Jonas, H. A., Burger, H. G., Cumming, I. A., Findlay, J. K., and de Kretser, D. M.,** Radioimmunoassay for luteinizing hormone-releasing hormone (LH-RH): its application to the measurement of LH-RH in ovine and human plasma, *Endocrinology,* 96, 384, 1975.

261. **Sandow, J., Keptner, W., and Vogel, H. G.,** Studies on in vivo inactivation of synthetic LH-RH, in *Hypophysiotropic Hormones,* Int. Congr. Ser. No. 263, Gall, C. and Rosemberg, E., Eds., Excerpta Medical Foundation, Amsterdam, 1973, 64.

262. **Clemens, L. E., Kelch, R. P., Markovs, M., Westhoff, M. H., and Dermody, W. C.,** Analysis of the radioimmunoassay for gonadotropin-releasing hormone (GnRH): studies on the effect of radioiodinated GnRH, *J. Clin. Endocrinol. Metab.,* 41, 1058, 1975.

263. **Nett, T. M. and Adams, T. E.,** Further studies on the radioimmunoassay of gonadotropin-releasing hormone: effect of radioiodination, antiserum and unextracted serum on levels of immunoreactivity in serum, *Endocrinology,* 101, 1135, 1977.

264. **Sonntag, W. E., Gerall, A. A., King, J. C., Dunlap, J. L., and Arimura, A.,** unpublished data, 1978.

265. **de la Cruz, K. G., Arimura, A., and Bettendorf, G.,** Radioimmunoassay (RIA) for luteinizing hormone releasing hormone (LHRH): plasma LHRH levels in normal ovarian cycles of women, in *Endocrinol. Proc. 5th Int. Congr. Endocrinol.,* (Abstr.), Vol. 1, Int. Congr. Ser. No. 402, Excerpta Medical Foundation, 1977, 128.

266. **Sonntag, W. E. and Arimura, A.,** unpublished observations, 1979.

267. **Griffiths, E. C., Hooper, K. C., Jeffcoate, S. L., and Holland, D. T.,** The presence of peptidases in the rat hypothalamus inactivating luteinizing hormone-releasing hormone (LH-RH), *Acta Endocrinol. (Copenhagen),* 77, 435, 1974.

268. **Griffiths, E. C., Hooper, K. C., Jeffcoate, S. L., and Holland, D. T.,** The effects of gonadectomy and gonadal steroids on the activity of hypothalamic peptidases inactivating luteinizing hormone-releasing hormone (LH-RH), *Brain Res.,* 88, 384, 1975.

269. **Kuhl, H. and Taubert, H. D.,** Short-loop feedback mechanism of luteinizing hormone: LH stimulates hypothalamic L-cystine arylamidase to inactivate LH-RH in the rat hypothalamus, *Acta Endocrinol. (Copenhagen),* 78, 648, 1975.

270. **Kuhl, H., Frey, W., Rosniatowski, C., Dericks-Tan, J. S. E., and Taubert, H. D.,** The effect of prostaglandins on hypothalamic L-cystine arylamidase activity and on luteinizing hormone secretion in the rat, *Acta Endocrinol. (Copenhagen),* 82, 15, 1976.

271. **Johansson, K., Hooper, F., Sievertsson, H., Currie, B. L., Folkers, K., and Bowers, C. Y.,** Biosynthesis in vitro of the luteinizing releasing hormone by hypothalamic tissue, *Biochem. Biophys. Res. Commun.,* 49, 656, 1972.

272. **Moguilevsky, J. A., Enero, M. A., Szwarcfarb, B., and Dosoretz, D.,** Effect of castration and testosterone in vitro, on the hypothalamic synthesis of different peptide fractions, *J. Endocrinol.,* 64, 155, 1975.

273. **Johansson, K. N., Currie, B. L., Folkers, K., and Bowers, C. Y.,** Biosynthesis of the luteinizing hormone releasing hormone in mitochondrial preparations and by a possible pantetheine-template mechanism, *Biochem. Biophys. Res. Commun.,* 53, 502, 1973.

274. **Reichlin, S. and Mitnick, M.,** Biosynthesis of hypothalamic hypophysiotrophic hormones, in *Frontiers in Neuroendocrinology,* Ganong, W. F. and Martini, L., Eds., Oxford Press, New York, 1973.

275. **Seyler, L. E., Mitnick, M. A., Gordon, J., and Reichlin, S.,** Hypothalamic LRF biosynthesis in vitro and plasma LRF in orchidectomized, hypophysectomized estrogen treated rats, in *Prog. 55th Annu. Meet. Am. Endocrinol. Soc. (Abstr.),* Chicago, Ill., 1973.

276. **Hall, R. W. and Steinberger, E.,** Synthesis of LH-RH by rat hypothalamic tissue in vitro. I: Use of specific antibody to LH-RH for immunoprecipitation, *Neuroendocrinology,* 21, 111, 1976.

277. **Sundberg, D. K. and Knigge, K. M.,** Luteinizing hormone-releasing hormone (LH-RH) production and degradation by rat medial basal hypothalami in vitro, *Brain Res.,* 139, 89, 1978.

278. **Clemens, J. A., Smalstig, E. B., and Sawyer, B. D.,** Studies on the role of the preoptic area in the control of reproductive function in the rat, *Endocrinology,* 99, 728, 1976.

279. **Clemens, J. A. and Bennett, D. R.,** Do aging changes in the preoptic area contribute to loss of cyclic endocrine function? *J. Gerontol.,* 32, 19, 1977.

280. **Hsu, H. K. and Peng, M. T.,** Hypothalamic neuron number in old female rats, *Gerontology,* 24, 434, 1978.

281. **Peng, M. and Peng, Y.,** Uptake of ^{3}H-estradiol in hypothalamus and pituitary of old female rats, *Fertil. Steril.,* 23, 535, 1972.

282. **Kanungo, M. S., Patnaik, S. K., and Koul, O.,** Decrease in 17β-oestradiol receptor in brain of ageing rats, *Nature (London),* 253, 366, 1975.

283. **Finch, C. E.,** The regulation of physiological changes during mammalian aging, *Q. Rev. Biol.,* 51, 49, 1976.

284. **Finch, C. E.,** Catecholamine metabolism in the brains of aging male mice, *Brain Res.,* 52, 261, 1973.

285. **Jones, V. J. and Finch, C. E.,** Senescence and dopamine uptake by subcellular fractions of the C57BL/6J male mouse brain, *Brain Res.,* 91, 197, 1975.

286. **Huang, H. H., Simpkins, J. W., and Meites, J.,** Hypothalamic norepinephrine (NE) and dopamine (DA) turnover and relation to LH, FSH and prolactin release in old female rats, *Prog. 59th Annu. Meet. Am. Endocrinol., Soc., (Abstr.),* 1977, 540.

287. **McCann, S. and Moss, R.,** Putative neurotransmitters involved in discharging gonadotropin-releasing neurohormones and the action of LH-releasing hormone on the CNS, *Life Sci.,* 16, 833, 1976.

Chapter 6

ENDOCRINE REGULATION OF THE TESTIS IN THE AGED MALE

Gail D. Riegle

TABLE OF CONTENTS

I. INTRODUCTION

Aging effects on male reproductive function has historically received a great deal of attention by gerontologists. Although age effects on male reproductive function are more variable in mammalian males than the almost inevitable infertility that accompanies aging in females, a progressive decline in both behavioral and physiological parameters of reproduction is characteristic of those species for which significant data are available.

II. PSYCHOLOGICAL-BEHAVIORAL EFFECTS ON MALE REPRODUCTION IN AGING

In a recent review, Butler[1] points out that societal attitudes towards sexuality of the aged affects reproductive function in older men. These societal attitudes are reinforced with personal concerns of deterioration of physiological function and negative body images among older men. Current understanding of specific neuroendocrine mechanisms involved with reproductive control systems affirm that such psychological variables can affect neural and endocrine control system components involved with reproductive control systems. Psychological factors, therefore, can clearly be involved with problems of impotence and infertility in older men.

Age-related changes in parameters of behavioral reproductive function have also been reported in other species. Mid-aged male rats (13 to 15 months) have been shown to have decreased noncopulatory erection responses compared to a group of 3-month-old control male rats.[2] Previous sexual experiences did not affect the numbers of erection responses of these mid-aged rats. The young male groups in this study also had higher serum testosterone concentrations than the mid-aged rats. The age-related reduction in erection responsiveness in the mid-aged rat could be reversed with testosterone treatments suggesting that this testicular hormone may be involved with the reduced erection response. In domesticated mammals, considerable data related to male reproduction has been obtained from cattle in association with the collection of semen for artificial insemination. The studies have shown that psychologic factors, environmental factors, and physical impairments affect sexual activities.[3,4]

Many of the anatomical, physiological, and behavioral changes in male reproduction occurring with increased age are consistent with a hypothesis of decreased testosterone secretion or reduced biological activity of testosterone in aged males. Changes in testosterone function in aging males could be related to multiple factors ranging from structural-functional alterations in the components of the testicular, pituitary, hypothalamic axis to alterations in tissue responsivenes to testosterone. Much of the remainder of this review will focus on the consideration of these variables.

III. THE AGED TESTIS

A. Anatomical Changes in the Aging Testis

Both gross and microscopic degenerative changes of the testes have been reported from aged males. Degenerative changes of the testes of aging men include progressive seminiferous tubule fibrosis, thickening of the seminiferous tubule basement membrane, reduction of the numbers of spermatogonia until only Sertoli cells remain, and eventual obliteration of the tubule.[5-7] Similar degenerative changes have been described in aging bulls.[8] Although the laboratory rat and mouse have been widely used in aging research, comparatively little data have been published regarding changes in testicular structure or spermatogonia function in these species. Progressive atrophy of the testes has been reported in aging Fischer 344 rats.[9] On the other hand, the weight of testes and fertility appears to be little affected by advancing age in the mouse.[10,11]

Although most of the changes in seminiferous tubule function in aged males could be related to reduced testosterone stimulation of this tissue, it is recognized that there are many individual differences in the type and amount of degenerative tissue change and the effect of age on fertility. To date, no conclusive correlations have been shown between indexes of age effects on spermatogenesis and measures of testosterone secretion. Another variable which could affect seminiferous tubule function in old age is the adequacy of the blood supply to this tissue. As fibrosis develops in the aged testes, the spermatogenic epithelium becomes increasingly separated from its capillary supply.[6] The microvascular of the aging human testes show thickening of arteriolar walls[12] and reduced testicular blood flow.[12,13] Similar vascular pathologies have been found in the testes of aged rabbits[14] and reduced blood flow has recently been reported in aged Wistar rat testes.[15] An inadequate microvascular blood supply to the testes could obviously affect hormone availability to the tissues in the testes, as well as affecting the adequacy of all other aspects of tissue maintenance.

Anatomical evidence of altered Leydig cell structure is not as uniform as changes in seminiferous tubule structure in aging males. The Leydig cells often appear morphologically normal in men with well advanced fibrosis of the testes.[3] However, numbers of Leydig cells per unit of testes volume have been shown to decrease in aged men[16,17] and the decrease in numbers of Leydig cells has been associated with reduced testosterone secretion.[18] These observations suggest that the testes of aged men may have less steroidogenic capacity than testes of younger men. In contrast to the effect of age on Leydig cells in the human, an increase in total Leydig cell numbers per testes with no change in average cell volume has been reported in 24-month-old Sprague-Dawley rats.[19] These data suggest that the decrease in seminiferous tubule function in the aged male rat may not be directly related to Leydig cell function.

Another condition which could affect testicular function in the aged is autoimmunization. Increased sperm autoantibodies have been reported in aged human males.[20] In addition, inflammatory cells have been found in and around areas of testicular degeneration.[12] Although at present it is difficult to determine whether the autoimmunity to testicular tissues is a primary cause of testicular dysfunction or whether the release of antibodies occurs after testicular degeneration, increased incidence of autoimmune disease of other endocrines is recognized to occur with aging and, thus, autoimmunity occurring in the testes may also be an important factor involved in the decline of testicular function with age.

B. Testicular Synthesis and Secretion of Testosterone

Several investigators have measured blood testosterone in aging men. Although the early data related to changes in blood androgens in aging men were often conflicting and controversial,[21-24] several recent studies involving large sample sizes indicate decreased average blood testosterone concentrations in aging men.[25-30] An additional important variable affecting the biological activity of testosterone was identified in the studies of Vermeulen[30] (Table 1). These data show sharply reduced plasma testosterone concentrations in men over 65 years of age compared to men under 50 years. This decrease in plasma testosterone was accompanied by an increase in plasma testosterone-binding capacity which resulted in a decrease in free testosterone from .106 ng/mℓ in the younger men to only .036 ng/mℓ in the aged group. These data point out that variables other than the commonly measured total blood concentration of a particular hormone can have a major affect on its biological activity during aging.

Although the laboratory mouse and rat have been proposed as a model of aging ef-

Table 1
TESTOSTERONE LEVELS, BINDING CAPACITY, AND FREE
TESTOSTERONE IN MALES

	Patient age		Statistical significance of
Variable	<50 years	>65 years	difference ρ
Plasma testosterone (ng/100 mℓ)	487	264	
	(407—583)	(210—331)	<0.001
Testosterone-binding	3.2	8.9	<0.001
capacity (10 *M*)	(2.3—83.6)	(7.3—11)	
Free testosterone fraction (%)	2.5	1.2	<0.001
	(2.4—2.6)	(1.0—1.4)	
Apparent free testosterone concentration	10.6	3.6	<0.001
(ng/100 mℓ)	(0.3—12.0)	(3.1—4.3)	

Note: Concentrations given as the mean; numbers in parentheses indicate 95 percentiles.

From Vermeulen, A., *Hypothalamus, Pituitary and Aging,* Everitt, A. V. and Burgess, J. A., Eds., Charles C Thomas, Springfield, Ill., 1976, 458. With permission.

fects on male reproduction, much less information is available concerning testicular endocrinology in these species. Several recent studies indicate decreased blood testosterone concentrations in aging male rats of several strains.[31-37] The affect of age on serum testosterone in male rats is illustrated by the data included in Figure 1 which show sharply reduced serum testosterone in serial blood samples collected from the aged control group compared to the young control rats. On the other hand, current available data suggest that the aged male mouse does not have similar decreases in blood testosterone concentrations.[10,38] In addition to measuring blood androgen concentrations, several laboratories have considered the effect of aging on testicular steroidogenesis in the rat. Although aged Long-Evans rats (from 12 to 24 months of age) were reported to have progressively reduced Δ^5-3β-hydroxysteroid dehydrogenase,[39] aged male Wistar rats had unimpaired function of this enzyme.[40]

C. Testicular Response to Gonadotropin Stimulation

These reports showing decreased blood testosterone concentration in aged male rats with apparently morphologically normal Leydig cells suggest that either the Leydig cells are less responsive to LH stimulation, or that these cells are receiving less LH stimulation that is required to maintain normal steroidogenesis. The author and colleagues initially tested the hypothesis of decreased Leydig cell responsiveness by subjecting groups of young (4 month) and aged (24 month) male Long-Evans rats to variable HCG stimulation (Figure 1). Groups of rats received intravenous injections 0.5 mℓ of saline containing 0, 1, 5, or 20 IU of HCG. Leydig cell responsiveness was measured in terms of the increase in serum testosterone from serial blood samples taken before HCG injection and at 45, 90 and 150 min following HCG treatment. Serum testosterone was increased in both young and aged groups following all three levels of HCG treatment. The increase in testosterone was smaller in the aged groups compared to the young group at each increment of HCG treatment tested and at all blood sampling intervals. The increase in serum testosterone concentration following the acute gonadotropin injection indicated that aged male rat Leydig cells retain their capacity to re-

EFFECT OF HCG ON SERUM TESTOSTERONE IN YOUNG AND AGED MALE RATS

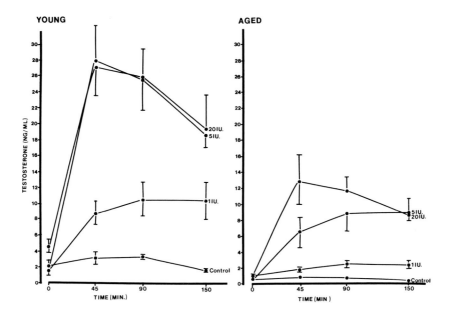

FIGURE 1. Effect of intravenous injection of 1, 5, and 20 IU of HCG on serum testosterone in young and aged male rats. Testosterone levels are shown as the group mean with
indicated SEM from blood samples taken under light ether anesthesia before and at 45,
90, and 150 min after HCG injection. (From Miller, A. E. and Riegle, G. D., *J. Gerontol.*,
33, 197, 1978. With permission.)

spond to gonadotropin and suggest that they are capable of sustaining higher concentrations of blood testosterone than that normally measured in these rats.

The author and colleagues next tested the capacity of aged male rat Leydig cells to
sustain testosterone secretion over a longer time interval. Groups of young (4 month)
and aged (24 to 28 month) male Long-Evans rats received daily subcutaneous injections
of physiological saline containing 0 to 5 IU HCG/100 g body weight (bw) for 7 days.
Control and treated young and aged groups received an intravenous injection of 0.2 or
2.0 IU of HCG/100 g bw 1 day following the last subcutaneous HCG injection. Serum
testosterone was measured in serial blood samples collected before the chronic subcutaneous administration of HCG, before the intravenous injection of HCG, and at 1,
2 and 3 hr after the intravenous hormone treatment.

The results of this experiment are presented in Figures 2 and 3. Basal testosterone
concentrations were again higher in young than aged male rats. Both the young and
aged groups which received the 7 days of subcutaneous HCG injections had much
higher testosterone concentrations at the end of this treatment regime. Posttreatment
serum testosterone concentrations were similar between the two age groups. Age differences in testicular responsiveness to intravenous HCG treatment were also abolished
by the chronic Leydig cell stimulation. Although the young control group receiving 2.0
IU HCG/100 g bw had a greater increase in serum testosterone following the HCG
treatment than in the aged control group, there were no differences in HCG responsiveness between young and aged groups which had received the chronic HCG treatment before this experiment (Figures 3). The results off this experiment confirm the
previous hypothesis that aged male rats are capable of sustaining much higher serum
testosterone concentrations than are normally measured in aged males and strongly sup-

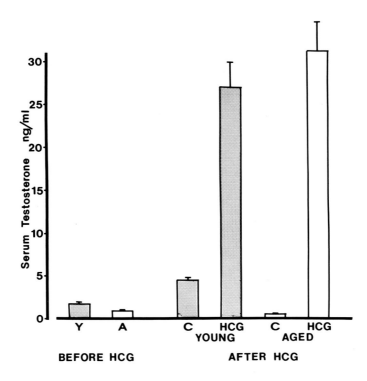

FIGURE 2. Effect of daily subcutaneous injection of HCG (5 IU HCG/ 100 g bw for 7 days) on serum testosterone levels in young (shaded bars) and aged (open bars) male rats. Blood samples were taken before HCG treatment was started and 24 hr after the final HCG injection. Young and aged control groups (C) received seven treatments of the injection vehicle. Testosterone levels are shown as the group mean with indicated SEM. (From Miller, and Riegle, G. D., *J. Gerontol.*, 33, 197, 1978. With permission.)

port the concept that inadequate gonadotropin stimulation of Leydig cell steroidogenesis is a primary factor resulting in their reduced serum testosterone. In addition, these data indicate that the understimulated Leydig cells of aged male rats are less responsive to initial gonadotropin stimulation and require gonadotropin stimulation over a longer duration to restore steroidogenic rates to levels typical of young male rat Leydig cells.

The author's data showing that testosterone secretion can be restored in aged male rats are supported by the results of similar experiments utilizing both in vivo and in vitro techniques from several other laboratories. Similar increases in serum testosterone concentrations have been stimulated by systemic HCG and LH treatments in several strains of young and aged rats.[31,36] Results from studies considering in vitro stimulation of testosterone secretion have not been as consistent. Although isolated Leydig cell suspensions from young (5 month) and mid-aged (12 month) Fischer 344 rats secreted similar amounts of testosterone following the addition of LH to their incubation medium, similar cell suspensions from aged (29 month) rats did not respond to the LH.[32] On the other hand, similar testosterone secretion was stimulated by HCG in isolated Leydig cells by young (3 month) and aged (26 to 28 month) Wistar rats.[31] The report of failure of response in these aged Fischer males[32] is contrary to other reported data suggesting a possible rat strain difference in this response or an age related change in vitro compared to in vivo testicular responsiveness.

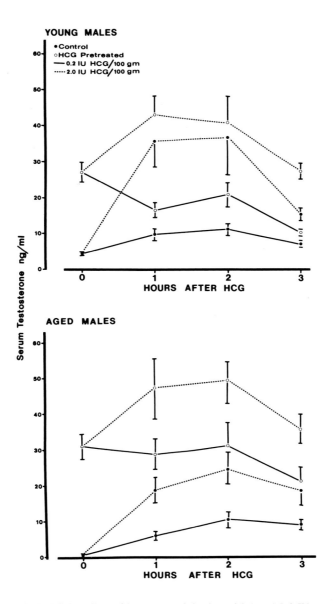

FIGURE 3. Effect of intravenous injection of 0.2 and 2.0 IU of HCG/100 g bw on serum testosterone levels in young and aged male rats pretreated with 0 and 5 IU HCG/100 g bw for 7 days. Testosterone levels are shown as the group mean with indicated SEM. (From Miller, A. E. and Riegle, G. D., *J. Gerontol.*, 33, 197, 1978. With permission.)

The ability of gonadotropins to stimulate Leydig cell function has also been tested in aged men. Although the pretreatment serum testosterone concentrations and the absolute testosterone levels after gonadotropin stimulation were lower in older men compared to younger men, the percentage increase in testosterone following HCG treatment was similar in young and aged men.[27,41] On the other hand, other groups have reported relative decreases in the proportional response of the testis of aged men to increase secretion of testosterone following HCG treatment.[28,42] The experiments showing reduced capacity of the testis to respond to gonadotropin stimulation suggest that a pri-

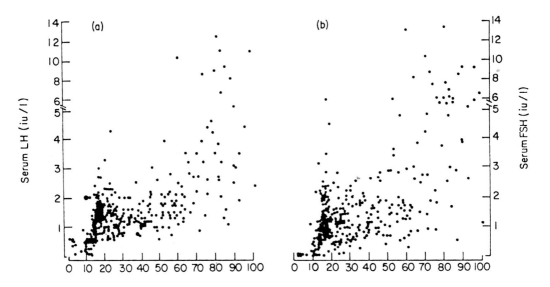

FIGURE 4. Serum LH (a) and FSH (b) as a function of age in normal males. (From Baker, H. W. G., Burger, H. G., deKretser, D. M., Hudson, B., O'Connor, S., Wang, C., Microvics, A., Court, J., Dunlop, M., and Rennie, G. C., *Clin. Endocrinol.*, 5, 349, 1976. With permission.)

mary loss of steroidogenic function in the aged men included in these studies is independent of secondary changes occurring because of altered pituitary secretions.

IV. THE AGED PITUITARY

A. The Effect of Age in Gonadotropin Secretion

The materials reviewed in the early sections of this chapter suggest age-related alterations in LH stimulation of the testes in men and rats. If the gonadal control system remains functional during aging, the previously mentioned decrease in testicular secretion and serum testosterone concentration should be detected by the brain-hypophyseal negative feedback systems and result in a compensatory increase in pituitary gonadotropin secretion. The relationships between the testes and the control of gonadotropin secretion has received considerable recent attention. Early studies of this control system in aging men showed that the increase in urinary gonadotropin with increasing age was much less than the increase which occurred in postmenopausal women.[42] Recent studies have demonstrated increased blood concentrations of LH and FSH in aging men.[25,28,29] These data show considerable individual variation in the affect of age on serum gonadotropins. It is not uncommon to find men of advanced age with gonadotropin concentration typical of those found in young in men. The changes in average serum gonadotropins in aged men are illustrated in Figure 4. Most of these studies showed a greater increase in serum FSH than in LH with increasing age, suggesting possible specificity in the effect of age on the control systems involving these gonadotropins.

The increase in serum LH in aged men suggests that the brain-pituitary feedback system is at least partially responsive to the decrease in blood testosterone in aged men. The previously mentioned studies show that Leydig cells in the testes of aged men can sustain higher concentrations of serum testosterone than that normally found in young males. It is not understood why the gonadotropin control mechanism does not stimulate enough gonadotropin secretion to restore sufficient testicular testosterone secretion to achieve equivalent biologically active serum testosterone concentrations as are found in young men.

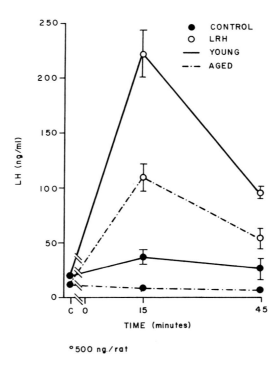

FIGURE 5. Effect of intravenous injection of 500 ng of LHRH on serum LH in young and aged male rats. Serum LH is shown as the group mean with indicated SEM from serial blood samples taken before and at 15 and 45 min after HCG injection. (From Riegle, G. D. and Meites, J., *Proc. Soc. Exp. Biol. Med.*, 151, 507, 1976. With permission.)

In contrast to the increase in serum gonadotropins found in aged men, there is no evidence for increased LH in aged male rats of several strains.[31,32,34,43-45] These data suggest a major difference in the responsiveness of the LH control systems in aged rats and men. Available data for aged male rats suggests that inadequate LH secretion is a primary factor responsible for the decrease in serum testosterone concentration.

B. Pituitary Responsiveness to GnRH Stimulation

The decrease in serum LH concentrations found in the aged male rat and the apparently insufficient increase in serum LH in response to reduced testosterone availability in men appear to be related to the reduced testosterone secretion in these species and also suggest a possible impairment in pituitary responsiveness to hypothalamic factors regulating gonadotropin synthesis and secretion. In recent years, several laboratories have measured pituitary responsiveness to stimulation by gonadotropin releasing hormone (GnRH) in the rat.

The author's studies of pituitary responsiveness to GnRH in aged male rats showed a smaller increase in serum LH following a single intravenous GnRH injection in aged compared to young rats[44] (Figure 5). This observation was supported by the finding of reduced pituitary LH content and a smaller increase in LH release following GnRH addition to pituitary incubates from aged compared to young male rats.[46] Although these studies suggested some impairment in LH secretion following acute GnRH stimulation in aged rats, aged rat pituitaries did respond to GnRH in both studies indicating that the aged male rat has functional capacity to sustain greater concentrations of serum LH than is normally found in these animals. In another study, the author and colleagues subjected young and aged male rats to multiple intravenous GnRH treatments[47] (three injections at 75-min intervals). Although the increase in serum LH was greater in the young than the aged rats following the first injection, similar LH concentrations were found in both age groups following the second and third GnRH treatments. Another study utilizing a different strain of rats and a different treatment regime showed smaller increases in absolute serum LH and FSH concentrations following a single subcutaneous GnRH injection in aged (21 month) compared to young (4 month) controls.[45] Although multiple subcutaneous GnRH injection in these rats induced increased serum LH and FSH in both young and aged groups, the absolute serum concentrations and the relative increase in LH and FSH from pretreatment hormone concentrations were less in the old group. In conclusion, these studies of male rat pituitary responsiveness to GnRH all indicate that the aged male rat can secrete a larger amounts of gonadotropin and that the reduced serum LH concentration found with aging is not due to an inability of the pituitary to secrete this hormone.

The current literature relating to the effect of GnRH stimulation on serum gonado-tropins in aging men contains inconsistancies and ambiguities. At least one group has reported similar increases in serum LH concentrations after GnRH treatment in young and aged men.[27] Others have found reduced pituitary responsiveness to GnRH in aged men.[28,48] The conclusion of reduced responsiveness was based on the observations that although aged men had higher pretreatment serum LH concentrations, serum LH levels were similar in young and aged men following the GnRH treatments. In addition, there are reports of decreased responsiveness of pituitary gonadotropins to LHRH in terms of both the magnitude of the increase in blood LH and the maximum concentration of LH attained following GnRH stimulation in aged compared to younger men.[49,50] De-creased pituitary responsiveness to GnRH in terms of the magnitude of increase in FSH concentration has also been reported.[49]

V. THE AGED HYPOTHALAMUS

A. Changes in Hypothalamic Sensitivity with Aging

In recent years, there has been growing recognition that the hypothalamus and other areas of the brain are invloved in regulation of pituitary gonadotropin secretion. It is now accepted that peptinergic neurons in the preoptic region of the hypothalamus syn-thesize GnRH. This hypothalamic hormone is transported to the median eminence where, upon appropriate stimulation, the pituitary regulating factor is released into the hypothalamic-hypophyseal portal vascular system and is transported to the anterior pi-tuitary gland.

Several independently working investigators have postulated significant age-related alterations in hypothalamic sensitivity to control input which affect hypothalamic reg-ulation of endocrine function. The current literature suggests that there can be either increased or decreased hypothalamic sensitivity to specific feedback control from sex steroids, decreased responsiveness to stress, and smaller changes in serum gonadotropin concentrations in response to drugs which affect neurotransmitter function in aged rats.[51-53]

The author's studies concerning aging effects on hypothalamic-hypophyseal control of LH secretion have shown that although acute stress results in a prompt increase in serum LH in young (3 to 5 month) male rats, presumably reflecting hypothalamic GnRH secretion, there is no increase in LH release in similarly stress-treated aged (24 month) rats.[44] In addition, the increase in serum LH following orchidectomy is slower and of smaller magnitude in aged compared to young male rats.[43] On the other hand, the author's work and experiments conducted by others show that aged gonadectomized male rats are more responsive to testosterone-negative feedback suppression of the postcastration elevation of serum LH.[43,54]

B. Effect of Aging on Hypothalamic Neurotransmitter Function

A large number of experiments from many different laboratories suggest that the neurotransmitters of the central nervous system regulate the secretion of GnRH from the hypothalamus. Studies indicating specific regulatory functions of the catecholamines have been particularly prominent in this regard. One of the first of these studies relating to neurotransmitter regulation of pituitary secretion showed the presence of dopamine containing neurons in the external layer of the median eminence by histochemical techniques.[55] These experiments suggested that dopamine release from these neurons was correlated with pituitary gonadotropin secretion. Subsequent studies have demonstrated high concentration of most known neurotransmitters in regions of the hypothalamus. In recent years, numerous experimenters have attempted to establish the precise role of specific neurotransmitters in the regulation of GnRH. Early experiments in this area showed stimulation of FSH release from rat anterior pituitary glands incubated with hypothalamic tissue in medium containing dopamine.[56] Other investigators found that third ventricle injection of this catecholamine stimulated FSH and LH secretion and inhibited prolactin (PRL) secretion in the rat.[57] On the other hand, data from additional experiments suggested that hypothalamic GnRH secretion may be specifically controlled by the activity of norepinephrine.[58,59] Most recent studies confirm norepinephrine as the amine involved specifically in triggering gonadotropin surges,[60] with the action of dopamine on gonadotropin release remaining controversial.[61] Although the effects of dopamine and norepinephrine on GnRH have been most extensively studied, there is convincing evidence that other neurotransmitters directly or indirectly affect hypothalamic secretion of this releasing hormone. Treatment of female rats with p-chlorophenylalanine, which depletes brain serotonin, will block the proestrus LH surge.[62] Treatment of these rats with 5-hydroxytryptamine, which restores serotonin without affecting norepinephrine function, reversed the p-chlorophenylalanine block on LH release. Results of more recent studies suggest that hypothalamic substances regulating gonadotropin and PRL secretion may also be influenced by factors which affect brain and hypothalamic activity of β-endorphin and met-enkephalin.[63,64]

There is growing evidence that alterations in specific hypothalamic neurotransmitter function may be involved with the changes in gonadotropin secretion, which presumably reflects changes in hypothalamic releasing hormone secretion, in aging rats. Much of the work to date has considered aging effects on neurotransmitter function in female rats. Systemic replacement of catecholamine precursors, such as L-dopa, can temporarily restore ovulation and ovarian cyclicity in aged constant estrous rats which do not have normal estrous cycles before treatment.[65,66] Also local application of L-dopa to the medial preoptic area can reinstate estrous cycles and ovulation in aged, constant estrous females.[67] In addition, pharmacological destruction of hypothalamic noradrenergic neurons using the neurotoxin 6-hydroxydopamine will block estrous cycles and induce the constant estrous state in young female rats.[68] More specifically, 6-hydroxydopamine induced depletion of norepinephrine in the suprachiasmatic region, but not the median eminence, was found to be capable of blocking progesterone-induced LH surges in estrogen-treated ovariectomized rats.[69] Another recent study shows that p-chlorophenylalanine-induced reduction of hypothalamic serotonin concentration blocked estrous cycles and also induced constant estrous states and alterations in hypothalamic mono-amine neurotransmitters in young female rats, which is similar to the changes in hypothalamic and reproductive function found in aged female rats.[70]

Changes in hypothalamic monoamine content and function which are consistent with the hypothesis of their involvement with gonadotropin and PRL secretion have been measured in aged male rats. In a preliminary study, the author and colleagues found decreased dopamine and norepinephrine content in a hypothalamic extract from aged (22 to 26 month) compared to young (4 to 6 month) male rats.[71] This report was confirmed and extended to show decreased hypothalamic content and turnover of dopamine and norepinephrine and increased serotonin turnover in old compared to young male rats.[72]

In the last few months, the author and colleagues have extended their initial studies of the effect of aging on catecholamine function in aged male rats.[73] In this study, blood concentrations of testosterone, LH, and PRL were compared to neuronal concentrations of dopamine and norepinephrine and to measures of dopaminergic neuronal activity in young (5 month) and aged (24 month) male rats. Rats were killed by decapitation after which the median eminence, posterior pituitary, striatum, nucleus accumbens, and hypothalamus were dissected from the brain, homogenized, and assayed for dopamine and norepinephrine content. Dopamine synthesis was estimated by measuring the concentration of dihydroxyphenylalanine (DOPA) 30 min after the administration of the DOPA decarboxylase inhibitor 3-hydroxybenzehydrazine.

Aged male rats had higher serum concentrations of PRL and lower concentrations of LH and testosterone, which is in agreement with the author's earlier studies.[73] Dopamine and norepinephrine concentrations of the tissues are shown in Table 2. Both dopamine and norepinephrine concentrations were reduced in the median eminence of aged male rats. The reduction in dopamine content suggests the loss of tuberoinfundibular dopaminergic neurons in this tissue. The biochemical index of dopaminergic nerve activity, DOPA accumulation (Table 3), was also reduced in the median eminence of aged rats. These data are consistent with the hypothesis of loss of tuberoinfundibular dopaminergic neurons with age and the age-related loss of this neurotransmitter function is believed to be related to the increase in PRL and decrease in LH and testosterone secretion in these rats. The dopamine concentration in the striatum, which receives terminals of the nigrostriatal dopaminergic neurons, was also reduced in the aged rat (Table 2), but the decrease was not accompanied by a similar decrease in DOPA accumulation (Table 3). In another portion of this study, age effects on nigrostriatal and tuberoinfundibular dopaminergic neurons were mimicked by intraventricular injections of the neurotoxin 6-hydroxydopamine into young male rats. In these treated rats, the decrease in dopamine in the median eminence was accompanied by a concomitant reduction in the rate of DOPA accumulation, whereas in the striatum, the reduction in the concentration of dopamine was not accompanied by reduced DOPA accumulation. These data confirm the changes in these neurons during aging and suggest that the loss of nigrostriatal dopaminergic neurons is accommodated for by a compensatory increase in the activity of the remaining nerves, whereas tuberoinfundibular dopaminergic nerves appear to be unable to compensate in a similar manner.

Evidence for changes in brain catecholamine function in aging rats is supported by some similar data from the mouse. Senescent C57BL/6J male mice have reduced hypothalamic metabolism of norepinephrine, reduced levels of catecholamine biosynthetic enzymes in selected brain regions, and impaired dopamine uptake by synaptasomes.[74,75] It is of interest that although these changes in brain catecholamine function with age in mice are similar to some of the previously discussed alterations in aged male rats,

Table 2
NOREPINEPHRINE AND DOPAMINE CONCENTRATIONS IN SELECTED
BRAIN REGIONS OF YOUNG AND AGED MALE RATS

	Norepinephrine		Dopamine	
	Young	Aged	Young	Aged
Striatum	—	—	102.8 ± 6.8	79.2 ± 6.1[a]
Nucleus accumbens	14.4 ± 1.8	14.9 ± 3.9	101.5 ± 7.8	103.2 ± 10.0
Hypothalamus	20.9 ± 1.2	17.9 ± 0.6	4.7 ± 0.6	4.1 ± 0.3
Median eminence	32.7 ± 3.2	26.4 ± 1.2[a]	113.9 ± 7.7	82.6 ± 5.3[a]
Posterior pituitary	1.7 ± 0.3	2.6 ± 0.3	8.3 ± 0.6	7.9 ± 0.8

Note: Each value (nanogram catecholamine per milligram protein) represents the mean ± SEM of eight determinations.

[a]Values which are significantly different ($p < 0.01$) from those in the young rat.

From Demarest, K. T., Riegle, G. D., and Moore, K. E., *Neuroendocrinology,* 31, 222, 1980. With permission.

Table 3
DOPA ACCCUMULATION IN SELECTED BRAIN REGIONS OF
YOUNG AND AGED MALE RATS

	Young	Aged
Striatum	9.6 ± 0.5	9.5 ± 0.5
Nucleus accumbens	7.4 ± 0.6	7.3 ± 0.8
Median eminence	10.4 ± 1.0	7.3 ± 0.4[a]
Posterior pituitary	1.3 ± 0.1	1.2 ± 0.2

Note: DOPA accumulation was estimated 30 min after the injection of NSD 1015 (100 mg/kg, i.p.). Each value represents the mean ± SEM of eight determinations expressed as nanogram DOPA/mg protein.

[a]Values in aged rats which are significantly different ($p < 0.01$ from those in young rats.

From Demarest, K. T., Riegle, G. D., and Moore, K. E., *Neuroendocrinology,* 31, 222, 1980. With permission.

the aged male mouse does not show the reduction in serum LH, FSH, and testosterone that are characteristic of the aging rat.

C. Hypothalamic GnRH Synthesis in the Aged Male
Alterations in the ability of the hypothalamic peptidergic neurons to synthesize or secrete releasing factors with increasing age is another variable of hypothalamic func-

tion which could affect the control of pituitary PRL and gonadotropin secretion. The author and colleagues determined the biological activity of hypothalamic extracts from young and aged male rats by measuring LH and PRL release from pituitary glands incubated in medium containing variable concentrations of hypothalamic extracts from young and aged rats.[51,76] Suppression of PRL secretion from incubated pituitaries was greater in hypothalamic extracts from young compared to aged male rats. This observation is consistent with the measured age differences in dopamine in the aged male rat median eminence reported previously. On the other hand, the author's work shows similar hypothalamic content of biologically active LH-releasing substances from young and aged rats. This similarity of LH-releasing activity was supported by a report showing similar GnRH activity measured by radioimmunoassay from young and aged female rat hypothalami.[77]

VI. SUMMARY

Evidence reviewed in this report indicates substantial deterioration in the reproductive function of aging mammalian males. Although current data suggest substantial qualitative and quantitative differences in the effect of age on reproductive processes within and between species, most studies show decreased fertility and alterations in the hypothalamic-pituitary-testicular endocrine regulatory system.

The effect of age on reproductive function in men and the labortory rat has been studied more extensively than on other species. Aging males of both these species show decreased fertility and alterations in the endocrine control system which regulates testicular function. Serum testosterone concentrations are reduced both in older men and aged rats. However, there are substantial differences in how the endocrine control system responds to the decrease in testosterone in these species. In the aged rat, the decrease in testosterone occurs secondarily to a reduction in LH stimulation of Leydig cell steroidogenesis. Although the responsiveness of the aged rat testes to LH and the pituitary to GnRH may be somewhat reduced in terms of both the response time and the magnitude of the increase in serum hormone concentration following stimulation, it is evident that the testes and pituitary are capable of maintaining much higher blood concentrations of LH and testosterone than normally occur in the aging male rat.

Although aged men also have reduced blood testosterone concentrations, their gonadotropin regulatory system responds to the decrease in testosterone with increased LH secretions. However, the increase in LH stimulation of Leydig cell steroidogenesis is not sufficient to restore blood testosterone to concentrations characteristic of young men. These findings suggest that the endocrine regulation of testicular function in aging men is characterized both by reduced Leydig cell responsiveness to LH and an insufficient increase in LH secretion in response to the reduction in blood testosterone concentration.

There is growing evidence that the responsiveness of the hypothalamus to control input is altered in the aging male. Although there is experimental support for a hypothesis of reduced hypothalamic responsiveness to many inputs that regulate GnRH secretion, the aged male rat appears to be more sensitive to the input of testosterone negative feedback than is the hypothalamus of the younger male.

Hypothalamic secretion of hormones which regulate pituitary PRL and gonadotropin secretion is believed to be controlled by the function of brain neurotransmitters. The hypothalamus and brain of aged male rats has substantial decreases in both the concentration and rate of secretion of dopaminergic and adenergic neurons. Both dopamine and norepinephrine are involved with the direct and indirect regulation of pituitary gonadotropin and PRL secretion. The decrease in LH and testosterone and increase in

PRL secretion characteristic of the aged male rat are consistent with the expected biological consequences of these reductions in catecholamine funtion. It is hypothesized that these reductions in hypothalamic norepinephrine and dopamine activites are a primary alteration in neuroendocrine regulation of function with increasing age and are directly involved with decreases in testicular function in the aging male.

REFERENCES

1. **Butler, R. N.,** Psychosocial aspects of reproductive aging, in *The Aging Reproductive System,* Schneider, E. L., Ed., Raven Press, New York, 1979, 1.
2. **Gray, G. D.,** Age related changes in penile erections and circulating testosterone in middle-aged male rats, in *Parkinson's Disease II, Aging and Neuroendocrine Relationships,* Finch, C. E., Potter, D. E., and Kenny, A. D., Eds., Plenum Press, New York, 1978, 149.
3. **Bishop, M. W. H.,** Aging and reproduction in the male, *J. Repro. Fert. Suppl.,* 12, 65, 1970.
4. **Fraser, A. F.,** The influence of psychological and other factors on reaction time in the bull, *Cornell Vet.,* 50, 126, 1960.
5. **Nelson, W. O. and Heller, C. G.,** Hyelinization of semiferous tubule associated with normal or failing Leydig cell function, *J. Clin. Endocrinol. Metab.,* 5, 13, 1945.
6. **Engle, E. T.,** The male reproductive system, in *Cowdry's Problems of Aging,* 3rd ed., Lansing, A. I., Ed., Williams & Wilkins, Baltimore, 1952, 708.
7. **De La Balze, F. A., Bar, G. E., Scarpa-Smith, F., and Irazu, J.,** Elastic fibers in tunica propria of normal and pathologic human testes, *J. Clin. Endocrinol. Metab.,* 14, 626, 1954.
8. **McEntee, K.,** Pathological conditions in old bulls with impaired fertility, *J. Am. Vet. Assoc.,* 132, 328, 1958.
9. **Coleman, G. L., Barthold, S. W., Osbaldiston, G. W., Foster, S. J., and Jonas, A. M.,** Pathological changes during aging in barrier reared Fischer 344 male rats, *J. Gerontol.,* 32, 258, 1977.
10. **Nelson, J. F., Lathum, K. R., and Finch, C. E.,** Plasma testosterone levels in C57BL/6J male mice: effects of age and disease, *Acta Endocrinol.,* 80, 744, 1975.
11. **Finch, C. E., Jonec, V., Wisner, J. R., Jr., Sinha, Y. N., deVellis, J. S., and Swerdloff, R. S.,** Hormone production by the pituitary and testes of male C57BL/6J mice during aging, *Endocrinology,* 101, 1310, 1978.
12. **Suoranta, H.,** Changes in the small blood vessels of the adult human testes in relation to age and some pathological conditions, *Virchows Arch. Pathol. Anat. Physiol.,* 352, 165, 1971.
13. **Sasano, N. and Ichigo, S.,** Vascular patterns of the human testes with special reference to its senile changes, *Tohuku J. Exp. Med.,* 99, 269, 1969.
14. **Ewing, L. L.,** Effect of aging on testicular metabolism in the rabbit, *Am. J. Physiol.,* 212, 1261, 1967.
15. **Pirke, K. M., Bofilias, I., Sinterman, R., Langhammer, H., Wolf, I., and Pabst, H. W.,** Relative capillary blood flow and Leydig cell function in old rats, *Endocrinology,* 105, 842, 1979.
16. **Sarjent, J. W. and McDonald, J. R.,** A method for the quantitative estimate of Leydig cells in the human testes, *Mayo Clin. Proc.,* 23, 249, 1948.
17. **Harbitz, T. B.,** Morphometric studies of the Leydig cells in elderly men with special reference to the histology of the prostate, *Acta Pathol. Microbiol. Scand.* 81, 301, 1973.
18. **Tillenger, K. G., Birke, G., Franksson, C., and Plantin, L. O.,** The steroid production of the testicules and its relation to numbers and morphology of Leydig cells, *Acta Endocrinol.,* 19, 340, 1955.
19. **Kaler, L. W. and Neeves, W. B.,** The androgen status of aging male rats, *Endocrinology,* 108, 712, 1981.
20. **Fjallbrant, B.,** Autoimmune human sperm antibodies and age in males, *J. Reprod. Fertil.,* 43, 145, 1975.
21. **Coppage, W. S. and Cooner, A. E.,** Testosterone in human plasma, *N. Engl. J. Med.,* 273, 902, 1965.
22. **Kent, J. R. and Acone, A. B.,** Plasa testosterone levels and aging in males, in *Androgens in Normal and Pathological Conditions,* Vermeulen, A. and Exley, D., Eds., Int. Congr. Ser. 101, Excerpta Medica Foundation, Amsterdam, 1966, 31.
23. **Hollander, N., and Hollander, V. P.,** The micro determination of testosterone in human spermatic vein blood, *J. Clin. Endocrinol.,* 18, 966, 1958.

24. **Gandy, H. M. and Peterson, R. F.,** Measurement of testosterone and 17 ketosteroids in plasma by double isotope dilution derivative technique, *J. Clin. Endocrinol. Metab.*, 28, 949, 1968.

25. **Baker, H. W. G., Burger, H. G., deKretser, D. M., Hudson, B., O'Connor, S., Wang, C., Microvics, A., Court, J., Dunlop, M., and Rennie, G. C.,** Changes in pituitary-testicular system with age, *Clin. Endocrinol.*, 5, 349, 1976.

26. **Greenblatt, R. B., Oettingen, M., and Bohler, C. S. S.,** Estrogen-androgen levels in aging men and women: therapeutic considerations, *J. Am. Geriatr. Soc.*, 24, 173, 1976.

27. **Mazzi, C., Riva, L. R., and Bernasconi, D.,** Gonadotropins and plasma testosterone in senescence, in *The Endocrine Function of the Human Testis*, Vol. 2, James V. H. T., Serio, M., and Martini, L., Eds., Academic Press, New York, 1974, 51.

28. **Rubens, R., Dhont, M., and Vermeulen, A.,** Further studies on Leydig cell function in old age, *J. Clin. Endocrinol. Metab.*, 39, 40, 1974.

29. **Stearns, E. L., MacDonald, J. A., Kauffman, B. J., Lucman, T. S., Winters, J. S., and Faiman, C.,** Declining testicular function with age: hormonal and clinical correlates, *Am. J. Med.*, 57, 761, 1974.

30. **Vermeulen, A.,** Leydig cell function in old age, in *Hypothalamus, Pituitary and Aging*, Everitt, A. V. and Burgess, J. A., Eds., Charles C Thomas, Springfield, Ill., 1976, 458.

31. **Pirke, K. M., Vogt, H. J., and Geiss, M.,** In vitro and in vivo studies on Leydig cell function in old rats, *Acta Endocrinol.*, 89, 393, 1978.

32. **Bethea, C. L. and Walker, R. F.,** Age-related changes in reproductive hormones and in Leydig cell responsivity in the male Fischer 344 rat, *J. Gerontol.*, 34, 21, 1979.

33. **Miller, A. E. and Riegle, G. D.,** Serum testosterone and testicular response to HCG in young and aged male rats, *J. Gerontol.*, 33, 197, 1978.

34. **Gray, G. D.,** Changes in the levels of luteinizing hormone and testosterone in the circulation of aging male rats, *J. Endocrinol.*, 76, 551, 1978.

35. **Chan, S. W. C., Leathem, J. H., and Esashi, T.,** Testicular metabolism and serum testosterone in aging male rats, *Endocrinology*, 101, 128, 1977.

36. **Harman, S. M., Danner, R. L., and Roth, G. S.,** Testosterone secretion in the rat in response to chorionic gonadotropin alterations with age, *Endocrinology*, 102, 540, 1978.

37. **Ghanadian, R., Lewis, J. G., and Chisholm, G. D.,** Serum testosterone and dihydrotestosterone changes with age in rats, *Steroids*, 25, 753, 1975.

38. **Eleftheriou, B. E. and Lucas, L. A.,** Age-related changes in testes, seminal vesicles and plasma testosterone levels in male mice, *Gerontologia*, 20, 231, 1974.

39. **Leathem, J. H. and Albrecht, E. D.,** Effect of age on testis Δ^5-3β-hydroxysteroid dehydrogenase in the rat, *Proc. Soc. Exp. Biol. Med.*, 145, 1212, 1974.

40. **Kobayashi, S. and Ichii, S.,** The effect of age on the activity of cholesterol side-chain cleavage in rat testis, *Endocrinol. Jap.*, 14, 134, 1967.

41. **Longcope, C.,** The effect of human chorionic gonadotropin on plasma steroid levels in young and old men, *Steroids*, 21, 583, 1973.

42. **Pedersen-Bjergaard, K. and Jonnesen, M.,** Sex hormone analysis: excretion of sexual hormones by normal males, impotent males, polyarthritics and prostatics, *Acta Med. Scand. Suppl.*, 213, 284, 1948.

43. **Shaar, C. J., Euker, J. S., Riegle, G. D., and Meites, J.,** Effects of castration and gonadal steroids on serum luteinizing hormone and prolactin in old and young rats, *J. Endocrinol.*, 66, 45, 1975

44. **Riegle, G. D. and Meites, J.,** Effects of aging on LH and prolactin after LHRH, L-Dopa, Methyl-Dopa, and stress in male rats, *Proc. Soc. Exp. Biol. Med.*, 151, 507, 1976.

45. **Bruni, J. F., Huang, H., Marshall, S., and Meites, J.,** Effects of single and multiple injections of synthetic GnRH on serum LH, FSH, and testosterone in young and old male rats, *Biol. Reprod.*, 17, 309, 1977.

46. **Riegle, G. D., Meites, J., Miller, A. E., and Wood, S. M.,** Effect of aging on hypothalamic LH-releasing and prolactin inhibiting activities and pituitary responsiveness to LHRH in the male laboratory rat, *J. Gerontol.*, 32, 13, 1976.

47. **Miller, A. E. and Riegle, G. D.,** Serum LH levels following multiple LHRH injections in aging rats, *Proc. Soc. Exp. Biol. Med.*, 157, 494, 1978.

48. **Hashimoto, T., Miyai, K., Izumi, K., and Kumahara, Y.,** Gonadotropin response to synthetic LHRH in normal subjects: correlation between LH and FSH, *J. Clin. Endocrinol. Metab.*, 37, 910, 1973.

49. **Snyder, P. J., Reitano, J. F., and Utiger, R. D.,** Serum LH and FSH responses to synthetic gonadotropin releasing hormone in normal men, *J. Clin. Endocrinol. Metab.*, 41, 938, 1975.

50. **Haug, E. A., Aakvaag, A., Sand, T., and Torjesen, P. A.,** The gonadotropin response to synthetic GnRH in males in relation to age, dose, and basal serum levels of testosterone, estradiol-17β and gonadotropins, *Acta Endocrinol.*, 77, 625, 1974.

51. **Aschheim, P.,** Aging in the hypothalamic-hypophyseal ovarian axis in the rat, in *Hypothalamus, Pituitary and Aging,* Everitt, A. V. and Burgess, J. A., Eds., Charles C Thomas, Springfield, Ill., 1976, 376.

52. **Riegle, G. D. and Miller, A. E.,** Aging effects on the hypothalamic-hypophyseal-gonadal control system in the rat, in *The Aging Reproductive System,* Vol. 4, Schneider, E. L., Ed., Raven Press, New York, 1978, 159.

53. **Meites, J., Huang, H. H., and Simpkins, J. W.,** Recent studies on neuroendocrine control of reproductive senescence in rats, in *The Aging Reproductive System,* Vol. 4., Schneider, E. L., Ed., Raven Press, New York, 1978, 213.

54. **Pirke, K. M., Geiss, M., and Sinterman, R.,** A quantitative study on feedback control of LH by testosterone in young adult and old male rats, *Acta Endocrinol.,* 89, 789, 1978.

55. **Fuxe, K. and Hokfelt, T.,** Catecholamines in the hypothalamus and pituitary gland, in *Frontiers in Neuroendocrinology,* Ganong, W. F. and Martini, L., Eds., Oxford University Press, Oxford, 1969, 47.

56. **Kamberi, I. A., Schneider, H. P. G., and McCann, S. M.,** Action of dopamine to induce release of FSH-releasing factor (FRF) from hypothalamic tissue in vitro, *Endocrinology,* 86, 278, 1970.

57. **Schneider, H. P. G., and McCann, S. W.,** Release of LH-releasing factor (LRF) into the peripheral circulation of hypophysectomized rats by dopamine and its blockage by estradiol, *Endocrinology,* 87, 249, 1970.

58. **Sawyer, C. H., Hilliard, J., Kanematsu, S., Scaramuzzi, R., and Blake, C. A.,** Effects on intraventricular infusion of norepinephrine and dopamine on LH release and ovulation in the rabbit, *Neuroendocrinology,* 15, 328, 1974.

59. **Cocchi, D., Fraschini, F., Jalanbo, H., and Mullers, E.,** Role of brain catecholamines in the postcastration rise in plasma LH of prepubertal rats, *Endocrinology,* 95, 1649, 1974.

60. **Sawyer, C. H.,** Some recent developments in brain-pituitary-ovarian physiology, *Neuroendocrinology,* 17, 97, 1975.

61. **McCann, S. M. and Moss, R. L.,** Putative neurotransmitters involved in discharging gonadotropin-releasing neurohormones and the action of LH-releasing hormone on the CNS, *Life Sci.,* 16, 833, 1976.

62. **Hery, M., LaPlante, E., and Kordong, C.,** Participation of serotonin in the phasic release of LH. I. Evidence from pharmacological experiments, *Endocrinology,* 99, 496, 1976.

63. **Lee, S., Panerai, A. E., Bellabarba, D., and Friesen, H.G.,** Effect of endocrine modifications and pharmacological treatments on brain and pituitary concentrations of β-endorphin, *Endocrinology,* 107, 245, 1980.

64. **Ieiri, T., Chen, H. T., Campbell, G. A., and Meites, J.,** Effects of naloxone and morphine on the proestrus surge of prolactin and gonadotropin in the rat, *Endocrinology,* 106, 1568, 1980.

65. **Quadri, S. K., Kledzik, G. S., and Meites, J.,** Reinitiation of estrous cycles in old constant-estrous rats by central acting drugs, *Neuroendocrinology,* 11, 248, 1973.

66. **Linnoila, M. and Cooper, R. L.,** Reinstatement of vaginal cycles in aged female rats, *J. Pharmacol. Exp. Ther.,* 199, 477, 1976.

67. **Cooper, R. L., Brandt, S. J., Linnoila, M., and Walker, R. F.,** Induced ovulation in aged female rats by L-dopa implants into the medial preoptic area, *Neuroendocrinology,* 28, 234, 1979.

68. **Benedetti, W. L., Sala, M. A., and Otegui, J. T.,** Persistent estrous in rats after anterolateral hypothalamic microinjections of L-hydroxydopamine, *Neuroendocrinology,* 21, 297, 1976.

69. **Simpkins, J. W., Advis, J. P., Hodson, C. A., and Meites, J.,** Blockage of steroid-induced luteinizing hormone release by selective depletion of anterior hypothalamic norephinephrine activity, *Endocrinology,* 104, 506, 1979.

70. **Walker, R. F., Cooper, R. L., and Timiras, P. S.,** Constant estrous: role of rostral hypothalamic monoamines in development of reproductive dysfunction in aging rats, *Endocrinology,* 107, 249, 1980.

71. **Miller, A. E., Shaar, C. J., and Riegle, G. D.,** Aging effects on hypothalamic dopamine and norepinephrine content in the male rat, *Exp. Aging Res.,* 2, 475, 1976.

72. **Simpkins, J. W., Mueller, G. P., Huang, H. H., and Meites, J.,** Evidence for depressed catecholamine and enhanced serotonin metabolism in aging male rats: possible relation to gonadotropin secretion, *Endocrinology,* 100, 1072, 1977.

73. **Demarest, K. T., Riegle, G. D., and Moore, K. E.,** Characteristics of dopaminergic neurons in the aged male rat, *Neuroendocrinology,* 31, 222, 1980.

74. **Finch, C. E.,** Catecholamine metabolism in the brains of aging, male mice, *Brain Res.,* 52, 261, 1973.

75. **Jonec, V. and Finch, C. E.,** Aging and dopamine uptake by subcellular fractions of the C57BL/6J male mouse brain, *Brain Res.,* 91, 197, 1975.

76. **Miller, A. E. and Riegle, G. D.,** Hypothalamic LH-releasing activity of young and aged intact and gonadectomized rats, *Exp. Aging Res.,* 3, 145, 1978.

77. **Steger, R. W., Huang, H. H., and Meites, J.,** Relation of aging to hypothalamic LHRH content and serum gonadal steroids in female rats, *Proc. Soc. Exp. Biol. Med.,* 161, 251, 1979.

Chapter 7

HYPOTHALMIC-PITUITARY REGULATION AND AGING

Arthur V. Everitt and Jennifer Wyndham

TABLE OF CONTENTS

I. INTRODUCTION

If aging is a regulated process related to growth and development then the site of control is likely to be in the hypothalamic-pituitary complex and associated suprahypothalamic areas. The main lines of evidence supporting this view come from long-term studies in rats demonstrating the anti-aging effects of surgical hypophysectomy[1-4] and dietary hypophysectomy[5,6] due to calorie restriction[7-18] or tryptophan deficiency,[19-21] and the aging effects of certain hypothalamic lesions.[22,23] These and related studies make use of classical techniques such as hypophysectomy, hormone and drug therapy, dietary manipulation, and hypothalamic lesions to modify the rate of aging in experimental animals.

II. CHOICE OF EXPERIMENTAL ANIMAL

For economic reasons, rats and mice are widely used in studies of hypothalamic-pituitary relationships to aging.

A. General Criteria of Selection in Aging Research

Mitruka et al.[24] have specified certain criteria for the choice of animals in gerontological research. They state that the ideal animal should have a well defined life span, be resistant to infectious diseases that cause high mortality or morbidity, easy to handle, and economical to maintain. Since data should be extrapolated to humans the animals should be similar to man in their anatomy, physiology, biochemistry, pathology, and nutritional requirements. Rats and mice are most widely used as models for gerontological research principally because of their short life span and low cost of maintenance.

However, they have some major deficiencies, especially with regard to their high susceptibility to chronic respiratory disease and resistance to atherosclerosis.

B. Aging and Disease

Longevity in rats is determined by the age of onset of disease.[25] In the aging rat there is a rising incidence of disease in most organs and there are strain differences in the pattern of disease.[25-31] The prevalence of these spontaneous lesions in old animals at autopsy should be defined for the strain being used in aging research, since many of the pathological changes could influence the interpretation of the study.[29] For example, in a life-long study of the role of the pituitary in aging, a strain of rat with a low incidence of pituitary tumors in old age should be used. Furthermore there should be multiple causes of death as in man. Certain inbred strains such as the NZB mouse are unsuitable for aging studies since death is usually due to a single cause, hemolytic autoimmune anemia.[30]

It is highly desirable to use germ-free or specific pathogen-free (SPF) animals in order to eliminate the effects of infectious diseases such as chronic respiratory disease, which can reduce life expectancy by up to 200 days in the male Wistar rat.[32] No strain of rat or mouse appears to be resistant to this highly infectious disease, which is due principally to the organism *Mycoplasma pulmonis*.[33-35] It is not possible to control this disease with antibiotics such as sulfamerazine or tetracycline.[33-35] One objection to the use of germ-free or SPF animals is the high cost of production and maintenance. Another criticism is that conventional rats rather than germ-free or SPF rats are more akin to the human situation of random exposure to infectious disease. However, with the control of acute infectious disease with antibiotics and better hygiene, man is approaching the germ-free state.

C. Selection for Specific Projects

The choice of rodent may ultimately be determined by the demands of the experimental technique. The anatomy of the area under study may be vital for the technique. Removal of the pituitary by the intra-aural technique of Koyama[36] can be achieved easily in the rat, but is more difficult in the hamster because the pituitary is smaller, flatter, and possesses lateral projections. For lesion studies in the hypothalamus, it is essential that an atlas of the anatomy of the hypothalamus exists for the species being used.

III. PITUITARY FACTORS IN AGING

The regulatory role of the pituitary in aging is relatively unexplored, being limited mainly to long-term studies showing the anti-aging effects of surgical and dietary hypophysectomy. In the rat or mouse surgical hypophysectomy lowers food intake dramatically[1,3] and retards aging processes in tail tendon collagen,[1-4,37-39] ovary,[40] kidney,[1,3,4,41] hind leg muscle,[42] skeleton,[43] immune functions,[44] and delays the development of age-associated pathology.[3,4] Similarly, hypopituitarism produced by the long-term feeding of diets deficient in calories or tryptophan delays many developmental and aging phenomena.[21]

A. Surgical Hypophysectomy
1. Technique in Rats
a. Animal Numbers and Age

The numbers of rats required for a study of the effects of hypophysectomy on life duration with periodic aging tests (not involving sacrifice of animals) are 25 completely

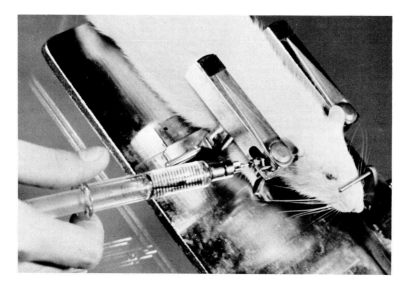

FIGURE 1. The technique of intra-aural hypophysectomy in the rat. An etherized rat is attached to the stereotaxic apparatus by insertion of ear bars into the external auditory canals. The suction needle is inserted through the right ear bar piercing the temporal bone and finally entering the pituitary, which is removed by gentle suction.

hypophysectomized and 25 sham operated rats. Since completeness of hypophysectomy can only be assessed with certainty at autopsy, it is essential to start with larger numbers of hypophysectomized rats. The accuracy of the technique depends on the skill and experience of the operator. For a technician performing 200 to 500 hypophysectomies in a year, a rejection rate of about 20% is found. Thus is is necessary to start with 35 hypophysectomies to yield 25 complete hypophysectomies.

At age 70 days and weight 200 to 250 g, male Wistar rats are of optimum size for the hypophysectomy instrument. It is possible to adjust this instrument to accept rats of other sizes, but the success rate is reduced.

At age 120 days, 50 days after operation, rats that are incompletely hypophysectomized are discarded on the basis of continued body growth and large testes. Further incomplete hypophysectomies are discarded at autopsy after the finding of pituitary fragments in the sella turcica, or the presence of large testes (two organs more than 350 mg), adrenals (two organs more than 25 mg), or thyroids (two organs more than 25 mg).

b. Intra-Aural Technique

A modification of the technique of Koyama[36] is used in this laboratory. An etherized rat is attached to the stereotaxic apparatus and a needle is inserted through the external auditory canal into the pituitary gland, which is removed by suction (Figure 1). The technique is as follows:

1. The hypophysectomy instrument (similar to the Hoffman-Reiter Hypophysectomy Instrument, H. Neuman & Co., Skokie, Ill.) must be preset for the size of animal being used. Carefully attach a dead rat to the apparatus (for details see items 5 and 6), remove the skull cap with bone cutters, gently lift up and remove the brain with a scalpel handle in order to expose the pituitary gland. Push the needle through

the hollow ear bar, and adjust the angle of the ear bar so that the tip of the needle is placed within the pituitary. Confirm the setting with a second rat before commencing a series of operations.

2. The rat is anesthetized in an ether jar, and is removed soon after collapsing. The animal may be numbered with an ear punch at this stage.

3. The anesthetized rat is transferred to the hypophysectomy apparatus and anesthesia maintained with a small pad wet with Penthrane® (methoxyflurane, Abbott Laboratories) placed in a nose cone at the head end. Penthrane® is less disagreeable than ether to the technician performing a large number of operations.

4. The external auditory canal is exposed on both sides and hair clipped from the area to improve visibility.

5. The head of the rat is placed in the head holder by inserting first the left and then the right ear bar into the appropriate auditory canal. It is important to ensure that the eyes are in the horizontal plane; if not, the ear bars are incorrectly located. When the ear bars are positioned properly, one should hear the snap of the tympanic membrane when it is pierced by the solid needle which clears a path to the pituitary gland.

6. The tooth bar is positioned in the mouth and the nose bar brought down. The tooth, nose, and ear bars are then locked. The entire head should be rigidly affixed as in any stereotaxic instrument, and the solid shaft of the right ear bar is now removed.

7. A 5-mℓ syringe with an 18-gauge 50-mm needle (Solila®, Luer Lok®) attached is filled with about 2 mℓ of 0.9% NaCl and the air is expelled.

8. With the bevel of the needle facing dorsally, it is slowly inserted into the hollow, right ear bar, but not to the full length. The tip of the needle should pierce the temporal bone and pass beneath the right trigeminal nerve. It should not be pushed so far that it pierces the cavernous sinus, since this results in bleeding, sometimes severe enough to warrant discarding the animal.

9. With 4 mm left to travel, the needle is rotated counter-clockwise 180° (bevel facing down ventrally) and slowly pushed in completely.

10. The pituitary in the capsule is broken up by rotating the needle in either direction.

11. With the bevel facing down ventrally, the pituitary is removed by gentle suction, applied in short strokes with rapid release of the syringe barrel.

12. When the pituitary is visible in the syringe, the syringe is disconnected from the needle which is left in position in the ear bar.

13. The fluid from the syringe is expelled onto a cotton pad and the amount, color, and consistency of the tissue collected is examined. It is possible to distinguish the adenohypophysis (pink) and the neurohypophysis (white). If the volume of the pituitary suggests incomplete removal, further suction may be applied to extract any remaining fragments.

14. The animal is released from the apparatus and injected subcutaneously with 2.5 mg of cortisone acetate suspension (0.1 mℓ of 25 mg cortisone per mℓ, Roussel Pharmaceuticals) and intraperitoneally with 1 mℓ of 1% terramycin (Pfizer Laboratories) in 5% glucose solution. It is then placed in a recovery cage.

The intra-aural or transauricular technique of hypophysectomy has been described by other workers.[45-47] This method of hypophysectomy is quicker and less error prone than the parapharyngeal approach of Smith.[48] The complete removal of all pituitary fragments requires considerable skill. Bilder and Denckla[44] refer to a formalin cauterization technique for the destruction of remaining fragments.

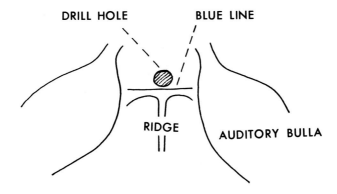

FIGURE 2. The basisphenoid area on the ventral surface of the skull showing landmarks for parapharyngeal hypophysectomy in the rat. With a dental drill, carefully make a hole just anterior to the blue line and then remove the pituitary with a suction tube applied to the hole.

c. Postoperative Care

1. Rats are housed four per cage on a wire grill floor of area 35 cm × 45 cm, and fed normal rat chow. The air-conditioned rat room is maintained at 28 ± 1°C, with a relative humidity of 60 ± 15% and 12 hr artificial light per day.
2. For the first week after operation, moistened, crushed rat chow is supplied in one petri dish per cage and 10% sucrose water is provided for drinking. Thereafter, normal food and water are provided.
3. Once per week rats are weighed, and injected subcutaneously with 1 mg (0.04 mℓ) of cortisone acetate suspension.

The mean life duration of hypophysectomized male Wistar rats housed at 28°C not receiving cortisone acetate injections is 515 ± 41 (SEM) and for those on corticosteroid replacement therapy it is 916 ± 46 days.[4]

d. Parapharyngeal Hypophysectomy
This laboratory has also used a modification of the technique of Smith[48] and other modifications have been described by several authors.[47,49,50]

1. An etherized rat weighing 130 to 150 g is placed on an operating board, ventral surface uppermost.
2. A longitudinal skin incision 2 cm long is made in the neck at the level of the thyroid gland and slightly to the right of the midline.
3. Using blunt dissection with fine forceps, penetrate the neck muscles, and locate the base of the skull, being careful not to damage the trachea or any blood vessels. If bleeding occurs, pack the wound with swabs and leave until the bleeding stops.
4. Retract the trachea, esophagus, and tracheal muscles to expose the base of the skull. With the aid of a binocular dissecting microscope find the ridge of the basisphenoid bone between the ear ossicles (auditory bulla) (Figure 2).
5. With a dental chisel make a slight depression just anterior to the blue line. Place the dental burr (#10-round, 30-mm shank) in the depression and carefully drill until the skull is perforated. The pituitary can be seen through the hole as a pinkish mass.

Use a dental drill with angled headpiece (Aesculap®) and attached light source.

6. The pituitary is removed by a suction tube applied to the hole. The fragments of pituitary can be collected in a small trap bottle placed in the suction line between the animal and the suction pump. Examination of the pituitary fragments collected in the bottle enables the operator to decide if further suction is required to remove any remaining pituitary. If bleeding occurs, apply a swab with a small piece of bone wax.

Surgical problems with the parapharyngeal technique are greater than with the intra-aural technique, since careless surgery or drilling can produce serious injury to the trachea, brain, or even mouth.

2. Hypophysectomy in the Mouse

The intra-aural method has been adapted for mice by Falconi and Rossi.[46] They use a smaller fixing plate than that for rats. A specially modified hypodermic needle sheathed in a tightly fitting steel tube is inserted into the auditory canal. The pituitary is removed by suction as before. The needle size is varied according to the size of the mouse. Postoperative care with a multivitamin solution containing vitamin K and 5% glucose injections is maintained throughout life.

The parapharyngeal technique in mice has been described by a number of workers.[51-55]

3. Replacement Therapy with Hormones

Untreated hypophysectomized rats have a shortened life duration.[1,2] Long-term replacement therapy with a single hormone enables the researcher to investigate the effect of that hormone on aging processes and life duration.

Cortisone in weekly subcutaneous injections of 1 mg (0.04 mℓ of 25 mg/mℓ cortisone acetate suspension in carboxymethyl cellulose, Roussel Laboratories) markedly prolongs the life of the male hypophysectomized rat.[3,4] These studies suggest that pituitary adrenocorticotropic hormone (ACTH) which stimulates the secretion of cortisone-like hormones by the adrenal cortex is a life-maintaining hormone.[56,57] This physiological dose of cortisone was found to accelerate the aging of collagen fibers in rat tail tendon[56] and to depress renal aging as measured by protein excretion.[3]

Pituitary growth hormone replacement (0.5 unit per day of Raben type hog pituitary, Nutritional Biochemicals Corporation) in male hypophysectomized rats restored normal growth and reduced mortality although mean life duration was still significantly less than that of intact rats.[58] Long-term growth hormone therapy accelerated many age-associated pathophysiological changes in the kidney,[59] as well as increasing protein-uria.[59]

Chronic thyroxine injections (2.5 μg/day) were found to accelerate all phases of skeletal growth and maturation in the female hypophysectomized rat.[43] In the absence of thyroxine, sketetal maturation is almost at a standstill.[43]

Denckla[242] has developed a hormone "cocktail" which is added to the drinking water of hypophysectomized rats fed regular laboratory chow. The mixture contains physiological amounts of cortisone succinate, desoxycorticosterone acetate, and triiodothyronine, along with subphysiological doses of estradiol, progesterone, and testosterone. The composition of the mixture was adjusted to normalize the immune competence of B cells and the contractility of the aortic strip. Hypophysectomized Sprague-Dawley rats receiving these hormones lived longer than controls, since at age 34 months, the survival was 20/95 hypophysectomized compared with only 2/125 controls.

B. Dietary Hypophysectomy

Calorie restriction has been found to depress most pituitary functions[5,6,60] as shown by decrements in serum levels[6] of growth hormone, prolactin, follicle stimulating hormone, luteinizing hormone, and thyroid stimulating hormone. Most studies indicate that adrenocorticotropic hormone (ACTH) secretion and adrenocortical functions are increased by acute calorie restriction, but may be decreased by prolonged restriction.[60,61] Since calorie restriction retards many aging phenomena,[7–18] it may act by reducing the secretion of one or more pituitary aging factors. Thus is becomes desirable to compare the antiaging effects of surgical hypophysectomy and calorie restriction, which appear to be very similar.[4]

1. Calorie Restriction

There are a number of techniques for restricting the intake of calories. Animals may be housed individually or in groups and fed once daily or fed less frequently, e.g., three times per week. In the authors' studies animals are usually restricted to the mean calorie intake of the male hypophysectomized rat, which is 7 g of commercial pelleted food, equivalent to 25 kcal/day.

a. Isolated and Fed Daily

Rats are housed individually either in metabolism cages with 18×18 cm square wire grill floor, or in three compartment cages, each compartment having a wire grill floor area of 20×15 cm. In the three compartment cages, the middle compartment was left unoccupied since rats attacked their neighbors. Rats are fed 7 g of pelleted food every day at 10 a.m. Pair feeding is desirable but impractable for life-long studies.

b. Isolated and Fed Three Times Weekly

This is the method most frequently used in this laboratory since it involves the least labor. Rats are fed 14 g of pelleted food on Monday and Wednesday morning, and 21 g late on Friday afternoon.

One serious objection to individual housing is that rats are normally housed in communities. When *ad libitum* fed rats or mice are isolated, they become aggressive,[62,63] hypertensive,[62–64] and overeat.[65] Thus it is desirable to calorie restrict animals in community cages.

c. Community Caged and Intermittently Fed

It is possible to achieve a mild food restriction of rats which significantly prolongs life by allowing a cage of six rats access to food for only 6 hr/day from 8 a.m. to 2 p.m.[66] One difficulty is that the more dominant rats eat more food than the submissive. When the degree of food restriction is increased to that of a hypophysectomized rat, the submissive animals die of starvation after a few weeks. One solution to this problem is to feed the animals daily in isolation cages and then return to community cages.

d. Hypopthalamic Lesions in the Feeding Center

Small bilateral lesions in the lateral hypothalamic feeding center depress food intake by about 20%, thereby leading to a slower rate of body growth.[67] The effects of such lesions on aging have not been investigated. One criticism of this technique is a possible lack of specificity since the lateral hypothalamus affects thirst and perhaps other functions.

2. Tryptophan Deficient Diet

The feeding of a tryptophan deficient diet to rats from an early age depresses pituitary and thyroid functions in a similar manner to calorie restricted diets.[20,21]

C. Pituitary Hormone Treatment

The administration of pituitary hormones to intact animals has been used to study aging phenomena in three ways: (1) to investigate hormone deficiencies in old age, (2) to induce age-associated diseases, and (3) to test for loss of tissue responsiveness and loss of receptors in the target tissues of aging animals.

1. Treatment of the Aging Syndrome

Evidence of a reduced hormone secretion in old age has been shown for certain pituitary hormones such as growth hormone[68] in man, and LH,[69,70] FSH,[70,71] and antidiuretic hormone[72] in the rat. The role of reduced hormone secretion in aging may be investigated by replacement therapy.

a. Growth Hormone

Daily intraperitoneal injections of growth hormone over a period of 200 days in middle aged male rats (commencing at age 400 days) stimulated body growth, but did not affect the course of physiological and pathological aging, nor life duration.[72] This study suggests that the aging syndrome in the rat is not due to a deficiency of growth hormone.

b. Gonadotropins

Aschheim[69,74] has reactivated senile ovaries of rats by intravenous LH injections, subcutaneous HCG infections, or by subcutaneous implantation of a rat pituitary. This study suggests that certain senile changes in the ovary of the rat are due to a deficiency of pituitary gonadotropins. This subject is discussed in more detail in Chapter 5.

c. Posterior Pituitary Hormones

Friedman and coworkers[75–77] found that the chronic administration of posterior pituitary extract to old rats normalized water and electrolyte balance, improved their health, and reduced mortality. There is evidence[78] that oxytocin may be the life-prolonging factor in posterior pituitary extract.

2. Induction of Age-Associated Diseases

There are studies showing that certain age-associated diseases may be induced in rats or mice with pituitary hormone injections.

a. Adrenocorticotropin (ACTH)

Daily injections of ACTH over a period of 10 days produces severe renal lesions in mice[79,80] which are similar to the glomerulosclerosis which accompanies aging in rats, mice, hamsters, and guinea pigs.

b. Growth Hormone

Growth hormone injections in guinea pigs, mice, and rats produce premature osteoarthrosis.[81,82] The chronic administration of growth hormone produces gigantism in female rats and an increased incidence of tumors in pulmonary, lymphatic, adrenal, and reproductive tissues.[83–83b] Growth hormone is also reported[84] to induce nephrosclerosis, periarteritis, and hypertension in unilaterally nephrectomized rats. Growth hormone increases the incidence of renal lesions in hypophysectomized rats.[59]

3. Test of Tissue Responsiveness and Receptors

In most tissues, with increasing age, progressively larger doses of hormones are needed to elicit a response. This is probably due in part to a loss of tissue receptors.[85]

Responsiveness to growth hormone in the rat is reduced with age with regard to body growth,[73,86] release of free fatty acids from adipose tissue,[87] and incorporation of H^3 cholesterol into aorta.[88] Studies of the binding of ^{125}I-labeled growth hormone to liver failed to reveal any age differences in the mouse.[89] The binding of ^{125}I-FSH to rat testes has been studied in young animals in relation to age.[90]

There are age decrements in the response of the adrenal cortex[91] of rats to ACTH and of the testis[92] of rats and ovary[93] of mice to gonadotropic hormones.

The relationship of age changes in hormone responsiveness to the age-related loss of tissue receptors is discussed in more detail in Chapter 4.

IV. HYPOTHALAMIC FACTORS IN AGING

The regulatory role of the hypothalamus in aging is now under investigation in a number of laboratories as described in Chapters 5, 6, and 8. The hypothalamus controls the vegetative functions of the body (temperature, feeding, endocrine and cardiovascular functions, sleep, and fluid balance) which are necessary to sustain life. As such, it provides mechanisms whereby environmental factors are able to modify vegetative functions and thus modulate the rate of aging and permit the survival of the organism. The hypothalamus regulates the rate of aging in at least three ways: by regulating the secretion of pituitary hormones, quantity of food eaten, and body temperature. A fourth mechanism proposed is that a biological clock in the hypothalamus precisely times the life program of developmnent, aging, and the onset of the diseases of senescence.

The classical methods of studying hypothalamic regulatory functions are electric stimulation of specific hypothalamic areas and electrolytic lesions in these regions. Electric stimulation is an acute technique which can be used to test the integrity of nervous connections in old age; for example, electric stimulation of the preoptic area of the hypothalamus can induce ovulation in old noncyclic female rats.[94] This shows that the hypothalamic-pituitary-ovarian neuroendocrine connections are intact in old rats. Hypothalamic lesions are used in chronic studies to show how the loss of a particular hypothalamic function can affect aging phenomena; for example, lesions in the preoptic area in young cycling female rats can induce repeated pseudopregnancies,[95] a condition commonly found in old female rats.

A. Lesions in the Lateral Hypothalamus

Since food intake is a major determinant of aging,[7–18] it is desirable to have a technique which will permanently reduce the food intake of the experimental animal. Bilateral electrolytic lesions in the lateral hypothalamus usually abolish feeding behavior resulting in death from starvation,[96,97] and can only be prevented by force feeding.[98] Studies in the authors' laboratory[99] showed that unilateral destruction of the feeding center only temporarily reduced food intake, which gradually rose to normal over a period of 30 days. However, a permanent depression of food intake can be achieved by placing small bilateral lesions in the lateral hypothalamus of the rat.[67]

1. Control Groups

It is necessary to have a number of controls to show that the effects observed are due to damage to the hypothalamic feeding centers. This is very difficult to prove since other structures along the electrode track are damaged and damage to one nucleus can also influence others. Suggested groups are

1. Unoperated controls of comparable weight and food intake to show that the experimental animals deviate from normal.
2. Shams with lesions in the cerebral cortex to show that trauma to the brain per se is not responsible for the effects observed.
3. Shams with hypothalamic lesions in the vicinity of the feeding center to show that partial destruction of the region does not account for the total effects observed in the fully lesioned animals. It has been shown that bilateral insertion of electrodes without passage of current can lead to aphagia.[100]
4. Experimental group with complete lesions in the lateral hypothalamus.

2. Preoperative Measurements

Studies of body weight and food intake are made for several weeks before hypothalamic lesioning.

3. Hypothalamic Lesioning Technique

Zarrow et al.[47] gives a good description of the technique. Described below is the technique used in the authors' laboratory.

1. A stereotaxic instrument with a head holder such as the Hoffman-Reiter Hypophysectomy Instrument with stereotaxic attachment is necessary.
2. The electrode is attached to a fixture which moves in three directions, anterior-posteriorily, laterally, and vertically.
3. The coordinates of hypothalamic nuclei are obtained from an atlas of the hypothalamus which is available for the rat[101-103] and mouse.[104,105] With the instrument used in the authors' laboratory, the incisor bar was 8.33 mm above the interaural line. For female Wistar descendents weighing 200 to 250 g, the coordinates of the lateral hypothalamus were 8.25 mm ventral to the brain surface, 6.75 mm anterior to the interaural line, and 2.0 mm lateral to the midline.
4. The rat is anesthetized in an ether jar and removed soon after collapsing.
5. The anesthetized rat is placed loosely in the stereotaxic apparatus and the anesthesia maintained with a small pad of Penthrane®.
6. The skin of the scalp and area beneath the ears are washed with 70% ethylalcohol and shaved.
7. Incisions are made in the skin flaps below the ears in order to reveal the external auditory meatus.
8. Ear bars are inserted into the meatus. Correct positioning is indicated by a crackling sound due to rupture of the tympanic membrane, blinking of the eyes, and finally visual inspection of the alignment of the head.
9. Anchor the incisor teeth with the incisor bar and test the rigidity of the preparation.
10. Clip the hair from the scalp and make a 3-cm midline incision. Scrape the surface of the skull to demonstrate the skull sutures.
11. Place the electrode over the position where the lesion is to be made and mark the skull by passing a current through the needle. This forms a black spot. Repeat on the other side of the midline for a bilaterial lesion.
12. With a dental drill and #1 burr, make a small hole through the skull. Clear the area of bone spicules so the electrode can pass in unimpeded.
13. Return the electrode to the desired position and lower to the correct depth.
14. The indifferent electrode is moistened in saline and inserted in the anus and connected to the earth terminal on the lesioning apparatus.
15. A current of 1 mA is passed for 10 sec.
16. Raise the electrode and repeat the lesioning on the other side.

17. Remove the electrode. Close the incision with wound clips. Place the animal in a warm recovery cage.

4. Verification of Lesion Placement

The accurate placement of lesions is the main problem in this procedure. Rats are checked at autopsy to see whether the lesion is in the lateral hypothalamus.

With an intracardiac (left ventricle) catheter in an etherized rat and descending aorta clamped, perfuse with 25 mℓ of warm 0.9% NaCl and then 50 mℓ of 10% formol saline. Carefully dissect out the brain and store in 10% formol saline.

Superficially placed lesions in the hypothalamus may often be observed from the external surface of the brain as a dark brown spot. Lesions in the lateral hypothalamus appear at the lateral margin of the tubercinerum, and destruction of the ventromedial nucleus is seen as a dark point in the middle of the tuber at the level of the infundibulum. This method for determining the location of lesions is quite precise. Further histological observations usually verify the accuracy of this superficial technique. This technique determines the lesion placement, but does not adequately measure the depth.

For the histological determination of the location of lesions, the brains are fixed in 10% saline for 48 hr and potassium ferrocyanide is added in order to stain any iron from anode electrodes. The tissue is then embedded in celloidin and serial sections in the coronal plane are cut at 25 μm. One in ten sections are stained for cells with Nissl's cresyl violet and, in selected specimens, Weigert's iron hematoxylin stain for fibers is used. A rapid method of verifying electrode localization in the brain using frozen sections has been described.[106]

5. Postoperative Care and Studies

In the living animal, a fall in food intake to a stable level is the best indication of correct lesion placement. Body growth is also inhibited. Therefore regular measurements of food intake and body weight are necessary for the duration of the study. Operative trauma caused by sham lesions in the cerebral cortex produces only minor temporary depression of food intake.[99]

B. Lesions in the Ventromedial Nucleus

Destruction of the ventromedial nucleus in the hypothalamus leads to overeating and obesity in the rat[107–110] and mouse.[111] A number of studies[112–115] associate overnutrition and obesity with an increased incidence of diseases of the cardiovascular-renal system, diabetes mellitus, and tumors. Thus rats with ventromedial lesions may be used to study the relationship between food intake and aging. Genetic obese rats[112,116,117] and mice[118] may serve the same purpose.

Coordinates for ventromedial lesions in male Wistar rats, using the authors' stereotaxic apparatus, were 5.7 mm anterior to the baseplate zero marking, 0.75 mm lateral to the midline, and 8.75 mm ventral to the surface of the dura mater. The bregma was used as the zero point in the midline. Other details of the technique are the same as for lateral hypothalamic lesioning.

In rats with unilateral lesions, food intake increases 60% after 1 week and remains at that level. Bilateral lesions double the food intake of adult rats.[119] Such rats become grotesquely fat and develop typical senile kidney lesions about 9 months earlier than unoperated controls.[22]

C. The Aging Center or Clock

A number of authors[56,120–122] have discussed the concept of a biological clock in the brain which times the aging process. Although this is an attractive hypothesis, there is no direct evidence to support it. Indirect evidence rests mainly on studies of catecholamine metabolism in the hypothalamus[19,122,123] and on studies showing that surgical hypophysectomy and dietary hypophysectomy (or food restriction) retard a whole range of aging phenomena. The belief is that an aging center in the hypothalamus controls the rate of pituitary hormone secretion and release of neurotransmitters by the autonomic nervous system and thus determines the rate of peripheral aging.[124-127] A number of biological clocks have been identified in the suprachiasmatic nucleus which control many biological rhythms.[128,129] Thus, a likely candidate for such a clock is the suprachiasmatic nucleus. In addition, there must be an integrating center which receives information from both the internal and external environments and after integration signals the clock to modify its setting or timing. The integrating center may be in the hypothalamus or in some suprahypothalamic region. It may take many years to find these cerebral centers which regulate aging.

V. MEASUREMENT OF AGING IN THE LIVING ANIMAL

There are two ways of studying aging, cross-sectional studies which compare groups of different aged animals at the same time, and longitudinal studies which make serial measurements on the same animals throughout life. Longitudinal studies are better controlled in terms of genetics and have been widely used in the authors' laboratory. Ideally tests should be simple and not involve killing the animal. If animals have to be killed during the test, then the numbers of animals in the study have to be increased accordingly.

The effect of a treatment of aging phenomena may be assessed[130] by studying (1) the impairment of physiological functions, (2) the onset of pathological changes, and (3) the life duration.

A. Body Weight

In the normal intact male Wistar rat body weight (Figure 3) increases rapidly during growth, reaching a peak at 500 days, plateaus for a variable period according to life duration, and then declines about 10 to 40% during the last 200 days.

Changes in body weight are a guide to the general health of the animal. A sick rat, when young, grows slowly, and when old loses weight. The senescent loss of body weight has been proposed as an index of aging in both the rat[131] and the mouse.[132,133]

Hypophysectomy at 70 days in rats weighing 200 g leads to an immediate loss of weight. This is followed by a stabilization at a level of about 80% of the initial weight (Figure 3). In completely hypophysectomized rats this weight remains relatively constant until the terminal phase, when body weight declines by 10 to 30% during the last 100 days. In partial hypophysectomized rats, remaining pituitary tissue secreting growth hormone causes a slow continuous growth.

Body weights are measured on a Mettler® P1000 balance at weekly intervals for 7 weeks after hypophysectomy and then at monthly intervals. It is important to measure body weight at the same time of the day, since body weight increases after feeding, which is mainly at night.

Body weight is not a perfect measure of growth. Measurements of body, tail, or tibia length[134] are better measures of bone growth. Lean body mass is better estimated by measuring urinary creatinine excretion per day.[135]

B. Food Intake

Food intake is a major determinant of aging and, as such, should be monitored periodically during a long-term study. For the healthy male Wistar rat, food intake rises

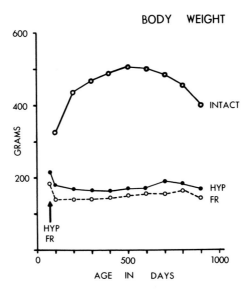

FIGURE 3. The effect of hypophysectomy (HYP) and food restriction (FR) begun at 70 days on body weight at different ages in conventional male Wistar rats. (Adapted from Everitt, A. V., Seedsman, J., and Jones, F., *Mech. Ageing Dev.*, 12, 161, 1980.)

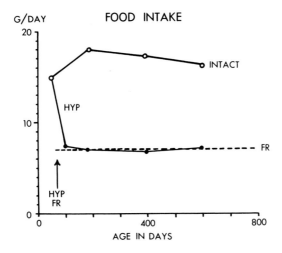

FIGURE 4. The effect of hypophysectomy (HYP) and food restriction (FR) begun at 70 days on the food intake of conventional male Wistar rats at different ages. (Adapted from Everitt, A. V., Seedsman, J., and Jones, F., *Mech. Ageing Dev.*, 12, 161, 1980.)

during early growth and in the adult remains relatively constant at about 20 g of standard laboratory chow per day (70 kcal/day) (Figure 4) until the terminal phase.[136] In the hypophysectomized rat, food intake falls rapidly to 7 g of food per day (25 kcal/day) and is maintained at that level until the terminal phase[1,3] (Figure 4).

For the measurement of food intake rats should be fully adapted to their cage environment. Rats transferred to new cages may have markedly variable food intakes for several weeks.

Food intakes are estimated over a 5-day period for groups of four to six rats housed in community cages equipped with wire grill floors and feces trays. Animals are supplied with a premeasured weight (say 1000 g) of pelleted food in their food hopper. Spilled food is collected on a metal sheet placed in the feces tray directly underneath the food hopper. At the end of the recording period, food dust and crumb spillage are separated from feces beneath the cage floor and weighed with the remaining food to determine food consumption. One problem is that spilled food may become damp with urine and hence its true weight may be different to estimate. Spilled food is usually less than 10% of the food consumed.

For rats adapted to living alone in metabolism cages, it is possible to measure food intake over 24-hr periods by a variation of the above procedure.

Food intake as such is not used as a measure of aging. However, the food intake of different experimental groups must be estimated because food intake is a major factor in aging.

C. Tail Tendon Collagen
1. Collagen Age Changes
Collagen is an extracellular protein which is not renewed during cell division and consequently accumulates age changes. During maturation and aging, the collagen content of most tissues increases and the collagen fibers become increasingly insoluble, more inert to the actions of enzymes and chemicals, and mechanically stronger. Age changes in the physical properties of collagen are usually attributed to the formation and accumulation of cross links between adjacent peptide chains.[137–139]

In 1955, Verzár[140] developed the first widely used test of biological aging using the isolated collagen fibers of rat tail tendon. He measured the tension developed during thermal contraction of collagen fibers in Ringer solution at 65°C and found that this increased markedly with age. Other tests of collagen aging measure contraction, relaxation, and rupture (or breaking) of the isolated collagen fiber in potassium iodide, sodium perchlorate, or urea solutions.[141]

2. Collagen Fiber Breaking Time in Urea
Elden and Boucek[142] found that the time to break an isolated collagen fiber under a load of 1 g in 10 M urea at 37°C increased greatly with age. This test was utilized by Olsen and Everitt[143] to demonstrate that hypophysectomy in the young rat slowed the rate of collagen aging in tail tendon of the adult.

a. Technique in the Rat

1. Tail tendon collagen fibers are extracted from rats under ether anesthesia, usually at 6-month intervals. There is no regeneration of collagen fibers.
2. With a razor blade, make an incision 2 cm from the tip of the tail, avoiding visible blood vessels. With small artery forceps, remove a bundle of collagen fibers and cut to 10 cm length.
3. With a dissecting needle or fine forceps, separate the bundle into individual fibers, being careful to handle only the ends of fibers. Large fibers may be immersed in 0.9% NaCl and carefully teased apart.
4. Allow the fibers to dry in air on a sheet of typing paper for 10 min. Weigh on a

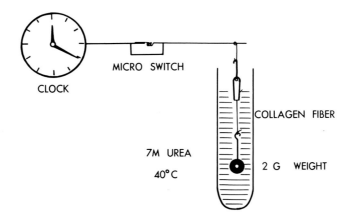

FIGURE 5. Apparatus for the measurement of the biological age of tail tendon collagen fibers removed from the rat at various ages. An isolated collagen fiber under a load of 2 g is immersed in 7 *M* urea solution at 40°C. The insertion of the loaded fiber actuates a micro-switch which turns on the electric clock. When the fiber breaks the clock is switched off.

10 mg Sauter® torsion balance. Use only fibers weighing between 1.7 and 2.3 mg for a 10 cm length.

5. The 7 *M* urea solution of pH 7.5 is prepared by dissolving 300 g urea in 450 mℓ of distilled water, assisted by heating but not boiling, and then adding 30 mℓ 0.1 *M* KH$_2$PO$_4$ and 20 mℓ 0.05 *M* sodium borate.

6. The urea solution is placed in 15 × 2.5-cm test tubes in a water bath maintained at 40.0 ± 0.1°C.

7. A 2 g weight is tied to one end of the fiber and the other end is inserted into a clamp (e.g., a split rubber stopper). The length of fiber between the weight and the clamp is adusted to 5 cm.

8. The loaded fiber held in the rubber stopper is lowered into a test tube containing 7 *M* urea at 40°C and the timing commenced.

9. The time of insertion into the urea solution and the time when the fiber breaks are recorded to the nearest minute. The difference is the breaking time. A stop watch may be used for short breaking times. Automatic recording is possible with an electric clock started by a microswitch when the loaded fiber is attached, and turned off when the fiber breaks and the weight falls (Figure 5).

10. In normal male Wistar rats the breaking time of isolated collagen fibers in 7 *M* urea at 40°C increases with age from about 10 min at 100 days to 100 min at 500 days and 300 min at 800 days (Figure 6). In rats hypophysectomized at 70 days or food restricted from the same age, breaking times are much less than intact, fully fed rats of the same age (Figure 6). Collagen fibers from an 800-day-old hypophysectomized rat break in about 80 min, which is similar to that for collagen fibers from a 400-day-old intact rat.

11. Collagen fibers from 2-year-old rats may require 200 min to break in 7 *M* urea at 40°C and so measurements are usually made at 50°C, when the breaking time becomes 70 min.

b. Technique in the Mouse

Harrison and Archer[144] have adapted the technique to mouse tail tendon collagen fibers.

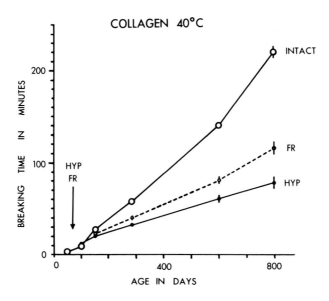

FIGURE 6. The effect of hypophysectomy (HYP) and food restriction (FR) begun at 70 days on the biological age of rat tail tendon collagen fibers, as measured by the breaking time in minutes (mean ± SEM) of a loaded isolated fiber in 7 *M* urea at 40°C. (Adapted from Everitt, A. V., *Proc. Aust. Assoc. Gerontol.*, 1, 127, 1971.)

1. The tail tendon fibers are extracted from the mouse after a local anesthetic, such as 0.05 mℓ of lidocaine hydrochloride, has been injected into the base of the tail, and placed in a petri dish containing saline or distilled water.
2. The fiber is attached to a 2.00-g weight and then suspended in urea solution maintained at 45.0 ± 0.1°C. The urea solution is held in 1000-mℓ beakers or in acrylite tanks 5 cm wide, 15 cm deep, and 60 m long. The water bath surrounding the urea container has a water level at least 1 cm higher than the urea level and its temperature is controlled so that variation is only 0.05°C. The solution in the water bath is kept well mixed and the volume of urea in its container is kept constant by refilling with distilled water whenever more than 5% has evaporated.
3. The time of fiber insertion is noted and a stop watch used to measure breaking time by listening for the sound of the weight hitting the bottom of the urea container.
4. The weight may alternatively be attached to a mercury switch (#AS412A1 made by Micro Switch, Freeport, Ill.) so that an electric clock is started when the weight is hung on it and stops when the fiber breaks, dropping the weight.

c. *Sources of Error*

1. Fiber thickness must be kept within a narrow range since breaking time is dependent on thickness. From each rat, four or five fibers are tested and their sizes selected to give a mean dry fiber weight of approximately 2.0 mg/10 cm.
2. Urea temperature must be maintained constant at the chosen temperature. The breaking times of mouse fibers decrease 5.4% for every 1°C increase in temperature between 41 and 51°C.[144]
3. Tail temperature affects collagen breaking time.[144] Fibers from cooler parts of the tail (mid-tail) have shorter breaking times than fibers from warmer parts (base). Rats

housed singly have lower tail temperatures and shorter breaking times than those housed in groups.[145]

3. Thermal Contraction of Collagen Fibers

Verzár[140] observed that isolated collagen fibers immersed in Ringer solution at 65°C shrink to about a quarter of their original length. The force which inhibits the thermal contraction increases with age from 1 g at 2 months to 10 g at 30 months. This method measures the isotonic thermal contaction of collagen fibers.

Isometric thermal contraction has been measured by Brocas and Verzár.[146] The collagen fiber is suspended in Ringers solution of pH 7.4 and the water bath surrounding the fiber in solution is heated to 70°C. The amount of tension is recorded by a tensimeter connected to a microammeter and the maximal tension is recorded just before the fiber breaks. The results give very similar values to those obtained by the isotonic contraction technique. Furthermore, there is excellent correlation between the isometric thermal contraction tension and the breaking time in 7 M urea at 40°C under a load of 2 g.[141]

4. Studies of Collagen Cross Links

The physical changes in collagen fibers with increasing age are due to the formation and accumulation of cross links, as shown by chromatography of collagen extracted from rats of different ages.[147–149] One of the cross links, the lysine-derived aldehyde cross link, exists in a labile and a stable form, and with increasing age the labile cross link changes into the stable form.[148] The labile form is cleaved by acid phosphate (NaH_2PO_4) washing of collagen fibers.[150] When urea breaking time tests are performed on acid-phosphate washed collagen fibers, the breaking time of collagen fibers from hypophysectomized rats remains at 1 min even at age 1000 days, while those from intact rats show a steady rise[151] after middle age at 500 days.

5. Collagen Aging in Other Tissues

A progressive increase occurs with age in the cross linkage of collagen in other tissues such as bone, skin, and artery.[152,153] Even though tail-tendon collagen is more soluble than collagen in other organs, it still undergoes cross linking as in other tissues. Thus it is possible that age changes in tail-tendon collagen, which is so accessible for biopsy, may reflect age changes in collagen in other sites.

D. Urinary Protein Excretion

The incidence of renal pathology rises progressively with age[25–29] and its development may be monitored by measuring protein excretion in urine which rises steadily with age in all rats.[135] Berg[154] notes that in the Sprague-Dawley rat of both sexes the degree of proteinuria corresponds roughly with the severity of renal lesions.

1. Technique in the Rat

a. Urine Collection

The "unadapted" rat is placed in a metabolism cage without food but with 50 mℓ of 10% sucrose as a supply of water and fuel. Urine is collected for exactly 24 hr.

Sucrose solution is used as an energy source because it is unwise to leave hypophysectomized rats without food for 24 hr; such animals may pass into a hypoglycemic coma and die. The problem of spillage of food containing protein into the urine being collected is also obviated by using 10% sucrose.

b. Protein Estimation

The trichloracetic acid dye method of Pesce and Strande[155] is used with minor modifications as follows:

1. Pipette 1.0 mℓ of urine into a centrifuge tube.
2. Add 5 mℓ of trichloracetic acid ponceau S working reagent.
3. Mix thoroughly.
4. Centrifuge for 10 min at 3500 rpm.
5. Remove the supernatant completely.
6. Dissolve the red precipitate completely in 10.0 mℓ of freshly prepared 0.8% NaOH.
7. After 30 min read the absorbance at 560 nm in a spectrophotometer. The color is stable for up to 6 hr.

c. Solutions

1. For ponceau S stock solution, dissolve 40 g of ponceau S (Sigma®) in 100 mℓ of distilled water.
2. For ponceau S working solution, add 2.0 mℓ of stock solution to 1 ℓ of 3% trichloroacetic acid solution. This solution is stable for 2 months at room temperature.

d. Standards

A calibration curve is constructed with standards containing 0 to 1000 μg of bovine serum albumin (Sigma®).

e. Age Change

In male Wistar rats longitudinal studies show a progressive rise in protein excretion throughout life in all animals. The average increase is from about 5 mg/day at age 100 days to 20 mg/day at 800 days (Figure 7). There are large animal differences, with some rats rapidly becoming nephrotic in middle age, while others show only a modest increase with age. Rats hypophysectomized at 70 days or food restricted from the same age show little or no increase in protein excretion with age.[3,4]

The rise in protein excretion with age is minimal for food intakes under 14 g/day, but increases rapidly with age with food intakes above 14 g/day.[156,157] At 900 days, protein excretion is 10 mg/day for rats eating 14 g of food per day rising to 150 mg/day for rats eating 21 g of food per day.[156] Rats with abnormally high food intakes (30 to 40 g/day), such as genetic obese rats or those with ventromedial lesions, rapidly develop nephrosis. However, obese hypophysectomized rats with a food intake of 15 g/day have low protein excretions even in old age.

2. Technique in the Mouse

The normal mouse, like the rat, excretes considerable quantities of protein in urine,[240] but there is little or no information about changes with age. Urine is collected under toluene from mice placed in metabolism cages for 24 hr with access to water but not food, and protein is precipitated with 5% trichloroacetic acid.

E. Other Urinary Excretion Parameters

Urine volume per day increases in old Wistar[136] and Sprague-Dawley[158] rats. The turnover of water (ratio of urine production: water intake) increases in old age.[72,159] The increased water turnover has been associated with renal lesions[158] and with the reduced secretion of antidiuretic hormone.[72] This hormone can be measured in urine or blood by bioassay of its antidiuretic action.[72,160]

Creatinine excretion declines in old rats[135,161] in association with the loss of muscle mass.[161] Urinary creatinine is a metabolite of muscle creatine.

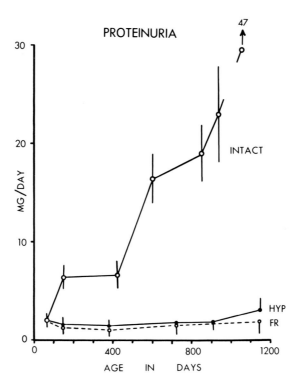

FIGURE 7. The effect of hypophysectomy (HYP) and food restriction (FR) begun at 70 days on the urinary excretion of protein in milligrams per day (mean ± SEM) at different ages in conventional male Wistar rats. Both hypophysectomy and food restriction inhibit the development of age-related renal disease, and suppress the rise in protein excretion. (Adapted from Everitt, A. V., Seedsman, J., and Jones, F., *Mech. Ageing Dev.*, 12, 161, 1980.)

F. Blood Parameters

Blood samples of up to 0.2 mℓ may be obtained from the tail of the rat. For collection of blood the rat is restrained in a holder. The tip of the tail is amputated with scissors and the first few drops of blood discarded. If the room temperature is less than 25°C it may be necessary to warm the rat in order to increase blood flow to the tail. This technique is satisfactory for blood counts and hemoglobin estimations.[162] Where plasma is required, tail blood is collected in heparinized microhematocrit tubes (Hawksley). The tubes are sealed at one end in a Bunsen flame and spun at 3000 rpm for 3 min. The tubes are broken so that only the plasma remains. The plasma from four tubes is blown into a small test tube, and 20- or 50-μℓ samples of plasma for analysis are measured with an Eppendorf® pipette.

For larger samples of 5 to 7 mℓ blood the rat has to be sacrificed. Grab the rat by the tail, stun by gently hitting its head on wood, decapitate with a guillotine (#30 decapitator, Harvard Apparatus Company, Millis, Mass.) and collect blood in a centrifuge tube. Incubate blood at 37°C for 2 hr for clotting and clot retraction. Centrifuge at 5000 rpm for 5 min. Carefully draw off serum with a Pasteur pipette and transfer to a labeled tube. Store at 0°C until required. An alternative procedure is to collect blood from the external jugular vein cut during pentobarbital anesthesia.

Blood counts of red and white cells and hemoglobin contents can be made using tail blood from rat and reveal significant age changes[162] and effects of hypophysectomy[1,3] and food restriction.[3] Similar techniques exist for the mouse.[163]

Blood chemistry age changes have been studied in the rat for protein,[164] cholesterol,[165,166] triglycerides,[167] glucose,[168] calcium,[169] and other electrolytes.[170]

Blood glucose can be measured in tail blood by transferring a large drop of blood to a Dextrostix® test strip. Time for exactly 60 sec. Wash off blood with a squirt of distilled water from a wash bottle. Blot dry on filter paper and insert in the Eyetone® reflectance meter (Ames). Blood glucose is read directly on the scale. This is a useful test in rats found dying in coma, since a number of hypophysectomized rats develop hypoglycemia.

Serum or plasma hormone level age changes in the rat are now being measured using radioimmunoassay techniques for pituitary hormones (FSH, LH, GH, TSH, and PRL) and also thyroid, adrenocortical, and gonadal hormones. Techniques are described in Chapters 5 and 6.

G. Blood Pressure

In longitudinal studies indirect measurement of blood pressure is usually achieved with a miniature pressure cuff[172] applied to the tail.

In cross-sectional studies where rats are being sacrificed, a catheter can be inserted into the carotid artery of the anesthetized rat and blood pressure measured directly with a manometer or pressure transducer.

Anesthesia may influence the blood pressure. Under ether or pentobarbital anesthesia, mean arterial presure is found to increase in the old rat[171] and the incidence of systolic hypertension (more than 140 mm Hg) rises with age.[172–173] In unanesthetized rats Rothbaum et al.[174] failed to show significant age differences in systolic blood pressure, but found significant decreases in cardiac output.

H. Electrocardiogram and Heart Rate

Heart rate is best estimated from the electrocardiogram which is usually recorded on the anesthetized rat. Under anesthesia heart rate is found to decrease with age,[171,176,177,179] but not in unanesthetized rats.[174] Hypophysectomy and food restriction lower heart rates by about 30%.[1,3]

The electrocardiogram in the old rat reveals increased frequency of arrhythmias,[178] left axis deviation,[176,177] and prolongation of PR and QRS intervals.[176,177]

I. Body Temperature

Body temperature, like food intake, is a major determinant of aging and for this reason should be measured in all experimental studies of aging.

Deep body or rectal temperature is readily measured in the unanesthetized rat with a fast responding thermister probe (Yellow Springs model No. 402) inserted into the rectum and temperature read on a digital thermometer (C.I.G. Medishield®). The rat is placed on a flat surface and held by the tail for taking temperature. Five measurements of temperature are made at the same time on different days. More reliable data may be obtained using a telethermometer.

Age changes in deep body temperature have been studied in rats[180–182] and mice.[183,184] Eleftheriou[183] has found an age-related decrement in rectal temperature which he associated with decreasing thyroid function.

J. Oxygen Consumption and Metabolic Rate

Like temperature, metabolic rate is an important determinant of aging and life duration. Denckla[185] has described a method for measuring the minimal oxygen consumption of the rat under pentobarbital anesthesia and at the thermoneutral temperature. The minimal oxygen consumtpion per 100 g fat-free body weight declines progressively with increasing age.[186]

K. Presence of Clinical Disease

Certain diseases of the rat can be observed without special tests. At 100-day intervals when weighed, rats are physically examined for respiratory disease (noisy or labored breathing, wet or bloody nostrils), eye disease (cataract, growths such as pterygium), dental disease (incisor tooth overgrowth), middle ear disease (head held on one side, twisting when held), gastrointestinal disease (diarrhea), skin disease (insects, baldness, sores), hind leg paralysis (impaired walking, dragging hind limbs), and tumors (skin, mammary glands, large abdominal growths, bones, testis). A marked loss of weight indicates the presence of serious disease.

VI. LIFE DURATION

Life duration is the most generally acceptable parameter of aging. Any experimental procedure which retards the rate of aging or reduces the vulnerability to the diseases of old age will extend the life span of outbred animals dying from multiple causes. Extension of the maximum life duration is the real test because an increase in mean life duration may be due to prevention of early deaths without affecting the rate of aging. This has occurred in human populations in the Western World during the last century. A Gompertz plot[187,188] of mortality rate against age is needed to distinguish between a change in aging rate (lines of different slope) and a change in vulnerability to disease (lines of same slope but displaced).

The mean life duration reported for the conventional outbred male rat[4,28,32,66,134,190,191,194,196,197] lies between 715 to 785 days and for the female rat,[28,66,134,190,192,194,195,197] 715 to 900 days. The maximum life duration reported for males is 996 to 1201 days and for females 1166 to 1300 days. SPF rats have similar life durations.[189] Inbred Fischer rats[193] appear to be shorter lived. There is a wider range of life expectancy in different inbred strains of mice[198–201] varying from a mean of 276 days for AKR/J females to 919 days for C57BL/6J females.

Life duration is normally based on the number alive when weaned at 3 weeks, since the mortality may be excessive during the first 3 weeks of life.[30] Hollander[30] recommends that both the 50% survival time (mean life duration) and the maximum age be reported in publications, since this makes it possible to estimate the slope of the mortality curve and to decide whether animals described as "old" are really old.

The life duration of a rodent depends on its strain; whether it is inbred, hybrid, or outbred; whether it is conventional, germ-free, or specific pathogen-free; and on animal house conditions and husbandry such as temperature, nutrition, isolated or community housing, and hygiene.

In a recent study[4] of outbred conventional male Wistar rats housed at 28°C and fed a commercail rat diet *ad libitum*, the mean life duration (±SEM) was 785 (±34) days with a maximum of 1120 days. The survival curve is shown in Figure 8. Over a 25-year period the maximum survival was 1201 days. Hypophysectomy at 70 days followed by weekly injections of cortisone increased mean life duration to 916 (±46) days,[4] with a maximum of 1282 days. Continuous severe food restriction (35% of *ad*

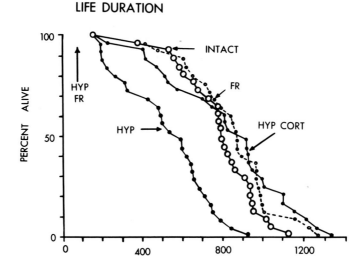

FIGURE 8. The effect of hypophysectomy (HYP) and food restriction (FR) begun at 70 days on the life duration of conventional outbred male Wistar rats. Hypophysectomized rats receiving 1 mg cortisone acetate per week in subcutaneous injections (HYP. CORT.) lived longer than intact rats (INTACT). (Adapted from Everitt, A. V., Seedsman, J., and Jones, F., *Mech. Ageing Dev.*, 12, 161, 1980.)

libitum intake) to the food intake of hypophysectomized rats increased mean life duration to 858 ± 38 days, with a maximum of 1342 days. The longest lived hypophysectomized rat has survived to 1352 days and food restricted to 1515 days. Ross[191] reported that his longest lived food restricted rat died at age 1750 days.

VII. AUTOPSY

At death the duration of life is determined and the body is examined for pathological lesions. Burek[28] has described the pathology of the old rat and emphasizes the higher incidence of disease in animals dying naturally compared with those that are killed. The pathology of the laboratory rat and mouse is also described in the earlier monograph of Cotchin and Roe.[202] Berg and Simms[25–27] have made extensive studies of the pathology of the old Sprague-Dawley rat. Due to limited histopathological resources this laboratory has been heavily dependent on the gross appearance and weight of organs for pathological assessment.

A. Method

1. Cages are examined daily (except Sundays) both morning and afternoon for dead or dying rats. Autopsies are performed as soon as possible. If necessary, bodies are frozen until convenient. Autopsy data are recorded in an autopsy book with columns ruled for each item, date, rat number, age, body weight, organ weights, gross pathology, etc.
2. The dead rat is weighed. There is a gradual loss of weight in old rats.[131] Severe weight loss is indicative of a serious disease. Body weight may increase due to the presence of a large tumor.
3. The rat is attached to an operating board by pushing a pin through each leg. With

a rule, measure the lengths of body and tail. Body and tail lengths increase during growth and show little or no decrease in old age.[134]

4. Examine the skin for tumors, parasites, sores, and hair loss.
5. Examine the nose, mouth, teeth, ears, urethra, and anus for abnormalities such as blood or other discharges.
6. Make a midline abdominal incision to expose the viscera. Look for the presence of fluid (suggesting renal, cardiovascular, or nutritional disease) or blood (due to hemorrhage from a tumor, cardiovascular accident, or trauma).
7. Examine abdominal organs for abnormalities such as tumors or infections.
8. Weigh the testes, seminal vesicles, kidneys, adrenals, spleen, and liver. Table 1 gives the mean ±SD for the weights of organs in 12 controls, 18 hypophysecto-mized, and 13 food restricted rats dying at age 800 days or more. Data from 32 healthy rats killed at mean age of 505 days are used as a basis for determining abnormal enlargment, arbitrarily set at 50% greater than the organ weight at 500 days.
9. Cut through the rib cage and diaphragm with large scissors. Look for fluid or blood.
10. Remove the heart free of auricles, squeeze out blood and clots as completely as possible and weigh.
11. Carefully dissect out the thymus and weigh. Although atrophic, the thymus can still be found in very old rats.
12. Remove the lungs and examine for congestion and abscesses. In this conventional Wistar rat colony, only about 25% of rats are free of gross respiratory disease
13. Dissect out the thoracic aorta from the aortic arch to the diaphragm. Strip off the adventitia by blunt dissection and transfer to 0.9% NaCl in a petri dish. Cut the aorta longitudinally with fine scissors. Estimate wet weight after immersion in 0.9% NaCl and blotting of excess fluid with moistened filter paper. Repeat until constant weight is obtained. Carefully lay out the aorta on graph paper and measure its length and width. Calculate aorta thickness in centimeters by dividing the wet weight in millligrams by the density of 1060 mg/cm^3 and the area in cm^2. The thickness increases with age from 0.018 cm at 200 days to 0.028 cm at 1000 days.
14. Make a midline incision on the neck to locate the trachea. With fine scissors dissect out the thyroid glands and weigh.
15. With coarse scissors cut through the skin to expose the skull cap. Using bone cutters carefully remove the skull cap. With a scalpel handle transfer the brain to filter paper and weigh. Be careful not to disturb the pituitary.
16. Using fine forceps, remove the pituitary and weigh. In hypophysectomized rats and fossa is checked for pituitary fragments. If any are present the animal is discarded from the study.
17. Cut the skin away from the left hind leg to display the muscles. With fine scissors dissect out and weight the gastrocnemius muscle and also the tibialis anterior and extensor digitorum longus muscles. The latter two muscles can be dissected out with precision; the gastrocnemius is more difficult to isolate.

B. Tumors

Approximately 40% of conventional male Wistar rats aged 800 days or more were found to have endocrine tumors when grossly examined at autopsy (Table 2). In 108 rats the percentages of rats bearing pituitary tumors were 19%, thyroid 23%, adrenal 29%, and testis 19%. For histopathological examination, tissues are fixed in 10% formol saline and sections stained with hematoxylin and eosin.

The incidence of these endocrine tumors is reduced to a low level (2 to 8%) by life-long food restriction or hypophysectomy early in life (Table 2).

Table 1
WET ORGAN WEIGHTS ± SD IN CONVENTIONAL MALE WISTAR RATS OF THE UNIVERSITY OF SYDNEY STRAIN, FREE OF GROSS TUMORS

	Controls		Hypophysectomized (at 70 days)	Food restricted (from 70 days)
	Middle aged, killed[a]	Old, died[b]	Old, died[b]	Old, died[b]
Age (days)	505 ± 64	906 ± 95	977 ± 109	982 ± 202
Number of rats	32	12	18	13
Body weight (g)	447 ± 35	316 ± 85	184 ± 4.2	142 ± 25
Body length (cm)	24.8 ± 0.8	23.8 ± 1.3	19.2 ± 1.1	19.8 ± 1.1
Brain (g)	1.89 ± 0.13[c]	1.82 ± 0.14	1.68 ± 0.16	1.69 ± 0.12
Pituitary (mg)	10.7 ± 2.3	12.8 ± 4.2	0	4.5 ± 2.0
Two thyroids (mg)	29.1 ± 8.7[c]	32.2 ± 8.6	20.7 ± 5.1	18.2 ± 5.6
Thymus (mg)	322 ± 52[c]	209 ± 91	149 ± 54	102 ± 38
Heart ventricles (mg)	1088 ± 109	1322 ± 310	762 ± 130	640 ± 221
Thoracic aorta (mg)	59 ± 19	87 ± 18	36 ± 7	51 ± 9
Liver (g)	17.7 ± 3.6	13.4 ± 4.4	4.8 ± 1.4	3.4 ± 1.4
Spleen (mg)	1126 ± 419	811 ± 351	388 ± 164	249 ± 80
Two kidneys (g)	3.16 ± 0.28	3.23 ± 0.91	1.29 ± 0.26	1.52 ± 0.21
Two adrenals (mg)	55.4 ± 11.2	99.8 ± 25.8	18.9 ± 6.6	47.1 ± 17.8
Two seminal vesicles (mg)	745 ± 228[c]	420 ± 227	39 ± 14	131 ± 58
Two testes (g)	3.77 ± 0.57	2.71 ± 1.39	0.28 ± 0.09	1.08 ± 0.51
Gastrocnemius muscle (mg)	1295 ± 47[c]	456 ± 165[d]	394 ± 107[e]	362 ± 120[f]
Tibialis anterior muscle (mg)	969 ± 116[c]	473 ± 116[d]	402 ± 133[e]	343 ± 82[f]
Extensor digitorum longus muscle (mg)	202 ± 20[c]	118 ± 48[d]	75 ± 20[e]	69 ± 17[f]

[a] Healthy rats.
[b] Rats dying spontaneously.
[c] Twelve rats.
[d] Six rats.
[e] Nine rats.
[f] Ten rats.

Table 2
NUMBER OF ANIMALS BEARING GROSS TUMORS IN CONVENTIONAL
MALE WISTAR RATS OF THE UNIVERSITY OF SYDNEY STRAIN
DYING AT AGE 800 DAYS OR MORE

	Controls	Hypophysectomized (at 70 days)	Food restricted (from 70 days)
Number of rats	108	68	38
Pituitary	21 (19%)	0	2 (5%)
Thyroid	25 (23%)	1	0
Adrenal	31 (29%)	0	1
Testis	21 (19%)	0	0
Endocrine	45 (42%)	1 (2%)	3 (8%)
Endocrine (excluding pituitary)	38 (35%)	1 (2%)	1 (3%)
Mammary	7 (6%)	0	1 (3%)
Other Tumors[a]	22 (20%)	3 (4%)	3 (8%)
Nonendocrine	29 (27%)	3 (4%)	4 (11%)
Any tumor	69 (64%)	4 (6%)	7 (18%)
Any tumor (excluding pituitary)	62 (57%)	4 (6%)	5 (13%)

[a]Brain, ear, lung, thymus, liver, pancreas, kidney, bladder, leg, skin.

Nonendocrine tumors (skin, bone, mammary, ear, lung, liver, kidney, brain, bladder) are seen in 27% of intact rats coming to autopsy at age 800 days or more, and in 11% of food restricted and 4% of hypophysectomized rats (Table 2).

There are a number of reports on the incidence of different tumors in old rats[14,15,28-30,203-208] and mice.[199,209,210] Spontaneous neoplasms are particularly high in inbred strains of mice[209] approaching 100% for specific tumors. Leukemia plays a major role in the premature death of short lived mice.[200]

C. Chronic Respiratory Disease

The most common disease of the conventional rat is chronic respiratory disease. In the authors' colony this disease is seen grossly in 75% at age 800 days or more, and microscopically in 95% of animals. Neither hypophysectomy in early life nor food restriction throughout life affect the gross incidence (Table 3). Nelson[35] describes the clinical and pathological features of this disease. The gray to red lesions are sometimes confined to a part of one lobe, but usually affect one whole lobe or several lobes. In late lesions whole lobes may be filled with caseous material and superficially resemble abscesses.

D. Hemorrhage

Blood may be found in a small percentage of rats at autopsy and usually occurs in the thoracic cavity. Berg[27] reported a fatal hemorrrhage occurring after rupture of an aneurysm in a rat with polyarteritis nodosa. The authors have observed two cases of hemorrhage into the pericardium.

E. Cardiac Enlargement

Left ventricular hypertrophy has been reported in old Sprague-Dawley rats in association with hypertension.[173] This condition can be recognized in the living rat from left axis deviation in the electrocardiogram.[176,177] At autopsy the left ventricles are enlarged.

Table 3
INCIDENCE OF DISEASE IN CONVENTIONAL MALE WISTAR RATS OF THE UNIVERSITY OF SYDNEY STRAIN DYING AT AGE 800 DAYS OR MORE

	Controls	Hypophysectomized (at 70 days)	Food restricted (from 70 days)
Number of rats	108	68	38
Lung disease	81 (75%)	44 (65%)	24 (63%)
Thoracic hemorrhage	13 (12%)	9 (13%)	6 (16%)
Cardiac ventricular enlargement[a]	21 (19%)	0	0
Adrenal enlargement[a]	89 (82%)	0	4 (11%)
Renal enlargement[a]	8 (7%)	0	0
Hind limb paralysis	72 (67%)	0	0

[a]Organ weight more than 50% greater than the mean weight in controls at age 500 days when body growth has ceased.

Histologically there are areas of fibrosis and degeneration of cardiac muscle fibers.[26,27,211,212] Cardiac hypertrophy is usually accompanied by hypertension or chronic renal disease.[211]

The authors[4] have arbitrarily defined abnormal cardiac enlargement as heart ventricle weight in excess of 1.7 g which is 50% greater than the mean weight of 1.1 g in normal rats aged 500 days, when growth has ceased. Applying this criterion to autopsy data, 19% of controls aged 800 days or more were found to have cardiac enlargment (Table 3). Cardiac enlargement was not seen in any rat hypophysectomized when young or continuously food restricted from early life.[4]

F. Aortic Wall Thickening

With increasing age in the rat, the thoracic aortic wall thickens[4] and aortic weight increases. There is an increase in the thickness of both the adventitia[215] and the media[215,216] and a loss of elasticity.[217] In the authors' male Wistar rats,[4] thoracic wall thickness increased from 0.18 mm at 70 days, to 0.24 mm at 500 days and 0.28 mm at 1000 days. Wet thoracic weight increased from 59 mg at 500 days and 87 mg at 900 days (Table 1). Hypophysectomized and food restricted rats showed much less thickening with increasing age.

G. Renal Disease

With the progression of age-associated renal disease there is enlargement of the kidneys in the rat.[213,214] Histologically the disease develops early in life as a thickening of the basement membranes of the glomerulus followed by dilation of adjacent convoluted tubules which become filled with proteinaceous casts.[25-27] It is possible to monitor the development of the disease by measuring protein excretion in urine.[135,154]

The authors[4] have arbitrarily defined abnormal renal enlargement as the weight of both kidneys in excess of 4.7 g, which is 50% greater than the mean weight of 3.16 in normal rats aged 500 days when growth has ceased. Using this value they find that about 7% of rats coming to autopsy aged 800 days or more have abnormal renal enlargement (Table 3). Renal enlargement was not seen in any rat hypophysectomized early in life or food restricted throughout life.[4]

H. Adrenal Enlargement

The adrenal glands continue to increase in size after the cessation of body growth at 500 days (Table 1). Adrenal enlargement (more than 50% greater than weight in middle age) was found in 82% of intact, 11% food restricted, and no hypophysectomized rats (Table 3).

I. Fluid in Thoracic and Peritoneal Cavities

The presence of fluid in the thorax (hydrothorax) or in the peritoneal cavity (ascites) is usually due to advanced renal disease.[27] It can also be caused by heart or liver disease, cancer, and other diseases which interfere with normal fluid balance.

J. Hind Limb Paralysis

Skeletal muscle degeneration in the hind limbs of the rat involves the gastrocnemius and adductor muscles, which undergo severe atrophy.[27,218] This disease develops later than other diseases and affects 70% of rats by age 1000 days.[42] Once the disease has developed there is severe wasting of the hindquarters and associated muscles. The weight of the gastrocnemius muscle decreases markedly in old rats. This disease has not been seen in any hypophysectomized[42] or food restricted rat, even up to the age of 1500 days.[4]

VIII. HISTOLOGY

Histological studies are performed ideally on healthy animals sacrificed at ages dictated by the study. Since most very old (1000 day) animals have multiple pathology, material obtained from moribund animals may be just as good as that from apparently healthy animals of the same age. In the case of food-restricted and hypophysectomized rats of this age, there is usually no macroscopic evidence of pathology and, hence, the use of moribund animals may be satisfactory. The presence of disease in old animals should be reported in the histological study, and in younger age groups only disease-free animals should be used.

Material may also be obtained after death. In this case there may be tissue autolysis, but this is no serious drawback if important information such as the type of tumor or the extent of renal degeneration is revealed by histological examination under the light microscope.

The electron microscope has brought to light a mass of data about age changes in the ultrastructure of tissues.

A. Electron Microscopy

The multivolume work of Glauert[219] describes in detail electron microscopic techniques. Summarized below are the methods currently in use in the present authors' laboratory.

1. Fixation

Two general procedures are available for fixation, perfusion of the whole animal with a fixative or immersion of a specimen (volume 1 to 2 mm^3) from a single organ in a fixative.

a. Perfusion

The perfusion apparatus (Figure 9) consists of a cannula for insertion into an artery or heart, connected by a polyethylene tube with a tap and bubble trap to a storage bottle

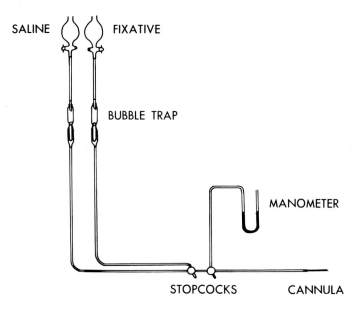

FIGURE 9. Apparatus for whole animal perfusion, consisting of a cannula for insertion into the left ventricle of the heart, connected via a polyethylene tube with stopcock and bubble trap to a storage bottle of fixative. The height of the bottles of fixative and saline is adjusted so that the perfusion pressure equals the blood pressure of the animal. The circulating blood is first flushed out with 0.9% NaCl and then the animal is perfused with fixative.

of fixative, maintained at a height corresponding to the animal's blood pressure. A second bottle contains 0.9% NaCl which is used to flush blood out of the circulation. The cannula for insertion into the left ventricle consists of a steel tube made from a 19-gauge hypodermic needle with both ends removed.

The fixative is 3% glutaraldehyde in 0.1 M cacodylate buffer at pH 7.4, prepared by diluting 120 mℓ of 25% glutaraldehyde solution (or 43 mℓ of 70% solution) to 1 ℓ with cacodylate buffer. The buffer is prepared by dissolving 42.8 g of sodium cacodylate in water and diluting to 1 ℓ. The pH of the buffer solution is adjusted by adding either 0.1 M NaOH or 0.1 M HCl.

Steps in perfusion are

1. Clean surgical instruments.
2. Fill the bottles with fixative and 0.9% NaCl warmed to 37°C.
3. Adjust the height of the bottles of fixative and saline so that the fluid in the bubble trap is 140 cm above the animals. This corresponds to a pressure of about 100 mm Hg.
4. Anesthetize the rat by intraperitoneal injection of pentobarbital (40 mg/kg body weight for a healthy old male rat).
5. When anesthetized, pin down ventral side uppermost to the operating board. With coarse scissors open the chest cavity and expose the heart.
6. With fine scissors, make a small incision in the left ventricle and insert the cannula. Secure with an artery clamp. Be sure that the cannula can move freely inside the heart.
7. Make a small incision in the right atrium.

8. Turn the tap so as to perfuse with 0.9% sodium chloride. About 50 mℓ of saline will flush out the circulating blood.
9. If an organ required for light microscopy must not be perfused with glutaraldehyde, then it is possible to clamp the artery to that organ (e.g., the kidney) and remove for immersion in formol saline or other fixative.
10. To perfuse the animal, turn the tap to the fixative. Perfuse with 250 mℓ of glutaraldehyde. This takes about 20 min in a large animal weighing 400 g, increasing to 45 min in a small animal weighing 100 g.
11. Following perfusion, tissues are removed and placed in 3% glutaraldehyde in 0.1 M sodium cacodylate buffer of pH 7.4 for 1 hr at 4°C.

b. Immersion

While perfusion of the whole animal may be desirable, acceptable results may be obtained by immersion in fixative of a specimen removed from the animal under anesthesia. The authors have used this technique in studies of sketetal muscle in hind leg.

The rat is anesthetized by an intraperitoneal injection of pentobarbital sodium (2.5 mg/100 g of body weight) followed by an intramuscular injection of ketamine (Ketalar®, Parke Davis, 7.5 mg/100 g of body weight). When deeply anesthetized biopsies are taken of the soleus, biceps femoris, and gastrocnemius muscles. Fixatives used for muscle are 1% osmium tetroxide in veronal buffer[220] for 40 min, 2 to 4% glutaraldehyde in cacodylate buffer[221] for 60 min, Karnovsky's formaldehyde glutaraldehyde[222] for 50 min, or 3% paraformaldehyde for 25 min. With the latter three fixatives it is necessary to postfix in 1% osmium tetroxide for 2 hr.

2. Collection of Specimens after Perfusion

From the perfused animal remove organs and prepare specimens of suitable size for electron microscopy.

a. Kidney

Remove the kidney and bisect longitudinally with a single-edge razor blade or scalpel. Cut pieces of kidney cortex or medulla of volume 1 to 2 mm^3 and place in glutaraldehyde fixative in a labeled specimen tube for 1 hr at 4°C.

b. Aorta

Place the thoracic aorta on a cork mat. Immerse in cacodylate buffer and strip off the adventitia by blunt dissection. Cut a 5-mm length of aorta from the thoracic aorta just caudal to the arch. Section longitudinally and lay out flat on the cork mat. With a razor blade cut strips 5 × 1 mm and return to glutaraldehyde fixative in a labeled specimen tube. Leave for 1 hr at 4°C. Abdominal aorta specimens are treated likewise.

3. Postfixation with Osmium Tetroxide

1. Remove specimen tubes from the refrigerator at 4°C.
2. With a pasteur pipette remove the glutaraldehyde.
3. Replace with 1 to 2 mℓ sodium cacodylate buffer and wash by movement of the tube in an angled slow motion rotor for 10 min.
4. Make two further washes in cacodylate buffer.
5. Remove cacodylate and replace with 1 to 2 mℓ 2% osmium tetroxide in 0.2 M collidine buffer. Leave for 1 hr on the rotor.
6. With a pasteur pipette transfer the osmium tetroxide into an osmium residue bottle.
7. Wash three times with sodium cacodylate buffer as above.

Osmium tetroxide-collidine buffer[223] is prepared by mixing 24 mℓ 2% OsO_4 in distilled water, 12 mℓ 0.2 M collidine buffer, 1.8 g sucrose, and four drops of 1% $CaCl_2$.

Collidine buffer is prepared by adding 2.67 mℓ of 2, 4, 6 trimethylpyridine to 50.0 mℓ double-distilled water plus 9 mℓ 1.0 N-HCl and diluting to 100 mℓ with double-distilled water. Adjust pH to 7.4.

4. Dehydration

Dehydrate the specimen in the tube in the slow speed rotor in a fume cupboard with progressively increasing concentrations of ethyl alcohol as follows:

1. 10 min with 30% acetone.
2. 10 min with 50% acetone.
3. 10 min with 70% acetone (can be left overnight).
4. Four changes each for 10 min with 100% acetone.

5. Infiltration with Embedding Media

Still using the rotor in the fume cupboard, infiltrate with Spurr's low viscosity embedding media[224] (Polysciences, Inc., Warrington, Penn.) as follows:

1. 1 hr in mixture of one part of Spurr's media plus two parts of 100% acetone.
2. 1 hr in mixture of two parts Spurr's media plus one part of 100% acetone.
3. Overnight in 100% Spurr's media at room temperature.

6. Embedding

In the fume cupboard, infiltrated specimens are embedded in fresh Spurr's embedding media in Beem capsules (Polaron Equipment Ltd., Watford, England). Specimens are positioned for sectioning in the desired plane. A paper label giving details in pencil is also positioned inside the capsule.

Specimens in Beem capsules on a tray are placed in an oven at 70°C for hardening of embedding media. About 4 hr are necessary.

Hardened blocks are removed by cutting the Beem capsules with a scalpel and stored.

7. Sectioning

The block is trimmed close with a stainless-steel razor blade and cut on an ultra microtome into sections 1 μm thick. These are stained with methylene blue and the features examined under a light microscope.

Particular features of the block can now be pinpointed for further study in the electron microscope. When these features are decided upon, the block is further trimmed around them.

Sections of the required thickness (100 nm or less) are cut with a glass knife, floated out on a water bath, and transferred to a grid for staining with lead citrate or uranyl acetate prior to examination under the electron microscope.

8. Ultrastructural Age Changes

Examination of the glomerulus of the old rat shows thickening of the basement membrane and fusion of the podocyte processes.[225] The proximal tubules also reveal marked age-related thickening of basement membranes.[3,226] These changes do not develop to the same extent in hypophysectomized or food-restricted rats.[3]

The aortic tunica media of old rats contain hypertrophic muscle cells and thin elastic laminae with branched fibers.[216] These changes are less marked in hypophysectomized rats.[227]

Associated with atrophy of hind leg muscles is progressive fiber degeneration with eventual phagocytosis and varying accumulation of lipid vacuoles, lipofuscin pigment, and autophagic vacuoles.[42,228] Hypophysectomized rat muscles of the same age possess relatively normal morphology with little or no degeneration.[42]

B. Light Microscopy

The techniques of light microscopy are well described in a number of texts.[229-232] The methods currently used in the authors' laboratory are summarized.

1. Fixation
a. Perfusion

The same perfusion procedure may be used as previously described above with 10% formol saline substituted for 3% glutaraldehyde.

In a number of tissues it is possible to use glutaraldehyde-perfused material for paraffin-embedded light microscopy such as lungs and brain. However, it is not satisfactory for kidney.

In this case, one kidney may be removed under anesthesia (after ligating the renal artery) and then immersed in formol saline for light microscopy, while the second kidney may be perfused with glutaraldehyde as for electron microscopy.

b. Immersion

The rat is killed with an overdose of pentobarbital sodium (6 mg/100 g of body weight) and the organ removed as soon as breathing stops.

For example, the kidney is removed, quickly weighed, bisected longitudinally, and placed in 10% formol saline at room temperature for 24 hr or longer. Organs may be stored in formol saline for long periods providing the fixative is changed every 3 months. Neutral buffered 10% formalin (3.5 g NaH_2PO_4, 6.5 g Na_2HPO_4, 100 mℓ of formalin, and 900 mℓ of distilled water) is recommended by many workers because it prevents the formation of the post-mortem precipitate which occurs in formol saline as it becomes acid.

Organs may be immersed in special fixatives, such as Helly's fixative for muscle.

c. Freezing

Where chemical fixatives may distort the structure excessively for the study in question, frozen sections can be cut from fresh tissue frozen on a microtome with the aid of carbon dioxide.

2. Dehydration

The specimen, along with a pencil-marked label, is transferred into a tissue capsule (Peel-a-way Scientific, South El-Monte, Calif.) and washed in running water for 12 to 24 hr.

The specimen (in the tissue capsule) is dehydrated by passing through a series of alcohols of increasing concentration (70% ethanol, 1 hr; 95% ethanol, 1 hr; 100% [absolute] ethanol, 1 hr).

3. Clearing

Alcohol is removed by immersing the specimen (in the tissue capsule) in chloroform for 1 hr, followed by chloroform overnight.

4. Infiltration with Paraffin

The tissue capsule is opened in a fume cupboard and the chloroform is allowed to evaporate.

With forceps the specimen and its label are transferred to a vial containing molten Paraplast® Plus (Sherwood Medical Industries, St. Louis, Mo.) at 58°C and left for 2 hr, Paraplast® changed, and left a further 2 hr.

5. Embedding

Molten Paraplast® is poured into a disposable plastic-tissue embedding mold (Peel-a-way, South El-Monte, Calif.).

With heated forceps the specimen is quickly transferred from the vial to the mold, so that no solidification of wax occurs on the specimen. The specimen is positioned for cutting by pressing into the Paraplast® which is beginning to solidify on the floor of the mold. The label is pressed part way into the solidifying wax at the surface of the mold.

The mold is refrigerated at 4°C until hard. This requires about 1 hr. When solid, the mold is torn off and the labeled blocks stored.

6. Section Cutting

Sections 5 to 6 μm thick are cut on a rotary microtome, floated onto a water bath at 48°C, and thence onto a labeled microscope slide. A few drops of horse serum added to the water bath of volume 3 ℓ adheres sections to the slide.

Slides are stored on end in an air oven at 58°C overnight to drain off excess Paraplast®.

7. Staining

Tissues may be stained with a general stain such as hematoxylin and eosin, or a specific stain such as Periodic acid Schiff (PAS)[233] stain for kidney, Nissl[234] stain for brain, Gomori aldehyde fuchsin[235] stain followed by a counterstain of picro-indigo-carmine for aorta, or Masson trichrome[236] stain for muscle.

8. Microscopic Age Changes

In the kidney of the old rat, the most striking age-associated changes[13,25,26,237,238] are proteinaceous casts in tubules, reduced numbers of glomeruli per field, increased glomerular diameter, thickening of the basement membranes of the glomerulus and proximal tubules, and thickening of Bowman's capsule. In hypophysectomized[3] and in food-restricted[11,13,15,157] rats, proteinaceous casts are seen only rarely and other changes are not so well developed even in extremely old animals of 1300 days.

Age-related thickening of the tunica media of the thoracic aorta and associated hypertrophy of muscle cells[216] occurs at a slower rate in hypophysectomized or food-restricted rats compared with *ad libitum* fed controls.[4,227]

Skeletal muscles in the hind leg of old rats undergoing atrophy[239] exhibit large variation in muscle fiber diameter, marked fiber degeneration, and increased collagenous fibrosis.[42] Hypophysectomized rats display normal muscle morphology even in extreme old age.[42]

IX. CONCLUSION

In the rat it is possible with the use of classical techniques such as hypophysectomy, food restriction, and hypothalamic lesioning to demonstrate changes in the rate of aging in a number of tissues (tail tendon, kidney, muscle, and artery) when studied by relatively simple techniques. Such methods permit investigation of the role of hypothalamic and pituitary factors in aging.

REFERENCES

1. **Everitt, A. V. and Cavanagh, L. M.,** The ageing process in the hypophysectomized rat, *Gerontologia,* 11, 198, 1965.
2. **Verzár, F. and Spichtin, H.,** The role of the pituitary in the aging of collagen, *Gerontologia,* 12, 48, 1966.
3. **Everitt, A. V.,** Hypophysectomy and aging in the rat, in *Hypothalamus, Pituitary and Aging,* Everitt, A. V. and Burgess, J. A., Eds., Charles C Thomas, Springfield, Ill., 1976, chap. 4.
4. **Everitt, A. V., Seedsman, J., and Jones, F.,** The effects of hypophysectomy and continuous food restriction, begun at ages 70 and 400 days, on collagen ageing, proteinuria, incidence of pathology and longevity in the male rat, *Mech. Ageing Dev.,* 12, 161, 1980.
5. **Mulinos, M. G. and Pomerantz, L.,** Pseudo-hypophysectomy, a condition resembling hypophysectomy produced by malnutrition, *J. Nutr.,* 19, 493, 1940.
6. **Campbell, G. A., Kurcz, M., Marshall, S., and Meites, J.,** Effects of starvation in rats on serum levels of follicle stimulating hormone, luteinizing hormone, thyrotropin, growth hormone and prolactin; response to LH releasing hormone and thyrotropin releasing hormone, *Endocrinology,* 100, 580, 1977.
7. **McCay, C. M., Maynard, L. A., Sperling, G., and Barnes, L. L.,** Retarded growth, life span, ultimate body size and age changes in the albino rat after feeding diets restricted in calories, *J. Nutr.,* 18, 1, 1939.
8. **McCay, C. M., Sperling, G., and Barnes, L. L.,** Growth, aging, chronic diseases and life span in rats, *Arch. Biochem.,* 2, 469, 1943.
9. **Carlson, A. J. and Hoelzel, F.,** Apparent prolongation of the life-span of rats by intermittent fasting, *J. Nutr.,* 31, 363, 1946.
10. **Riesen, W. H., Herbst, E. J., Walliker, C., and Elvehjem, C. A.,** The effect of restricted calorie intake on the longevity of rats, *Am. J. Physiol.,* 148, 614, 1947.
11. **Saxton, J. A., Jr. and Kimball, J. C.,** Relation of nephrosis and diseases of albino rats to age and to modifications of diet, *Arch. Pathol.,* 32, 951, 1941.
12. **Ross, M. H.,** Protein, calories and life expectancy, *Fed. Proc. Fed. Am. Soc. Exp. Biol.,* 18, 1190, 1959.
13. **Bras, G. and Ross, M. H.,** Kidney disease and nutrition in the rat, *Toxicol. Appl. Pharmacol.,* 6, 247, 1964.
14. **Ross, M. H. and Bras, G.,** Lasting influence of early caloric restriction in prevalence of neoplasms in the rat, *J. Natl. Cancer Inst.,* 47, 1905, 1971.
15. **Berg, B. N. and Simms, H. S.,** Nutrition and longevity in the rat. II. Longevity and onset of disease with different levels of food intake, *J. Nutr.,* 71, 255, 1960.
16. **Chvapil, M. and Hrůza, A.,** The influence of ageing and undernutrition on chemical contractility and relaxation of collagen fibres in rats, *Gerontologia,* 3, 341, 1959.
17. **Everitt, A. V.,** Food intake, growth and the ageing of collagen in rat tail tendon, *Gerontologia,* 17, 98, 1971.
18. **Holečková, E., Fabry, P., and Poupa, O.** Studies in the adaptation of metabolism. VIII. The latent period of explanted tissue of rats adapted to intermittent starvation, *Physiol. Bohemoslov.,* 8, 15, 1959.
19. **Segall, P. E., Ooka, H., Rose, K., and Timiras, P. S.,** Neural and endocrine development after chronic tryptophan deficiency in rats. I. Brain monoamine and pituitary responses, *Mech. Ageing Dev.,* 7, 1, 1978.
20. **Ooka, H., Segall, P. E., and Timiras, P. S.,** Neural and endocrine development after chronic tryptophan deficiency. II. Pituitary-thyroid axis, *Mech. Ageing Dev.,* 7, 19, 1978.
21. **Segall, P. E.,** Interrelations of dietary and hormonal effects in aging, *Mech. Ageing Dev.,* 9, 515, 1979.
22. **Kennedy, G. C.,** Effects of old age and overnutrition on the kidney, *Br. Med. Bull.,* 13, 67, 1957.
23. **Clemens, J. A. and Bennett, D. R.,** Do aging changes in the preoptic area contribute to loss of cyclic endocrine function? *J. Gerontol.,* 32, 19, 1977.
24. **Mitruka, B. M., Rawnsley, H. M., and Vadehra, D. V.,** *Animals for Medical Research. Models for the Study of Human Disease,* John Wiley & Sons, New York, 1976, chap. 12.
25. **Simms, H. S. and Berg, B. N.,** Longevity and the onset of lesions in male rats, *J. Gerontol.,* 12, 244, 1957.
26. **Berg, B. N.,** Longevity studies in rats. II. Pathology of ageing rats, in *Pathology of Laboratory Rats and Mice,* Cotchin, E. and Roe, F. J. C., Eds., Blackwell Scientific, Oxford, 1967, 749.
27. **Berg, B. N.,** Pathology and aging, in *Hypothalamus, Pituitary and Aging,* Everitt, A. V. and Burgess, J. A., Eds., Charles C Thomas, Springfield, Ill., chap. 3.

28. **Burek, J. D.,** *Pathology of Aging Rats,* CRC Press, Boca Raton, Fla., 1978.
29. **Cohen, B. J., Anver, M. R., Ringler, D. H., and Adelman, R. C.,** Age-associated pathological changes in male rats, *Fed. Proc. Fed. Am. Soc. Exp. Biol.,* 37, 2848, 1978.
30. **Hollander, C. F.,** Animal models for aging and cancer research, *J. Natl. Cancer Inst.,* 51, 3, 1973.
31. **Coleman, G. L., Barthold, S. W., Osbaldiston, G. W., Foster, S. J., and Jonas, A. M.,** Pathological changes during aging in barrier-reared Fischer 344 male rats, *J. Gerontol.,* 32, 258, 1977.
32. **Everitt, A. V. and Cavanagh, L. M.,** The effect of chronic lung disease on the course of ageing in the male rat, *Gerontologia,* 8, 1, 1963.
33. **Lindsey, J. R., Baker, H. J., Overeash, R. G., Cassell, G. H., and Hunt, C. E.,** Murine chronic, respiratory disease. Significance as a research complication and experimental production with *Mycoplasma pulmonis, Am. J. Pathol.,* 64, 675, 1971.
34. **Innes, J. R. M., Garner, F. M., and Stookey, J. L.,** Respiratory disease in rats, in *Pathology of Laboratory Rats and Mice,* Cotchin, E. and Roe, F. J. C., Eds., Blackwell Scientific, Oxford, 1967, 229.
35. **Nelson, J. B.,** Respiratory infections of rats and mice with emphasis on indigenous mycoplasma, in *Pathology of Laboratory Rats and Mice,* Cotchin, E. and Roe, F. J. C., Eds., Blackwell Scientific, Oxford, 1967, 259.
36. **Koyama, R.,** Simple method of hypophysectomy in rats (Koyama's external auditory canal method), *Endocrinol. Jpn.,* 4, 321, 1962.
37. **Everitt, A. V., Olsen, G. G., and Burrows, G. R.,** The effect of hypophysectomy on the aging of collagen fibers in tail tendon of the rat, *J. Gerontol.,* 23, 333, 1968.
38. **Delbridge, L. and Everitt, A. V.,** The effect of hypophysectomy and age on the stabilization of labile cross-links in collagen, *Exp. Gerontol.,* 7, 413, 1972.
39. **Everitt, A. V. and Delbridge, L.,** The role of the pituitary and the thyroid in the aging of collagen in rat tail tendon, in *Hypothalamus, Pituitary and Aging,* Everitt, A. V. and Burgess, J. A., Eds., Charles C Thomas, Springfield, Ill., 1976, chap. 11.
40. **Jones, E. C. and Krohn, P. L.,** The effect of hypophysectomy on age changes in the ovaries of mice, *J. Endocrinol.,* 21, 497, 1961.
41. **Everitt, A. V. and Duvall, L. K.,** The delayed onset of proteinuria in ageing hypophysectomized rats, *Nature (London),* 205, 1015, 1965.
42. **Ficarra, M. A. and Everitt, A. V.,** Morphological age changes in rat skeletal muscle. Effect of hypophysectomy, submitted for publication.
43. **Asling, C. W., Simpson, M. E., Li, C. H., and Evans, H. M.,** The effects of chronic administration of thyroxine to hypophysectomized rats on their skeletal growth, maturation and response to growth hormone. *Anat. Record,* 119, 101, 1954.
44. **Bilder, G. E. and Denckla, W. D.,** Restoration of the ability to reject xenografts and clear carbon after hypophysectomy of adult rats, *Mech. Ageing Dev.,* 6, 153, 1957.
45. **Sato, M. and Yoneda, S.,** An efficient method for transauricular hypophysectomy in rats, *Acta Endocrinol. (Copenhagen),* 51, 43, 1966.
46. **Falconi, G. and Rossi, G. L.** Transauricular hypophysectomy in rats and mice, *Endocrinology,* 74, 301, 1964.
47. **Zarrow, M. X., Yochim, J. M., and McCarthy, J. L.,** *Experimental Endocrinology. A Sourcebook of Basic Techniques,* Academic Press, New York, 1964, chap. 10.
48. **Smith, P. E.,** Hypophysectomy and replacement therapy in the rat, *Am. J. Anat.,* 45, 205, 1930.
49. **Ingle, D. J. and Griffith, J. Q.,** Surgery of the rat, in *The Rat in Laboratory Investigation,* 2nd ed., Farris, E. J. and Griffith, J. Q., Eds., Lippincott, Philadelphia, 1949, chap. 16.
50. **Brolin, S. E., Carstensen, H., and Hellman, B.,** Remarks on the performance and control of hypophysectomy in the rat, *Acta Endocrinol. (Copenhagen),* 22, 68, 1956.
51. **Bahner, F. and von Graff, H.** The Technique and results of hypophysectomy in the mouse, *Acta Endocrinol. (Copenhagen),* 24, 333, 1957.
52. **Young, S.,** Experiences with hypophysectomy in mice: histology of pituitary remnants, *Br. J. Cancer,* 13, 208, 1959.
53. **Young, S. and Fraser, L. F.,** Experiences with hypophysectomy in mice: criteria of complete removal, *Br. J. Cancer,* 14, 285, 1960.
54. **Bolkainy, El M. N.,** Technique for hypophysectomy of the mouse, *J. Natl. Cancer Inst.,* 30, 1077, 1963.
55. **Lostroh, A. and Jordan, C. W., Jr.,** Improved procedure for hypophysectomy of the mouse, *Proc. Soc. Exp. Biol. Med.,* 90, 267, 1955.
56. **Everitt, A. V.,** The hypothalamic-pituitary control of ageing and age-related pathology, *Exp. Gerontol.,* 8, 265, 1973.

57. **Everitt, A. V.,** Conclusion: aging and its hypothalamic-pituitary control, in *Hypothalamus, Pituitary and Aging,* Everitt, A. V. and Burgess, J. A., Eds., Charles C Thomas, Springfield, Ill., 1976, chap. 34.

58. **Everitt, A. V. and Burgess, J. A.,** Growth Hormone and aging, in *Hypothalamus, Pituitary and Aging,* Everitt, A. V. and Burgess, J. A., Eds., Charles C Thomas, Springfield, Ill., 1976, chap. 23.

59. **Everitt, A. V.,** Pituitary function and aging, in *Aging: A Challenge to Science and Social Policy,* Vol. 1, Danon, D. and Shock, N. W., Eds., Oxford University Press, Oxford, 1981, 249.

60. **Everitt, A. V. and Porter, B.,** Nutrition and aging, in *Hypothalamus, Pituitary and Aging,* Everitt, A. V. and Burgess, J. A., Eds., Charles C Thomas, Springfield, Ill., 1976, chap. 30.

61. **Bouillé, C. and Assenmacher, I.,** Effects of starvation on adrenal cortical function in the rabbit, *Endocrinology,* 87, 1390, 1970.

62. **Valzelli, L.,** The isolation syndrome in mice, *Psychopharmacologia,* 31, 305, 1973.

63. **Gardiner, S. M. and Bennett, T.,** Factors affecting the development of isolation-induced hypertension in rats, *Med. Biol.,* 56, 277, 1978.

64. **Bennett, T. and Gardiner, S. M.,** Corticosteriod involvement in the changes in noradrenergic responsiveness of tissues from rats made hypertensive by short term isolation, *Br. J. Pharmacol.,* 64, 129, 1978.

65. **Fiala, B., Snow, F. M., and Greenough, W. T.,** "Impoverished" rats weigh more than "enriched" rats because they eat more, *Dev. Psychobiol.,* 10, 537, 1977.

66. **Drori, D. and Folman, Y.,** Environmental effects on longevity in the male rat: exercise, mating, castration and restricted feeding, *Exp. Gerontol.,* 11, 25, 1976.

67. **Mitchell, J. S. and Keesey, R. E.,** The effects of lateral hypothalamic lesions and castration upon the body weight and composition of male rats, *Behav. Biol.,* 11, 69, 1974.

68. **Finkelstein, J. W., Roffwarg, H. P., Boyar, R. M., Kream, J., and Hellman, L.,** Age-related change in the twenty-four-hour spontaneous secretion of growth hormone, *J. Clin. Endocrinol.,* 35, 665, 1972.

69. **Aschheim, P.,** Aging in the hypothalamic-hypophyseal ovarian axis in the rat, in *Hypothalamus, Pituitary and Aging,* Everitt, A. V. and Burgess, J. A., Eds., Charles C Thomas, Springfield, Ill., 1976, chap. 19.

70. **Simpkins, J. W., Mueller, G. P., Huang, H. H., and Meites, J.,** Evidence for depressed catecholamine and enhanced serotonin metabolism in aging male rats; possible relation to gonadotropin secretion, *Endocrinology,* 97, 543, 1975.

71. **McPherson, J. C., Costoff, A., Mahesh, V. B.,** Effects of aging on the hypothalamic-hypophyseal-gonadal axis in female rats, *Fertil. Steril.,* 28, 1365, 1977.

72. **Turkington, M. R. and Everitt, A. V.,** The neurohypophysis and aging with special reference to the antidiuretic hormone, in *Hypothalamus, Pituitary and Aging,* Everitt, A. V. and Burgess, J. A., Eds., Charles C Thomas, Springfield, Ill., 1976, chap. 7.

73. **Everitt, A. V.,** The effect of pituitary growth hormone on the aging male rat, *J. Gerontol.,* 14, 415, 1959.

74. **Aschheim, P.,** La réactivation de l'ovaire des rattes séniles en oestrus permanent au moyen d'hormones gonadotropes ou de la mise à l'obscruité, *C.R. Acad. Sci.,* 260, 5627, 1965.

75. **Friedman, S. M. and Friedman, C. L.,** Effect of posterior pituitary extracts on the life span of old rats, *Nature (London),* 200, 237, 1963.

76. **Friedman, S. M. and Friedman, C. L.,** Prolonged treatment with posterior pituitary powder in aged rats, *Exp. Gerontol.,* 1, 37, 1964.

77. **Friedman, S. M., Friedman, C. L., and Nakashima, M.,** Effect of pitressin on old age changes of salt and water metabolism in the rat, *Am. J. Physiol.,* 199, 35, 1960.

78. **Bodanszky, M. and Engel, S. L.,** Oxytocin and the life-span of male rats, *Nature (London),* 210, 751, 1966.

79. **Christian, J. J.,** Effects of β^{1-24} synthetic corticotrophin on reproductive tract and kidneys of immature mice, *Acta Endocrinol. (Copenhagen),* 55, 62, 1967.

80. **Christian, J. J.,** Anterior pituitary in relation to renal disease, in *Hypothalamus, Pituitary and Aging,* Everitt, A. V. and Burgess, J. A., Eds., Charles C Thomas, Springfield, Ill., 1976, chap. 16.

81. **Silberberg, R.,** The pituitary in relation to skeletal aging and disease, in *Hypothalamus, Pituitary and Aging,* Everitt, A. V. and Burgess, J. A., Eds., Charles C Thomas, Springfield, Ill., 1976, chap. 12.

82. **Reinhardt, W. O. and Li, C. H.,** Experimental production of arthritis in rats by hypophyseal growth hormone, *Science,* 117, 295, 1953.

83. **Moon, H. D., Simpson, M. E., Li, C. H., and Evans, H. M.,** Neoplasms in rats treated with pituitary growth hormone, I, *Cancer Res.,* 10, 297, 1950.

83a. **Moon, H. D., Simpson, M. E., Li, C. H., and Evans, H. M.,** Neoplasms in rats treated with pituitary growth hormone, II, *Cancer Res.,* 10, 364, 1950.
83b. **Moon, H. D., Simpson, M. E., Li, C. H., and Evans, H. M.,** Neoplasms in rats treated with pituitary growth hormone, III, *Cancer Res.,* 10, 549, 1950.
 84. **Selye, H.,** Role of somatotrophic hormone in the production of malignant nephrosclerosis, periarteritis nodosa and hypertensive disease, *Br. Med. J.,* 1, 263, 1951.
 85. **Roth, G.,** Hormone receptor and responsiveness changes during aging: genetic modulation, in *Genetic Effects on Aging,* Bergsma, D. and Harrison, D. E., Eds., Alan R. Liss, New York, 1978, 365.
 86. **Emerson, J. D.,** Development of resistance to growth promoting action of anterior pituitary growth hormone, *Am. J. Physiol.,* 181, 390, 1955.
 87. **Jelinkova, M. and Hruza, Z.,** Decreased effect of norepinephrine and growth hormone on the release of free fatty acids in old rats, *Physiol. Bohemoslov.,* 13, 327, 1964.
 88. **Hruza, Z.,** Lipid metabolism and aging. Endocrine role, in *Hypothalamus, Pituitary and Aging,* Everitt, A. V. and Burgess, J. A., Eds., Charles C Thomas, Springfield, Ill., 1976, chap. 24.
 89. **Sorrentino, R. N. and Florini, J. R.,** Variations among individual mice in binding of growth hormone and insulin to membranes from animals of different ages, *Exp. Aging Res.,* 2, 191, 1976.
 90. **Thanki, K. H. and Steinberger, A.,** Effect of age and hypophysectomy on FSH binding by rat testes, *Andrologia,* 10, 195, 1978.
 91. **Hess, G. D. and Riegle, G. D.,** Effect of chronic ACTH stimulation on adrenocortical function in young and aged rats, *Am. J. Physiol.,* 222, 1458, 1972.
 92. **Miller, A. E. and Riegle, G. D.,** Serum testosterone and testicular response to HCG in young and aged male rats, *J. Gerontol.,* 33, 197, 1975.
 93. **Green, J. A.,** Some effects of advancing age on the histology and reactivity of the mouse ovary, *Anat. Record,* 129, 333, 1957.
 94. **Clemens, J. A., Amenomori, Y., Jenkins, T., and Meites, J.,** Effects of hypothalamic stimulation, hormones and drugs on ovarian function in old female rats, *Proc. Soc. Exp. Biol. Med.,* 132, 561, 1969.
 95. **Clemens, J. A. and Bennett, D. R.,** Do aging changes in the preoptic area contribute to loss of cyclic endocrine function? *J. Gerontol.,* 32, 19, 1977.
 96. **Anand, B. K.,** Nervous regulation of food intake, *Physiol. Rev.,* 41, 67, 1961.
 97. **Anand, B. K. and Brobeck, J. R.,** Hypothalamic control of food intake in rats and cats, *Yale J. Biol. Med.,* 24, 123, 1951.
 98. **Ballie, P. and Morrison, S. D.,** The nature of the suppression of food intake by lateral hypothalamic lesions in rats, *J. Physiol. (London),* 165, 227, 1963.
 99. **Gray, R. H. and Everitt, A. V.,** Hypophagia and hypodipsia induced by unilateral hypothalamic lesions in the rat, *Am. J. Physiol.,* 219, 398, 1970.
100. **Morrison, S. D. and Mayer, J.,** Effect of sham operations in the hypothalamus on food and water intake in the rat, *Am. J. Physiol.,* 191, 255, 1957.
101. **de Groot, J.** *The Rat Forebrain in Stereotoxic Coordinates, Tweede Raeks,* Decl. L11, No. 4, N. V. Noord-Hollandsche Uitgevers Maatschciapprij, Amsterdam, 1959.
102. **Albe-Fessard, D., Stutinsky, F., and Libouban, S.,** *Atlas Stéréotaxique du Diencéphale du Rat Blanc,* 2. ed., Centre National de la Recherche Scientifique, Paris, 1971.
103. **Sherwood, N. M. and Timiras, P. S.,** *A Stereotaxic Atlas of the Developing Rat Brain,* University of California Press, Berkeley, 1970.
104. **Sadman, L. R., Angevine, B. J., and Pierce, T. E.,** *Atlas of the Mouse Brain and Spinal Cord,* A Commonwealth Fund Book, Harvard University Press, Cambridge, Massachusetts, 1971.
105. **Lehmann, A.,** *Atlas Stereotaxique du Cerveau de la Souris,* Editions du Centre National de la Recherche Scientifique, Paris, 1974.
106. **Powell, E. W.,** A rapid method of intracranial electrode localization using unstained, frozen sections. *EEG Clin. Neurophysiol.,* 17, 432, 1964.
107. **Brobeck, J. R.,** Mechanism of the development of obesity in animals with hypothalamic lesions, *Physiol. Rev.,* 26, 541, 1946.
108. **Brobeck, J. R., Tepperman, J., and Long, C. N. H.,** Experimental hypothalamic hyperphagia in the albino rat, *Yale J. Biol. Med.,* 15, 831, 1943.
109. **Kennedy, G. C.,** The hypothalamic control of food intake in rats, *Proc. Roy. Soc. B.,* 137, 535, 1950.
110. **Hetherington, S. W. and Ranson, S. W.,** Hypothalamic lesions and adiposity in the rat, *Anat. Rec.,* 78, 149, 1940.
111. **Pasley, J. N. and Powell, E. W.,** Reproductive organs, obesity and central hypothalamic nuclei in the male mouse, *Psychoneuroendocrinology,* 3, 311, 1979.

112. **Koletsky, S.**, Pathologic findings and laboratory data in a new strain of obese hypertensive rats, *Am. J. Pathol.*, 80, 129, 1975.
113. **Schimert, G. C.**, Cardiovascular consequences of obesity, *Triangle*, 13, 31, 1974.
114. **Mann, G. V.**, The influence of obesity on health, I, *New Engl. J. Med.*, 291, 178, 1974.
114a. **Mann, G. V.**, The influence of obesity on health, II, *New Engl. J. Med.*, 291, 226, 1974.
115. **Stunkard, A. J.**, Nutrition, aging and obesity, in *Nutrition, Longevity and Aging*, Rockstein, M. and Sussman, L. M., Eds., Academic Press, New York, 1976, 253.
116. **Bray, G. A. and York, D. A.**, Genetically transmitted obesity in rodents, *Physiol. Rev.*, 51, 598, 1971.
117. **Zucker, L. M.**, Hereditary obesity in the rat associated with hyperlipemia, *Ann. N.Y. Acad. Sci.*, 131, 447, 1965.
118. **Heston, W. E. and Vlahakis, G.**, Genetic obesity and neoplasia, *J. Natl. Cancer Inst.*, 29, 197, 1962.
119. **Kennedy, G. C.**, The development with age of hypothalamic restraint upon the appetite of the rat, *J. Endocrinol.*, 16, 9, 1957.
120. **Blumenthal, H. T.**, Preface, in *The Regulatory Role of the Nervous System in Aging, Interdisciplinary Topics in Gerontology*, Vol. 7, S. Karger, Basel, 1970.
121. **Comfort, A.**, *The Biology of Senescence*, 3rd ed., Churchill Livingstone, Edinburgh, 1979, chap. 9.
122. **Samorajski, T.**, Central neurotransmitter substances and aging—a review. *J. Am. Geriatr. Soc.*, 25, 337, 1977.
123. **Finch, C. E.**, Neuroendocrine and autonomic aspects of aging, in *Handbook of the Biology of Aging*, Finch, C. E. and Hayfleck, L., Eds., Van Nostrand Reinhold Company, New York, 1977, chap. 11.
124. **Everitt, A. V. and Huang, C. Y.**, Hypothalamus, neuroendocrine and autonomic nervous system in aging, in *Handbook on Mental Health and Aging*, Birren, J. and Sloane, R. B., Eds., Prentice Hall, Englewood Cliffs, N.J., 1980, chap. 5.
125. **Everitt, A. V.**, Neuroendocrine theories of ageing, in *Ageing in Australia*, Donald, J. M., Everitt, A. V., and Wheeler, P. J., Eds., Australian Association of Gerontology, Sydney, 1979, 93.
126. **Everitt, A. V.**, The neuroendocrine system and aging, *Gerontology*, 26, 108, 1980.
127. **Everitt, A. V.**, Pacemaker mechanisms in aging and the diseases of senescence, in *Handbook of the Diseases of Aging*, Blumenthal, H. T., Ed., Van Nostrand Reinhold Company, New York, in press.
128. **Moore, R. Y.**, Central neural control of circadian rhythms, in *Frontiers in Neuroendocrinology*, Ganong, W. F. and Martini, L., Eds., Raven Press, New York, 1978, chap. 7.
129. **Krieger, D. T.**, Factors influencing the circadian periodicity of ACTH and corticosteroids, *Med. Clin. N. Am.*, 62, 251, 1978.
130. **Everitt, A. V.**, The nature and measurement of aging, in *Hypothalamus, Pituitary and Aging*, Everitt, A. V. and Burgess, J. A., Eds., Charles C Thomas, Springfield, Ill., 1976, chap. 5.
131. **Everitt, A. V.**, The senescent loss of body weight in male rats, *J. Gerontol.*, 12, 382, 1957.
132. **Robertson, T. B. and Ray, L. A.**, Experimental studies on growth. X. The late growth and senescence of the white mouse, *J. Biol. Chem.*, 37, 377, 1919.
133. **Lindop, P. J.**, Growth rate, lifespan and causes of death in SAS/4 mice, *Gerontologia*, 5, 193, 1961.
134. **Berg, B. N. and Harmison, C. R.**, Growth, disease and aging in the rat, *J. Gerontol.*, 12, 370, 1957.
135. **Everitt, A. V.**, The urinary excretion of protein, non-protein nitrogen, uric acid and creatinine in ageing male rats, *Gerontologia*, 2, 33, 1958.
136. **Everitt, A. V.**, The change in food and water consumption and in faeces and urine production in ageing male rats, *Gerontologia*, 2, 21, 1958.
137. **Verzár, F.**, Aging of the collagen fiber, *Int. Rev. Connect. Tissue Res.*, 2, 243, 1964.
138. **Bailey, A. J., Robins, S. P., and Balian, G.**, Biological significance of the intermolecular crosslinks of collagen, *Nature (London)*, 251, 105, 1974.
139. **Hall, D. A.**, *The Ageing of Connective Tissue*, Academic Press, London, 1976.
140. **Verzár, F.**, Veränderungen der thermoelastischen Eigenschaften von Sehnenfasern bei Alten, *Experientia*, 11, 230, 1955.
141. **Boros-Farkas, M. and Everitt, A. V.**, Comparative studies of age tests on collagen fibres, *Gerontologia*, 13, 37, 1967.
142. **Elden, H. R. and Boucek, R. J.**, Investigation of the aging process by physical-chemical means, in *Biological Aspects of Aging*, Shock, N. W. Ed., Columbia University Press, New York, 1962, 34.

143. **Olsen, G. G. and Everitt, A. V.**, Retardation of the aging process in collagen fibres from the tail tendon of the old hypophysectomized rat, *Nature (London)*, 206, 307, 1965.

144. **Harrison, D. E. and Archer, J. R.**, Measurement of changes in mouse tail collagen with age: temperature dependence and procedural details, *Exp. Gerontol.*, 13, 75, 1978.

145. **Everitt, A. V., Porter, B. D., and Steele, M.**, Dietary, caging and temperature factors in the aging of collagen fibres in rat tail tendon, *Gerontology*, 27, 37, 1981.

146. **Brocas, J. and Verzár, F.**, Measurement of isometric tension during thermic contraction of collagen fibres, *Gerontologia*, 5, 223, 1961.

147. **Delbridge, L. and Everitt, A. V.**, Age changes in the polymer composition of collagen using molecular sieve chromatrography, *Gerontologia*, 18, 169, 1972.

148. **Bailey, A. J.**, Stabilization of the intramolecular crosslink of collagen with ageing, *Gerontologia*, 15, 65, 1969.

149. **Robins, S. P., Shimokomaki, M., and Bailey, A. J.**, Chemistry of the collagen cross-links, *Biochem. J.*, 131, 771, 1973.

150. **Delbridge, L., Everitt, A. V., and Steele, M. G.**, The effect of acid phosphate on the solubility of collagen, *Conn. Tissue Res.*, 1, 311, 1972.

151. **Delbridge, L. and Everitt, A. V.**, The effect of hypophysectomy and age on the stabilization of labile cross-links in collagen, *Exp. Gerontol.*, 7, 413, 1972.

152. **Mechanic, G. L., Gallop, P. M., and Tanzer, M. L.**, The nature of crosslinking in collagens from mineralized tissues, *Biochem. Biophys. Res. Commun.*, 45, 644, 1971.

153. **Heikkinen, E. and Kulonen, E.**, Age factor in the maturation of collagen. Intramolecular linkages in mildly denatured collagen, *Experientia*, 20, 310, 1964.

154. **Berg, B. N.**, Spontaneous nephrosis with proteinuria, hyperglobulinemia, and hypercholesterolemia in the rat, *Proc. Soc. Exp. Biol. Med.*, 119, 417, 1965.

155. **Pesce, M. A. and Strande, C. S.**, A new micromethod for determination of protein in cerebrospinal fluid and urine, *Clin. Chem.*, 19, 1265, 1973.

156. **Everitt, A. V.**, The thyroid gland, metabolic rate and aging, in *Hypothalamus, Pituitary and Aging*, Everitt, A. V. and Burgess, J. A., Eds., Charles C Thomas, Springfield, Ill., 1976, chap. 26.

157. **Everitt, A. V. and Porter, B.**, Effects of calorie intake and dietary composition on the development of proteinuria, age-associated renal disease and longevity in the rat, *Gerontology*, in press.

158. **Foley, W. A., Jones, D. C. L., Osborn, G. K., and Kimeldorf, D. J.**, A renal lesion associated with diuresis in the aging Sprague Dawley rat, *Lab. Invest.*, 13, 439, 1964.

159. **Friedman, S. M., Friedman, C. L., and Nakashima, M.**, Adrenal-neurohypophyseal regulation of electrolytes and work performance age related changes in the rat, in *Endocrines and Aging*, Gitman, L., Ed., Charles C Thomas, Springfield, Ill., 1967, 142.

160. **Guzek, J. W. and Lesnik, H.**, The bioassay of vasopressin through its antidiuretic effect, *Endokrinologie*, 53, 201, 1968.

161. **Neumaster, T. D. and Ring, G. C.**, Creatinine excretion and its relation to whole body potassium and muscle mass in inbred rats, *J. Gerontol.*, 20, 379, 1964.

162. **Everitt, A. V. and Webb, C.**, The blood picture of the aging male rat, *J. Gerontol.*, 13, 255, 1958.

163. **Leuenberger, H. G. W. and Kunstyr, I.**, Gerontological data of C57BL/6J mice. II. Changes in blood counts in the course of natural aging, *J. Gerontol.*, 31, 648, 1976.

164. **Salatka, K., Kresge, D., Harris, L., Jr., Edelstein, D., and Ove, P.**, Rat serum protein changes with age, *Exp. Gerontol.*, 6, 25, 1971.

165. **Hrůza, Z. and Wachtlová, M.**, Decrease of cholesterol turnover in old rats, *Exp. Gerontol.*, 4, 245, 1969.

166. **Grad, B. and Hoffman, M. M.**, Thyroxine secretion rates and plasma cholesterol levels of young and old rats, *Am. J. Physiol.*, 182, 497, 1955.

167. **Reaven, G. M.**, Effect of age and sex on triglyceride metabolism in the rat, *J. Gerontol.*, 33, 368, 1978.

168. **Klimas, J. E.**, Oral glucose tolerance during the life-span of a colony of rats, *J. Gerontol.*, 23, 31, 1968.

169. **McBroom, M. J. and Weiss, A. K.**, A longitudinal and comparative study of the soft tissue calcium levels throughout the life-span of highly inbred rats, *J. Gerontol.*, 28, 143, 1973.

170. **Nachbaur, J., Clark, M. R., Provost, J. P., and Dancla, J. L.**, Variations of sodium, potassium, and chloride plasma levels in the rat with age and sex, *Lab. Anim. Sci.*, 27, 972, 1977.

171. **Lee, J. C., Karpeles, L. M., and Downing, S. E.**, Age-related changes of cardiac performance in male rats, *Am. J. Physiol.*, 222, 432, 1972.

172. **Medoff, H. S. and Bongiovanni, A. M.**, Age, sex and species variations on blood pressure in normal rats, *Am. J. Physiol.*, 143, 297, 1945.

173. **Berg, B. N. and Harmison, C. R.,** Blood pressure and heart size in aging rats, *J. Gerontol.,* 10, 416, 1955.

174. **Rothbaum, D. A., Shaw, D. J., Angel, C. S., and Shock, N. W.,** Cardiac performance in the unanesthetized senescent rat, *J. Gerontol.,* 28, 287, 1973.

175. **Baskin, S. I., Roberts, J., and Kendrick, Z.,** Effect of age on body weight, heart rate and blood pressure in pair-caged, male, Fischer 344 rats, *Age,* 2, 47, 1979.

176. **Berg, B. N.,** The electrocardiogram in aging rats, *J. Gerontol.,* 10, 420, 1955.

177. **Everitt, A. V.,** The electrocardiogram of the aging rat, *Gerontologia,* 2, 204, 1958.

178. **Jones, D. C., Osborn, G. K., and Kimeldorf, D. J.,** Cardiac arrhythmias in aging male rats, *Gerontologia,* 13, 211, 1967.

179. **Everitt, A. V.,** Systolic blood pressure and heart rate in relation to lung disease and life duration in male rats, *J. Gerontol.,* 12, 378, 1957.

180. **Finch, C. E., Foster, J. R., and Mirsky, A. E.,** Aging and the regulation of cell activities during exposure to cold, *J. Gen. Physiol.,* 54, 690, 1969.

181. **Rapaport, A.,** L'adaptation du comportement du rat jeune et âgé aux variations de la température ambiante I. Adaptation au froid, *Gerontologia,* 13, 14, 1967.

182. **Kibler, H. H. and Johnson, H. D.,** Temperature and longevity in male rats, *J. Gerontol.,* 21, 52, 1966.

183. **Eleftheriou, B. E.,** Changes with age in protein bound iodine (PBI) and body temperature in the mouse, *J. Gerontol.,* 30, 417, 1975.

184. **Leto, S., Kokkonen, G., and Barrows, C. H.,** Dietary proteins, life span and physiological and biochemical variables in female mice, *J. Gerontol.,* 31, 144, 1976.

185. **Denckla, W. D.,** Minimal O_2 consumption as an index of thyroid status: standardization of a method, *Endocrinology,* 93, 61, 1973.

186. **Denckla, W. D.,** Role of the pituitary and thyroid glands in the decline of minimal O_2 consumption with age, *J. Clin. Invest.,* 53, 572, 1974.

187. **Sacher, G. A.,** Life table modification and life prolongation, in *Handbook of the Biology of Aging,* Finch, C. E. and Hayflick, L., Eds., Van Nostrand Reinhold Company, New York, 1977, chap. 24.

188. **Simms, H. S.,** Longevity studies in rats. I. Relation between life span and age of onset of specific lesions, in *Pathology of Laboratory Rats and Mice,* Cotchin, E. and Roe, F. J. C., Eds., Blackwell Scientific, Oxford, 1967, chap. 22.

189. **Jones, D. C. and Kimeldorf, D. J.,** Life span measurements in the male rat, *J. Gerontol.,* 18, 316, 1963.

190. **Verzár, F.,** Discussion, in *The Lifespan of Animals. CIBA Foundation Colloquia on Aging,* Vol. 5, Wolstenholme, G. E. W. and O'Connor, M., Eds., Churchill, Livingstone, London, 1959, 82.

191. **Ross, M. H.,** Length of life and nutrition in the rat, *J. Nutr.,* 75, 197, 1961.

192. **Miller, D. S. and Payne, P. R.,** Longevity and protein intake, *Exp. Gerontol.,* 3, 231, 1968.

193. **Jacobs, B. B. and Huseby, R. A.,** Neoplasma occurring in aged Fischer rats, with special reference to testicular, uterine and thyroid tumors, *J. Natl. Cancer Inst.,* 39, 303, 1967.

194. **French, C. E., Ingram, R. H., Uram, J. A., Barron, G. P., and Swift, R. W.,** The influence of dietary fat and carbohydrate on growth and longevity in rats, *J. Nutr.,* 51, 329, 1953.

195. **Schroeder, H. A. and Mitchener, M.,** Life-term studies in rats: effects of aluminium, barium, beryllium, and tungsten, *J. Nutr.,* 105, 421, 1975.

196. **Schroeder, H. A., Balassa, J. J., and Vinton, W. H., Jr.,** Chromium, cadmium and lead in rats: effects on lifespan, tumors and tissue levels, *J. Nutr.,* 86, 51, 1965.

197. **French, C. E., Uram, J. A., Ingram, R. H., and Swift, R. W.,** The effects of high levels of terramycin and streptomycin on longevity in the rat, *J. Nutr.,* 54, 75, 1954.

198. **Sacher, G. A. and Duffy, P. H.,** Genetic relation of life span to metabolic rate for inbred mouse strains and their hybrids, *Fed. Proc. Fed. Am. Soc. Exp. Biol.,* 38, 184, 1979.

199. **Storer, J. B.,** Longevity and gross pathology at death in twenty-two inbred mouse strains, *J. Gerontol.,* 21, 204, 1966.

200. **Goodrick, C. L.,** Life-span and inheritance of longevity of inbred mice, *J. Gerontol.,* 30, 257, 1975.

201. **Fasting, M. F. W. and Blackmore, D. K.,** Life span of specified-pathogen-free (MRC category 4) mice and rats, *Lab. Anim.,* 5, 179, 1971.

202. **Cotchin, E. and Roe, F. J. C.,** *Pathology of Laboratory Rats and Mice,* Blackwell Scientific, Oxford, 1967.

203. **Berg, B. N. and Simms, H. S.,** Nutrition and longevity in the rat. III. Food restriction beyond 800 days. *J. Nutr.,* 74, 23, 1961.

204. **Thompson, S. W., Huseby, R. A., Fox, M. A., Davis, C. L., and Hunt, R. D.,** Spontaneous tumors in the Sprague Dawley rat, *J. Natl. Cancer Inst.,* 27, 1037, 1961.

205. **Pollard, M. and Teah, B. A.,** Spontaneous tumors in germ-free rats, *J. Natl. Cancer Inst.,* 31, 457, 1963.
206. **Ross, M. H. and Bras, G.,** Influence of protein under- and overnutrition on spontaneous tumor prevalence in the rat, *J. Nutr.,* 103, 944, 1973.
207. **Boorman, G. A. and Hollander, C. F.,** Spontaneous lesions in the female WAG'/Rij' (Wistar) rat, *J. Gerontol.,* 28, 152, 1973.
208. **Pollard, M. and Luckert, P. H.,** Spontaneous liver tumors in aged germ free Wistar rats, *Lab. Anim. Sci.,* 20, 74, 1979.
209. **Hoag, W. C.,** Spontaneous cancer in mice, *Ann. N.Y. Acad. Sci.,* 108, 805, 1963.
210. **Andervont, H. B. and Dunn, T. B.,** Occurrence of tumors in wild house mice, *J. Natl. Cancer Inst.,* 28, 1153, 1962.
211. **Wilens, S. L. and Sproul, E. E.,** Spontaneous cardiovascular disease in the rat. I. Lesions of the heart, *Am. J. Pathol.,* 14, 177, 1938.
212. **Wexler, B. C.,** Myocardial infarction in young vs. old male rats: pathophysiological changes, *Am. Heart J.,* 96, 70, 1978.
213. **Durand, A. M. A., Fisher, M., and Adams, M.,** Histology in rats as influenced by age and diet. I. Renal and cardiovascular systems, *Arch. Pathol.,* 77, 268, 1964.
214. **Kennedy, G. C.,** Age and renal disease, *CIBA Found. Colloq. Ageing,* 4, 250, 1958.
215. **Wilens, S. L. and Sproul, E. E.,** Spontaneous cardiovascular disease in the rat. II. Lesions of the vascular system, *Am. J. Pathol.,* 14, 201, 1938.
216. **Cliff, W. J.,** The aortic tunica media in ageing rats, *Exp. Mol. Pathol.,* 13, 172, 1970.
217. **Gillman, T. and Hathorn, M.,** Sex incidence of vascular lesions in ageing rats in relation to previous pregnancies, *Nature (London),* 183, 1139, 1959.
218. **Berg, B. N.,** Muscular dystrophy in aging rats, *J. Gerontol.,* 11, 134, 1956.
219. **Glauert, A. M.,** *Practical Methods in Electron Microscopy,* North Holland, Amsterdam, 1975.
220. **Palade, G. E.,** A study of fixation in electron microscopy, *J. Exp. Med.,* 95, 285, 1952.
221. **Sabatini, D. D., Bensch, K., and Barnett, R. J.,** Cytochemistry and electron microscopy—the preservation of cellular ultrastructure and enzymatic activity by aldehyde fixation, *J. Cell Biol.,* 17, 19, 1963.
222. **Karnovsky, J. J.,** A formaldehyde-glutaraldehyde fixative of high osmolarity for use in electron microscopy, *J. Cell Biol.,* 27, 137, 1965.
223. **Bennett, H. S. and Luft, J. H.,** *S*-Collidine as a basis for buffering fixatives, *J. Biophys. Biochem. Cytol.,* 6, 113, 1959.
224. **Spurr, A. R.,** Low viscosity epoxy resin embedding medium for electron microscopy, *J. Ultrastruct. Res.,* 26, 31, 1969.
225. **Couser, W. G. and Stilmant, M. M.,** Mesangial lesions and focal glomerular sclerosis in the aging rat, *Lab. Invest.,* 33, 491, 1975.
226. **Christensen, E. I. and Madsen, K. M.,** Renal age changes. Observations on the rat kidney cortex with special reference to structure and function of the lysosomal system in the proximal tubule, *Lab. Invest.,* 39, 289, 1978.
227. **Everitt, A. V.,** Cardiovascular aging and the pituitary, in *Hypothalamus, Pituitary and Aging,* Everitt, A. V. and Burgess, J. A., Eds., Charles C Thomas, Springfield, Ill., 1976, chap. 14.
228. **Fujisawa, K.,** Some observations on the skeletal musculature of aged rats. Part 2. Fine morphology of diseased muscle fibres, *J. Neurol. Sci.,* 24, 447, 1975.
229. **Bancroft, J. D. and Stevens, A.,** *Histopathological Stains and Their Diagnostic Uses,* Churchill Livingstone, Edinburgh, 1975.
230. **Baker, J. R.,** *Cytological Technique,* Chapman and Hall, London, 1975.
231. **Bradbury, S.,** *Peacock's Elementary Microtechnique,* 4th ed., Arnold, London, 1973.
232. **Sanders, B. J.,** Animal histology techniques, in *Handbook of Laboratory Animal Science,* Vol. 2, Melby, E. C., Jr. and Altman, N. H., CRC Press, Cleveland, Ohio, 1974, 119.
233. **McManus, J. F. A.,** Histological and histochemical uses of periodic acid, *Stain Technol.,* 23, 99, 1948.
234. **Fernstrom, C. R.,** A durable Nissl stain for frozen sections, *Stain Technol.,* 33, 175, 1958.
235. **Gomori, G. L.,** Aldehyde-fuchsin: a new stain for elastic tissue, *Am. J. Clin. Pathol.,* 20, 665, 1950.
236. **Lillie, R. D.,** *Histopathological Technic,* Blakiston, Philadelphia, 1948, 196.
237. **Hirokawa, K.,** Characterization of age-associated kidney disease in Wistar rats, *Mech. Ageing Dev.,* 4, 30, 1975.
238. **Bras, G.,** Age-associated kidney lesions in the rat, *J. Infect. Dis.,* 120, 131, 1969.

239. **Fujisawa, K.,** Some observations on the skeletal musculature of aged rats. Part 1. Histological aspects, *J. Neurol. Sci.,* 22, 353, 1974.
240. **Finlayson, J. S. and Bauman, C. A.,** Mouse proteinuria, *Am. J. Physiol.,* 192, 69, 1958.
241. **Finlayson, J. S. and Bauman, C. A.,** Protein bound sterols in rodent urine, *Am. J. Physiol.,* 190, 297, 1957.
242. **Denckla, W. D.,** personal communication.

Chapter 8

THYMUS-NEUROENDOCRINE INTERACTIONS DURING DEVELOPMENT AND AGING

 N. Fabris and L. Piantanelli

TABLE OF CONTENTS

I. INTRODUCTION

The idea that the thymus might be considered as an endocrine gland integrated in the complex hormonal mechanism regulating the growth and the internal homeostasis of high organisms was first suggested by the observations that this organ seemed to be functionally active only before puberty, when the majority of endocrine glands are involved in body development and that alterations of its growth pattern was frequently accompanied by modifications of the growth rate of the whole organism.[1]

The trials to give an experimental support to these observations, although they were quite numerous at that time, failed however to help the main hypothesis. Neither experiments correlating thymus to developmental growth[2] nor those trying to involve the thymus in basic metabolic processes, such as glucose metabolism,[3] offered substantial evidence to the general idea.

Although a few "fans" of that hypothesis continued to work in the field and demonstrated, through classical endocrinology experimental designs, a number of possible functional links between thymus and sexual glands or thyroid or adrenals,[4] the biological impact of their findings has been frustrated by the impossibility of measuring thymus activity in other ways than by its weight.

The discovery, in the early 1960s, of the immunological role of thymus,[5,6] by giving, besides the intrinsic biological information, a way to experimentally measure its activity has obscured all the previous work. Furthermore, the great importance of the immune system for the body defense, which was realized shortly after the first discovery, brought forth the idea that the thymus and its cellular products were a kind of task force against external noxae, totally autonomous and independent of physiological alterations in the "internal milieu."[7]

A number of observations in recent years have, however, demonstrated that, although the thymus-dependent immunity has an highly sophisticated autoregulatory mechanism,[8] much of its efficiency is influenced by extraimmunological homeostasis mechanisms.[9] Central and autonomic nervous system, endocrine balance, and metabolic turnover have been shown to play a role in the development and maintenance of the immune system.[9] These observations have gained further support from the finding that receptors for protein hormones and for catecholamines are certainly present on the membrane of lymphocytes, although their concentration may be different according to the subsets of lymphocytes under investigation.[10]

On these findings have been based the idea that the potentiality of the immune system in a given moment or period of life is under the influence of complex neuroendocrine homeostatic regulation, which may be, therefore, a kind of second regulation level superimposed on the intrinsic mechanism of self-regulation of the immune system.[9]

The comprehensive picture of these integrative mechanisms still waits, however, for a systematic experimental approach which should take into consideration not only the fact that the majority of homeostatic regulation mechanisms are interdigitated with each other, but also of the discovery, or, better, rediscovery of a consistent endocrine activity of the thymus.[11]

This point is of striking biological importance since it introduces new humoral factor(s) which cannot be considered as depleted of physiological relevance for the whole neuroendocrine system. Although such interactions between endocrine thymus activity and neuroendocrine balance are based on relatively few observations, mainly indirect and sometimes controversial, it is worthwhile to try to order them within the scope, at least, of a consistent working hypothesis.

With this aim, findings which support, at present, the functional relationships between the thymus and the neuroendocrine system and their impact on the efficiency

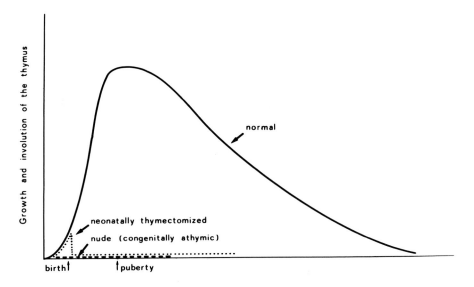

FIGURE 1. Scheme on the differences among athymic nude, neonatally thymectomized, and old normal mice in relation to thymic function.

either of the immune system or of other body organs and apparati will be summarized.

Moreover, due to the precociousness in life of functional involution of the thymus and of its endocrine activity, which precedes the majority of age-related disfunctional biases, an attempt will be made to reconsider the possible role of the thymus for aging processes, as already suggested for the age-related decline of immune function.[12]

II. THYMUS-NEUROENDOCRINE INTERACTIONS

The existence of a functional relationship between the thymus and the neuroendocrine system has been suggested by a number of observations dealing either with possible neurohormonal alterations following the removal of the thymus or with the modifications which may be induced within the thymus itself by different endocrine manipulations.

As in the majority of investigations carried out in experimental animals, the animal model chosen is quite relevant for the interpretation of the findings, particularly when they are supposed to evaluate functions critical only during limited periods of life. This concept is well illustrated by the differences which characterize the animal models used in order to demonstrate the influence of the thymus on the neuroendocrine balance. In this case all animal models shown in Figure 1, i.e., thymectomized mice, congenitally athymic nude animals, and old normal mice have been used on the rationale that all of them may be considered thymus-deprived animals. It is clear, however, that, according to the length of the period of life during which these animals have experienced the presence of their own thymus, they differ substantially from each other; few days of normal thymus activity (from first appearance of thymus around the 13th day of gestation till birth) in neonatally thymectomized mice, many months in old mice, and virtually no days in congenitally athymic nude mice.

If some thymus-neuroendocrine system interactions are critically exerted during a quite restricted time in ontogeny, then the differences among the animal models illustrated in Figure 1 might assume a great discriminatory capacity rather than representing a source of contradictory findings. Similar considerations may obviously apply also to animal models used to study the effect of the neuroendocrine system on thymus functioning. In fact, at least for tumor surveillance, it has been already substantiated that the nearly opposite findings obtained by using congenitally hypopituitary dwarf or adult-hypophysectomized mice may represent a means to distinguish the relevance of the hypophysis for the efficiency during ontogenesis or in adult life of immunological defense mechanisms against tumor growth[9-13] more than an experimental paradox on the hormone dependency of tumor growth.

In addition to these methodological premises, further attention must be paid to the kind of parameter used to measure a given functional interaction, since not all of them may have the same discriminatory power on the interaction under study.[14,15]

A. Effect of Thymus Hypofunctioning on Neuroendocrine Homeostasis

It has been reported already (in 1960) that wasting disease, a syndrome which follows neonatal thymectomy in rodents and usually causes death of animals within few months, is characterized, in addition to the more obvious immunological disturbances, by a number of pathological signs, which can hardly be linked to the direct effect of immune deficiencies themselves.[16]

Mice thymectomized at birth show a progressive impairment of body growth with reduced length of ears and tail, microsplancnia, microsomia, thinness of the skin and lack of subcutaneous fat, osseal alterations, particularly evident in the vertebrae with consequent hunched posture, and hypotrophy of various tissues including submaxillary gland, hair follicles, and bone marrow.[16]

In neonatally thymectomized rats, quite similar pictures have been reported[17,18] although in these species wasting disease occurs only in a minority of thymectomized animals. Nevertheless nonwasting neonatally thymectomized rats or rats thymectomized more than 2 days after birth also show modifications of some extraimmunological parameters such as deficient bone marrow myelopoiesis,[19] altered serum enzyme activity,[20] and defective liver regeneration after partial hepatectomy.[21]

These observations on thymectomized animals have been further confirmed in other thymus-deprived animals such as athymic nude mice(nu/nu)[22] and athymic nude rats(rnu/rnu),[23] both of which are characterized, in addition to the absence of hairs(nudity), by congenital aplasia of the thymus. The majority of pathological signs observed in thymectomized animals are present also in nude mutations;[22-23] however, some of them, including altered age/weight ratio, do not seem to appear when animals are maintained in germ-free conditions.

In all cases, these preliminary and indirect observations supporting the existence of thymus-neuroendocrine interactions have suggested investigation in a more direct way of the morphological and functional aspects of the neuroendocrine system in both thymectomized and nude animals. Although findings in this context are still incomplete, the observations which follow seem to be supported by a substantial body of experimental evidence.

1. Adenohypophysis

Neonatal thymectomy in mice causes a progressive degranulation of acidophylic cells in the hypophysis while leaving unaffected other pituitary cell lineages.[24]

The degranulated cells, according to their morphological features under EM examination, seem to belong to the growth hormone and prolactin-producing lineages.[24] In thymectomized rats a precocius and long-lasting stimulation of growth-hormone producing cells followed by similar, although frequently transient changes of β- and δ-cells, have been observed.[25]

Determination of blood levels of pituitary hormones in these animals is still fragmentary. In thymectomized mice, reduction of plasma levels of prolactin and increased levels of luteotropic hormone(LH) have been reported.[26] In thymectomized rats decreased levels of ACTH and increased blood concentrations of LH were observed. These alterations, however, are present only during early stages after thymectomy, being followed in adulthood by their normalization.[27]

Although the determination of plasma levels of growth hormone in thymectomized mice would have been of major interest according to the histological picture of the pituitary, unfortunately, until now it has not been done. A reduced synthesis of growth hormone in thymectomized mice is, however, indirectly supported by the fact that treatment with growth hormone can restore to normalcy the decreased body growth rate of thymectomized mice, although it does not prevent their death.[28]

In nude mutations findings are somewhat contradictory. In athymic nude mice degranulation and enlargement of endoplasmic reticulum in acidophilic growth-hormone producing cells, similar to those observed in thymectomized mice, has been reported,[29] while according to other authors,[30] the alterations consist mainly in a decreased size and number of those cells. Furthermore, determination of blood levels of pituitary hormones has revealed reduced prolactin and increased LH concentrations.[26] Moreover, the low levels of both T_3 and T_4 found in nude mice together with the experimental possibility of restoring them by exogenous administration of thyrotropic hormone(TSH), have suggested that TSH synthesis and/or release are also disturbed in nude mutation.[31] All these abnormalities, according to data from other laboratories, are not to be linked, however, to nude mutations per se, but to intercurrent viral or bacterial infections. While altered plasma levels of pituitary hormones, including growth hormone, have been in fact confirmed in nude mice reared under conventional conditions, they are not present in animals maintained in a germ-free environment.[32]

Finally, no differences in the morphology of the pituitary gland have been observed between nude rats and their heterozygous littermates.[23] Hormonal determinations in these animals have not been done thus far.

2. Thyroid

The picture of the thyroid in thymo-deprived animals is unclear. Transitory signs of stimulation have been observed in thymectomized guinea pigs and ascribed to pituitary involvement.[33] In nude mice[29,31] but not nude rats,[23] features of hypotrophy of the gland with reduced plasma levels of T_3 and T_4 have been reported, although this fact might depend on the housing environment of mice rather than on the nude mutation per se (see preceding).

In old normal mice, which are characterized by an involuted thymus (see Figure 1) and by low levels of T_3, the implantation of a neonatal syngeneic thymus under the kidney capsule induces a significant increment of plasma T_3 levels.[34]

3. Adrenals

Both neonatally thymectomized and nude mice have been reported to show an abnormal histological picture of adrenals[29] accompained by increased plasma levels of corticosterone at least during the first months of life.[31] Isolated adrenals of nude mice produce three times as much desoxycorticosterone as those of normal mice, while no difference is observed in the synthesis of other corticosteroids.[31] Similar pictures of adrenal stimulation have been observed in neonatally thymectomized guinea pigs[33] and rats.[35] High corticosterone levels have been recorded, however, in the blood of adrenal vein[36] rather than in the systemic circulation.[37]

According to other authors, neon. thymectomy in rats induces on the contrary reduction of corticosterone plasma levels, which, in the presence of the concomitant low levels of ACTH would suggest an action of the thymus on the adrenals via the hypo-physis.[27]

4. Gonads

Gonadal function in thymus-deprived animals has been deeply investigated since it was demonstrated that neonatal thymectomy in hamster had quite different end effects according to the sex (males undergo wasting diseases, females do not),[38] while in mice it was causing sterility in females, but not in males.[39] Moreover, it was also shown that the latter phenomenon occurred when thymectomy was performed at 3 days, but not at 7 days of life, thus suggesting the existence of a limited period of life during which thymus could influence the programming of gonadal functions.[40]

Following such a concept, further investigations in both thymectomized and athymic nude mice, have shown that both thymus-deprived conditions are characterized by a delayed vaginal opening time, with deeper sexual underdevelopment in nude mice than in thymectomized animals.[40] Thymectomy performed at 10 days of age was ineffective.

On the other hand, a neonatal thymus grafted very early in life was able to fully restore sexual development in both animal models, but it was ineffective when trans-planted after the 10th day of age. The likelihood that immunological function might mediate all these effects has been ruled out by the observation that injection of syn-geneic mature lymphocytes into newborn nude mice was able to reconstitute their im-munological efficiency, but not their defective ovarian development.[40]

Sex hormone determinations have revealed that in female nude mice the plasma con-centrations of both 17-β-oestradiol and progesterone are quite low particularly in post-pubertal age, while in female neonatal thymectomized mice only progesterone levels are found decreased when compared to the values observed in normal animals.[31] Un-expectedly, thymus implants into nude mice restore 17-β-oestradiol, but not proges-terone plasma level.[31] These findings, together with the observation that plasma levels of LH are increased in nude mice and return to normal by thymus grafts[26] and the fact that exogenous administration of LH to nude mice may induce an increment of their progesterone plasma levels,[31] strongly suggest that other factors of unknown origin should play some role and likely justify such a contradictory results.

Also data on neonatally thymecotmized male animals are somewhat unclear: testos-terone plasma levels are found to be reduced,[27,31] at least before puberty, and although concomitantly there is an increased level of LH, it does not seem that the action of the thymus should be regarded as directly exerted on the testis.[27]

In the intricate picture derived from such contradictory results, only one observation seems certainly well observable in all animals, including the nude rat: the sexual di-morphysm which characterizes submaxillary glands is absent in thymus-deprived ani-mals.[23,41]

5. Endocrine Pancreas

Very little is known in this field, although quite strict interactions exist between pituitary function and the endocrine activity of islands of Langerhans.

Determination of hormone blood levels in thymus-deprived animals have not been carried out thus far. Preliminary experiments in nude mice have however shown that while there are not differences in the basal levels of plasma insulin between nude and normal littermates the insulin-dependent esokinase pattern in the liver is strongly altered in nude animals.[42] More consistent findings include the observation that in old normal mice the abnormally high plasma level of insulin is restored to young values by trans-planting a syngeneic neonatal thymus.[34]

6. Low Molecular Weight Hormones

This field is likely one of the more relevant aspects to be investigated since it has been demonstrated that thymus-dependent humoral factors do act on cAMP via membrane receptor sites which are strictly linked to catecholaminergic sensitive membrane receptors.[43] With regard to thymus vs. neuroendocrine system interaction, only indirect evidence is as yet available.

Among this, the findings that some physiological reactions induced by the stimulation of beta-adrenergic receptors are reduced in nude, thymectomized, and old normal mice and that they can be restored to normalcy by syngeneic neonatal thymus transplants, represent the most consistent data at present.[34] Preliminary experiments suggest, furthermore, that such an action of the thymus on the beta-adrenergic receptor-adenyl cyclase-cAMP system is exerted through modification of the beta-adrenergic receptor density on the surface of target cells.[44]

B. Influence of the Neuroendocrine System on Thymus Activity

The idea that the thymus is under the influence of the neuroendocrine system stemmed mainly from the observation that endocrine imbalances may alter the growth pattern of the thymus.

Thus surgical removal of the hypophysis[45] in rats or congenital hypopituitarism as it occurs in dw/dw mice,[46] causes hypotrophy of the thymus, which can be restored to normal size by treatment with developmental hormones and particularly by growth hormone and thyroxine.[47] In humans, no similar pictures have been described; only in anencephalic fetuses hypertrophy of the thymus has been recorded and interpreted as being due to hypofunction of adrenals.[48]

Also the thyroid has great influence on the growth rate of the thymus: hypo- and hyperfunction of the gland cause respectively reduced or increased size of the thymus both in rodents[49] and in man.[50]

With regard to adrenal and sexual glands, enlargement of the thymus following the removal of these glands and hypotrophy after treatment with steroid hormones are well known phenomena.[51] Impressive modifications induced by sex hormone treatment have been reported to occur, in particular, at the level of the epithelial component of the thymus.[52] This last observation was one of the first which attempted to dissociate, among the effects induced by the neuroendocrine system on the thymus, those primarily directed on the epithelial cells. These cells were already at that time considered as responsible for the endocrine function of the thymus,[53] although direct evidence came only recently.[54] All the previous observations could well be interpreted, in fact, as being due to an hormonal effect directly exerted on thymocytes, which doubtless possess membrane receptors for various hormones.[55]

That the neuroendocrine system may effect the endocrine activity of the thymus has recently received some more direct experimental evidence. First, it has been shown that the amount of thymic hormone extractable from the thymus, according at least to the Bernardi-Comsa procedure, varies greatly depending on different hormonal balances. Thus, reduced thymic hormone content has been observed in hypophysectomized, thyroidectomized, and adrenalectomized rats, whereas increased amounts were recorded in castrated animals. Treatment of ectomized animals with substitutive hormonal therapy seemed to restore the physiological level of thymic hormone.[56]

Even more direct evidence came from experiments in which the level of circulating thymic factor, as measured by the procedure of Bach and Dardenne[57] has been determined in different experimental disendocrinopathies. By this method it has been demonstrated that in congenitally hypopituitary dwarf mice the level of circulating thymic factor (FTS) is significantly lower than in normal littermates[58] and it can be recovered to normalcy by treatment with thyroxine.[59] Among the other endocrinological situations evaluated, adrenalectomy and castration did not appreciably modify FTS level, whereas experimental diabetes causes strong reduction of it. The latter can be quickly corrected by treatment of diabetic mice with insulin.[59]

The complexity of the hormonal production of various endocrine glands and of the interactions among them, does not allow for the drawing of clear-cut conclusions from the in vivo experimental designs, previously reported. The best way to define interactions between the neuroendocrine system and production of humoral factors from the thymus would be that offered by the technical possibility of growing thymic epithelial cells in vitro and testing thymic humoral factors in the supernatant under stimulation with different hormones.[55] Unfortunately very little has been done in this field: it has been demonstrated only that some hypophyseal hormones, such as corticotropic and thyrotropic hormones, are able to increase the proliferation rate of thymic epithelial cells,[60] however no determinations of their effect on the in vitro production of thymic factors have been carried out to date.

Observations in man, at least in this context, are totally absent: FTS determinations have been in fact performed only in patients suffering from primary immunodeficiency diseases. However, the observation of low levels of FTS in patients affected by trisomy 21[61] who, in addition to a number of immunological alterations seem to suffer also from neuroendocrinological unbalances, may be relevant.

All this information, taken together, clearly indicates that the rate of synthesis and/or release of thymic factors depends on the neuroendocrinological balance, although the exent of such a dependence needs to be defined by further studies. Future work should, furthermore, try to investigate not only the effect of hormones on either the amount of thymic factor stored within the thymus or on the level of circulating FTS, but on the actual turnover of these factors, which, as it occurs for other hormones, is not always revealed by the amount stored in the gland or circulating in the blood.

III. THYMUS-NEUROENDOCRINE INTERACTIONS IN AGING

Since it has been demonstrated that modifications induced by experimental manipulation of the thymus alter the neuroendocrine system and vice versa, it may also be expected that the physiological decline with advancing age either of the thymus or of the neuroendocrine system has negative consequences on the other partner. Although the age-dependent variations of such interactions are still not well known, it is clearly defined that at least one component of these interactions, e.g., the thymic function, shows profound and precocious modifications with advancing age.

The thymus, in fact, attains its maximum size at puberty, after which it starts to pregressively involute and to be replaced by fat. This process is nearly complete in man by the 5th to 6th decade: the cortical areas are depleted of lymphoid cells and epithelial cells show cystic changes and reduction of intracellular granules.[62]

Measurement of circulating levels of thymic factors has demonstrated that both in animals and man the serum level of FTS declines relatively early in life. In rodents FTS is virtually undetectable in animals older than 15 months of age,[63] and in man in individuals over 50 years of age.[64] This last finding has been confirmed also by using a different technique, which likely measures another thymic factor (i.e., thymopoietin). However in this case a slightly longer survival of thymic endocrine activity results in man.[65]

A. Thymus vs. Neuroendocrine Function

Recent experimental work from the authors laboratory has demonstrated that the determination of some morphological and functional parameters of aging is clearly related to thymic involution. From a morphological point of view, the age-dependent increase in nuclear volume of hepatocytes, likely related to augmented ploidy, is corrected to young values by transplanting a neonatal thymus.[66] Although direct evidence is still lacking, it is likely that such an effect is exerted by the thymus through modification of the hormonal balance which is known to influence the mitotic activity of liver cells. Preliminary experiments have, in fact, demonstrated that, together with the correction of the nuclear volume of the hepatocytes, old animals grafted with a neonatal thymus show a substantial recovery of the abnormal serum level of some hormones such as T_3 and insulin.[34] Nevertheless a direct influence of some thymic factor on chromatin structure and template capacity, as reported by other authors in their in vitro experiments[66,68] cannot be excluded.

Also, functional parameters of aging are influenced by the thymus. Particularly susceptible are those parameters which measure adaptive responsiveness to different stimuli and whose quasi-linear decrease from puberty to old age parallels the age-dependent decline of thymic function. Thus, the decline of in vivo responses to beta-adrenergic stimulation evoked by a single injections of isoproterenol and measured either as the peak of DNA synthesis in submandibular glands 34 hr after stimulation or as amount of total water intake,[42] is corrected by transplanting a neonatal thymus 30 days before testing.

The interpretation of these findings should take into consideration that a common mechanism responsible for the observed age-dependent alterations of in vivo beta-adrenergic responses could be found at the level of beta-adrenergic receptors. As a matter of fact, a decrease of beta-adrenoceptor density with advancing age has been recorded in different tissues such as brain[69] and lymphocytes.[70] In submandibular glands the situation seems to be more complex since two functional populations of receptors displaying high and low affinity, respectively, have been characterized.[44] Experimental data are consistent either with a model where receptors can be found (low affinity) or coupled with the effector enzyme (high affinity) or with a model of receptor population eliciting "negative cooperativity" among binding sites, that is, receptors show a decreasing affinity for the ligand with increasing occupancy.[44] The high affinity population shows an age-dependent decrease quite similar to that found in other tissues. The presence of the low affinity population, however, may lead to a different hypothesis about the causes of the age-dependent changes in membrane receptors. In fact, a change in the functional high affinity population does not require a change in protein synthesis or catabolism, but a simple modification in the receptor enzyme coupling, due, in part, to a change in membrane fluidity.

With regard to the authors' model, preliminary experiments seem to demonstrate that a neonatal thymus transplanted into old recipients is able to increase the density of beta-adrenoceptors. Such a finding might well explain the recovery of the in vivo beta-adrenergic adaptive response achieved in old mice by the same grafting procedure. According to the hypothesis reported above, such a thymus dependent modulation of adrenoceptor might be due either to a direct effect of thymic factors or through the observed recovery of the hormonal balance. It is known, in fact, that membrane fluidity depends, to a reasonable extent, on the hormonal equilibrium. Thus, while thyroidectomy results in a decreased density of a high affinity population of adrenoceptors, a subsequent thyroxine injection causes a reversal of such an impairement.[71] Catecholamines are known to exert a regulatory role on their own receptors: increased levels of catecholamines lead to a decrease in high affinity receptor number and vice versa.[72] An increased receptor density is also known to be evoked by steroid hormone, although the mechanism is not yet clear.[73] The aforementioned recovery of T_3 and insulin serum levels in old mice by a neonatal thymus graft could be in agreement with this interpretation.[34]

All these findings, taken together, on one hand give further support to the idea that the thymus exerts a widespread influence on the neuroendocrine system. On the other hand, they strongly suggest that such an influence is operating throughout the whole span of life and that its deterioration may represent an important component of the aging process. Such an influence may likely be mediated through the action of the thymic factors, which have been extensively studied for their effect on the immune system, but which, for their impact with basic cellular and subcellular mechanisms, may be assumed to have a larger range of action.

B. Neuroendocrine vs. Thymic Function

The progressive decline of thymic endocrine activity with advancing age may be due either to alterations of epithelial cells which become unable to synthetize and/or release thymic factors or to alterations occurring in those extrinsic mechanisms which seem to control the function of the endocrine epithelium.[74] Experiments in mice have demonstrated that both intrinsic and extrinsic factors can play a role: in fact; thymuses from old mice, when grafted into adult thymectomized recipients, can partially restore the circulating FTS level of the recipients, whereas newborn thymuses are less efficient in restoring FTS levels in old recipients than in young adult thymectomized mice.[74]

Among the microenvironmental factors which may be responsible for these findings, neuroendocrine factors are certainly of primary relevance, either because some of them have been proven to act on thymus endocrine activity, or because a progressive deterioration of the neuroendocrine-balance is among the detrimental processes more frequently encountered in old age.[75]

Direct experimental evidence for this hypothesis comes from the recent observation that the circulating levels of FTS can be restored in old mice by treating them with thyroxine,[59] a hormone which, at least in mice, shows a progressive reduction in its turnover with advancing age.[76]

The recovery of FTS secretion in old mice is not a sterile event since it induces an increased functionality of the peripheral immune system as assessed by the reconstitution of the number of T-lymphocytes and of their responsiveness to mitogen stimulation, which are abnormally low in old mice.[76]

It is of interest to note that, in addition to the recovery of FTS level and to peripheral immune efficiency in old mice, thyroxine seems to rejuvenate the thymus, so that when such a thymus is transplanted into a young thymectomized recipient, its behavior more resembles that of a young thymus than of an old one. These findings, while on one hand clearly confirm the influence of the endocrine system on the thymic humoral activity, on the other hand strongly support the idea that the functional decline of thymic factor production is to a large extent a reversible phenomenom. From preliminary experiments it seems, however, that such reversibility disappears in very old age. Thyroxine treatment does not seem to be equally active in very old (over 26 months) mice. This fact does not exclude, however, the possibility that by neuroendocrinological manipulations other than thyroxine treatment, a recovery of thymic factor production in old mice may still be achieved.

Finally, it is to be noted that a number of quite connected clinical situations could help in understanding the regulatory control on FTS production. Precocius aging syndromes, such as those of the NZB strain of mice and of trisomy 21,[61] show an early

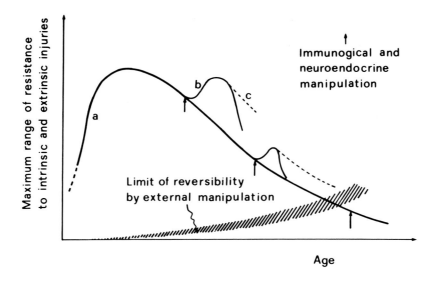

FIGURE 2. Hypothetical scheme on the age-dependent influence of thymus-neuroendocrine network on the resistance to external and internal injuries. The capacity of the organism to overcome injuries is depicted as a line (a) which reaches its maximum when the thymus-neuroendocrine network is fully established during development. Thereafter a reduction of such a capacity occurs progressively with advancing age. Concomitantly, it may be expected that an increasing amount of irreversible damage takes place (dashed zone), so as to reduce the corrective effect of any external manipulation until an age after which no correction is further achievable. Both immunological (thymus grafting) or endocrinological (hormonal treatment) manipulations performed before that age are able to ameliorate the physiological range of resistance, although such a correction is quantitatively less efficient as age increases. The correction achieved by one or the other manipulation does not shift all deterioration to the right, however, as would be expected in the case of a definite rejuvenating effect (line o). On the contrary, the increased resistance achieved by the manipulation of only one of the components of the network is not sustained for a long time, due to the deleterious influence of the other branches left unmodified (line b). It cannot be excluded, however, that by more complete manipulations of the thymus-neuroendocrine network, the corrective action might be maintained for longer periods, thus approaching a real rejuvenating treatment (line c).

loss of FTS activity when compared to age-matched controls. Whether the causes for such an early deterioration of thymic endocrine activity are identical to those responsible for physiological aging, remains to be investigated.

IV. CONCLUSIONS AND PERSPECTIVES

The idea of the thymus and the neuroendocrine system functionally connected by a number of physiological interrelationships has received consistent support from the discovery of an endocrine activity of the thymus. By means of this thymic endocrine activity it is by far easier, in fact, to explain how the neuroendocrine system may influence thymus-dependent immunity and how, on the other hand, the thymus may interfere in extraimmunological homeostatic mechanisms, such as endocrine balance or regulation by the autonomic nervous system. It is, at present, unknown, however, whether such a thymus-neuroendocrine network operates through the thymic humoral factors defined with immunological assays or if other factors also from thymic origin are involved. Also, the possibility that other forms of interactions might take place between the cellular product of the thymus, e.g., T-lymphocytes, and the neuroendocrine system, as suggested by other authors,[77] cannot be ruled out.

Another relevant concept which is supported by present data is that this thymus-neuroendocrine network is functioning throughout the life span. Experimentally induced alterations on one of the components of such a network, during ontogeny, impair the development of the others. Similarly during aging, disturbances occurring at thymic level seem to influence the deteriorations of the other systems and vice versa.

While findings are consistent with the idea that this thymus-neuroendocrine network does deteriorate with advancing age, it is difficult, at present, to define which component declines early in life and, therefore, may be considered as the primary cause for the aging of the whole network. The findings on thyroxine-dependent recovery of thymic endocrine functions in old animals clearly suggest that the older the animal, the lower the sensitivity of its thymus to hormonal correction. On the other hand, while doubtlessly a neonatal thymus graft can correct abnormalities in the neuroendocrine system in old age, it is unknown at present whether such a correction can be achieved at any time and, in all cases, how long it lasts. Preliminary experiments in this context have shown that the older the mouse, the shorter the functional survival of the grafted thymus.

A hypothetical schema of such concepts is represented in Figure 2, which suggests that any corrective manipulation on single components of the thymus-neuroendocrine network may only lead to transitory rejuvenating effects.

Yet, a difference seems to exists between these two experimental designs. While with hormonal reconstitution no recovery of thymic production is achieved in very old animals, suggesting no capacity for reversibility is left in the old thymus, a certain degree of reversibility is present in the neuroendocrine system. However, the recovery cannot be sustained for long time. Such different kinetics certainly are not enough to assign to the thymus the primary role in aging processes, but it may certainly justify reconsidering, at least at a speculative level, its possible role as a biological clock for physiological functions equally as important, such as immune and neuroendocrine homeostasis.

REFERENCES

1. **Chiodi, H.,** Influence de la thymectomie sur la croissance et le develement des rats blancs. *Seances Soc. Biol.,* 130, 298, 1939.
2. **Szent-Györgyi, A., Hegyeli, A., and McLaughlin, J. A.,** Constituents of the thymus gland and their relation to growth, fertility, muscle and cancer, *Proc. Natl. Acad. Sci. U.S.A.,* 48, 1439, 1962.
3. **Gudernatsch, F.,** The present status of the thymus problem, *Med. Rec.,* 146, 101, 1937.
4. **Comsa, J.,** Hormonal interactions of the thymus, in *Thymic Hormones,* Luckey, T. D., Ed., University Park Press., Baltimore, 1973.
5. **Miller, J. F. A. P.,** Immunological function of the thymus, *Lancet,* 2, 748, 1961.
6. **Good, R. A., Dalmasso, A. P., Martinez, C., Archer, O. K., Pierce, J. C., and Papermaster, B. W.,** The role of the thymus in development of immunologic capacity in rabbits and mice, *J. Exp. Med.,* 116, 773, 1962.
7. **Miller, J. F. A. P. and Osoba, D.,** Current concepts on the immunological function of the thymus, *Physiol. Rev.,* 47, 437, 1967.
8. **Cantor, H. and Boyse, E. A.,** Regulation of cellular and humoral immune responses by T cell subclasses, *Cold Spring Harbor Symp. Quant. Biol.,* 41, 23, 1976.
9. **Fabris, N.,** Body homeostasis mechanisms and immunological aging, in *Immunology of Aging,* Makinodan, T. and Kay, M. M. B., Eds. CRC Press, Boca Raton, Fla., 1981, 61.
10. **Gavin, J. R., III,** Polipeptide hormone receptor on lymphoid cells, in *Immunopharmacology,* Comprehensive Immunology No. 3, Hadden, J. W., Coffey, R. G., and Spreafico, F., Eds., Plenum Press, New York, 1977, 357.

11. **Goldstein, A. L., Guba, A., Zatz, M. M., Hardy, M. A., and While, A.,** Purification and biological activity of thymosin a hormone of the thymus gland, *Proc. Natl. Acad. Sci. U.S.A.,* 69, 1800, 1972.
12. **Burnet, F. M.,** An immunological approach to aging, *Lancet,* 2, 358, 1970.
13. **Piantanelli, L. and Fabris, N.,** Hypopituitary dwarf and athymic nude mice and the study of the relationships among thymus, hormones and aging, in *Genetic effects on Aging,* Harrison, D. E. and Bergsma, D., Eds. Sinauer Association, Suderland, Mass., 1978, 315.
14. **Fabris, N.,** The relevance of immunological parameters for the study of the hormone-dependency of lymphoid cells, in *Abstr. Symp. Immune Syst. 11th Int. Congr. Gerontol.,* 1978, 18.
15. **Fabris, N.,** Hormones and Aging, in *Immunology and Aging,* Comprehensive Immunology No. 3, Makinodan, T. and Yunis, E., Eds., Plenum Press, New York, 1977, 72.
16. **McIntire, K. R., Sell, S., and Miller, J. F. A. P.,** Pathogenesis of the post-neonatal thymectomy wasting syndrome, *Nature (London),* 204, 151, 1964.
17. **Waksman, B. H., Arnason, B. G., and Jankovic, B. D.,** Role of the thymus in immune reactions in rats. III. Changes in the lymphoid organs of thymectomized rats, *J. Exp. Med.,* 116, 187, 1962.
18. **Fachet, J., Stark, E., Palkovits, M., and Mihaly, K.,** Effect of neonatal thymectomy on endocrine and lymphatic organs, reticular elements and blood count. I. Finding in rats not suffering from wasting-syndrome. *Acta Med. Acad. Sci. Hung.,* 21, 297, 1965.
19. **Corsi, A. and Giusti, GV.,** Cellular distribution in the bone marrow after thymectomy, *Nature (London),* 216, 493, 1967.
20. **Fachet, J., Szabo, I., and Cseh, G.,** Effect of thymectomy on lipoprotein lipase activity in serum and heart of rats, *Experientia (Basel),* 20, 708, 1964.
21. **Fachet, J., Stark, E., Palkovits, M., and Vallent, K.,** Der Einfluss der Thymektomie, auf die Leberregeneration nach partieller Hepatektomie, *Zeitschr. F. Zellforsch.,* 60, 609, 1963.
22. **Gershwin, M. E., Merchant, B., Gelfand, M. C., Vickers, J., Steinberg, A. D., and Hansen, C. T.,** The natural history and immunopathology of outbred athymic (nude) mice, *Clin. Immunol. and Immunopathol.,* 4, 324, 1975.
23. **Vos, J. G., Berkvens, J. M., and Kruijt, B. C.,** The athymic nude rat, *Clin. Immunol. Immunopathol.,* 15, 213, 1980.
24. **Pierpaoli, W., Bianchi, H., and Sorkin, E.,** Modification of the growth-hormone producing cells in the hypophysis of neonatally thymectomized mice, *Clin. Exp. Immunol.,* 9, 889, 1971.
25. **Comsa, J., Philipp, E. M., and Leonhardt, H.,** Effects of thymectomy on the endocrines of the rat, *Isr. J. Med. Sci.,* 13, 354, 1977.
26. **Pierpaoli, W., Kopp, H. G., and Bianchi, E.,** Interdependence of thymic and neuroendocrine functions in ontogeny, *Clin. Exp. Immunol.,* 24, 501, 1976.
27. **Deschaux, P., Binimbi Massengo and Fontanges, R.,** Endocrine interaction of the thymus with the hypophysis, adrenals and testes: effect of two thymic extracts, *Thymus,* 1, 95, 1979.
28. **Fabris, N., Pierpaoli, W., and Sorkin, E.,** Hormones and the immune response, in *Development Aspects of Antibody formation and Structure,* Sterzl, J. and Riha, I., Eds. Czechoslovak Academy Press, Prague, 1970, 79.
29. **Pierpaoli, W. and Sorkin, E.,** Alterations of adrenal cortex and thyroid in mice with congenital absence of the thymus, *Nature (London) New Biol.,* 238, 282, 1972.
30. **Ruitenberg, E. J. and Berkvens, J. M.,** The morphology of the endocrine system in congenitally athymic (nude) mice, *J. Pathol.,* 121, 225, 1977.
31. **Pierpaoli, W. and Besedovsky, N. O.,** Role of the thymus in programming of neuroendocrine function, *Clin. Exp. Immunol.,* 20, 325, 1975.
32. **Outzen, H. C., Custer, R. P., Eaton, G. J., and Prehn, R. T.,** Spontaneous and induced tumor incidence in germfree "nude" mice, *J. Reticulo. Sci.,* 17, 1, 1975.
33. **Comsa, J.,** Thymic hormones, *Hormones,* 2, 226, 1971.
34. **Piantanelli, L., Basso, A., Muzzioli, M., and Fabris, N.,** Thymus-dependent reversibility of physiological and isoproterenol-evoked age-related parameters in athymic (nude) and old normal mice, *Mech. Ageing Dev.,* 7, 171, 1978.
35. **Fachet, J., Stand, E., Vallent, K., and Palkovits, M.,** Functional interaction between thymus and adrenal cortex, *Acta Med. Acad. Hung.,* 18, 461, 1962.
36. **Buntner, B. and Szymik, N.,** Effects of thymectomy on steroid secretion and adrenal venous blood in male rats, *Endocrinol. Exp.,* 8, 31, 1974.
37. **Sininsky, A. and Martin, C. R.,** Influence of thymectomy on plasma corticosterone in the rat, *Gen. Comp. Endocrinol.,* 8, 378, 1967.
38. **Sherman, J. D. and Dameshek, W.,** "Wasting disease" following thymectomy in the hamster, *Nature, (London),* 197, 469, 1963.
39. **Nishizuka, Y. and Sakakura, T.,** Thymus and reproduction: sex-linked dysgenesis of the gonad after neonatal thymectomy in mice, *Science,* 166, 753, 1969.

40. **Besedovsky, H. O. and Sorkin, E.,** Thymus involvement in female sexual maturation, *Nature (London),* 249, 356, 1974.
41. **Wortis, H. H.,** Pleiotropic effects of the nude mutation, in *Immunodeficiency in Man and Animals,* Bergsma, D., Ed., Sinauer Association, Suderland, Mass., 11, 528, 1975.
42. **Fabris, N. and Piantanelli, L.,** Thymus, homeostatic regulation and aging. Proceedings of the 11th International Congress on Gerontology, *Excerpta Med. Congr. Ser.,* 451, 1979.
43. **Goldstein, G., Scheid, M., Hammertring, U., Bose, E. A., Schlesinger, D. H., and Niall, H. D.,** Isolation of a polypeptide that has lymphocytes-differentiating properties and is probably represented universally in living cells, *Proc. Natl. Acad. Sci. U.S.A.,* 72, 11, 1976.
44. **Piantanelli, L., Fattoretti, P., and Viticchi, C.,** Beta-adrenoceptor changes in submandibular glands of old mice, *Mech. Ageing Dev.,* 14, 155, 1980.
45. **Duquesnoy, R. J., Mariani, T., and Good, R. A.,** Effect of hypophysectomy on the immunological recovery from X-irradiation, *Proc. Soc. Exp. Biol. Med.,* 132, 1176, 1969.
46. **Fabris, N., Pierpaoli, W., and Sorkin, E.,** Hormones and the immunological capacity. III. The immunodeficiency diseases of the hypopituitary Snell-Bagg dwarf mouse, *Clin. Exp. Immunol.,* 9, 209, 1971.
47. **Fabris, N., Pierpaoli, W., and Sorkin, E.,** Hormones and the immunological capacity. VI. Restorative effects of developmental hormones or of lymphocytes on the immunodeficiency syndrome of the dwarf mouse, *Clin. Exp. Immunol.,* 9, 227, 1971.
48. **Bearn, J. G.,** Influence of the pituitary-adrenal axis on development of the rat foetal thymus, *Proc. Soc. Exp. Biol. Med.,* 122, 273, 1966.
49. **Fabris, N.,** Immunodepression in thyroid-deprived animals, *Clin. Exp. Immunol.,* 15, 601, 1973.
50. **Simpson, J. F., Gray, E. S., and Beck, J. S.,** Age involution in the normal human adult thymus, *Clin. Exp. Immunol.,* 19, 261, 1975.
51. **Castro, J. E.,** Hormone mechanism of immunopotentiation in mice after castration, *J. Endocrinol.,* 62, 311, 1974.
52. **Cherry, C. I., Einstein, R., and Glucksmann, A.,** Epithelial cords and tubules of rat thymus: effects of age, sex, castration, thyroid and other hormones on their incidence and secretory activity, *Br. J. Exp. Pathol.,* 48, 90, 1968.
53. **Osoba, D.,** The effects of thymus and other lymphoid organs enclosed in millipore diffusion chambers on neonatally thymectomized mice, *J. Exp. Med.,* 122, 633, 1965b.
54. **Dardenne, M., Papiernik, M., Bach, J. F., and Stutman, O.,** Studies on thymus products. III. Epithelial origin of the serum thymic factor, *Clin. Exp. Immunol.,* 27, 299, 1974.
55. **Pyke, K. W. and Gelfand, E. W.,** Morphological and functional maturation of human thymic epithelium in culture, *Nature (London),* 251, 421, 1974.
56. **Comsa, J., Leonhardt, H., and Ozminski, K.,** Hormonal influences on the secretion of the thymus, *Thymus,* 1, 81, 1979.
57. **Bach, J. F. and Dardenne, M.,** Studies on thymus products. II. Demonstration and characterization of a circulating thymic hormone, *Immunology,* 25, 353, 1973.
58. **Pelletier, M., Montplaisir, S., Dardenne, M., and Bach, J. F.,** Thymic hormone activity and spontaneous autoimmunity in dwarf mice and their littermates, *Immunology,* 30, 783, 1976.
59. **Fabris, N. and Mocchegiani, E.,** Homeostatic control of thymic factor turnover, in Abstr. of the 4th Int. Congr. on Immunol., Paris, July 1980.
60. **Deschaux, P.,** Etude In Vivo et In Vitro des Interactions du Thymus avec Certaines Glandes Endocrines, Thesis, University of Lyon, Lyon, France, 1977.
61. **Franceschi, C., Licastro, F., Chiricolo, M., Bonetti, F., Zanotti, M., Fabris, N., Mocchegiani, E. Fantini, M. P., Paolucci, P., and Masi, M.,** Deficiency of autologous mixed lymphocyte reactions and serum thymic factor level in Down Syndrome, *J. Immunol.,* 126, 2161, 1981.
62. **Goldstein, G. and Mackay, I. R.,** *The Human Thymus,* William Heinemann, London, 1969, 128.
63. **Bach, J. F., Dardenne, M., Pleau, J. M., and Bach, M. A.,** Isolation, biochemical characteristics and biological activity of a circulating thymic hormone in the mouse and in the human, *Ann. N.Y. Acad. Sci.,* 249, 186, 1975.
64. **Bach, J. F., Dardenne, M., Papiernik, M., Barvis, A., Levasseur, P., and Lebrand, H.,** Evidence for a serum-factor secreted by the human thymus, *Lancet,* 2, 1056, 1972.
65. **Lewis, V. M., Twomey, J. J., Bealmear, P., Goldstein, G., and Good, R. A.,** Age, thymic involution, and circulating thymic hormone activity, *J. Clin. Endocrinol. Metab.,* 47, 145, 1978.
66. **Pieri, C., Giuli, C., Del Moro, M., and Piantanelli, L.,** Electron microscopic morphometric analysis of mouse liver II. Effect of ageing and thymus transplantation in old animals, *Mech. Ageing Dev.,* 13, 275, 1980.
67. **Gianfranceschi, G. L., Amici, D., and Guglielmi, L.,** Evidence for the presence in calf thymus of a peptidic factor controlling DNA transcription in vitro, *Biochim. Biophys. Acta,* 414, 9, 1975.

68. **Gianfranceschi, G. L., Amici, D., and Guglielmi, L.,** Restriction of template capacity of rat liver chromatin by a non-histone peptide from calf thymus, *Nature (London),* 262, 622, 1976.

69. **Greenberg, L. H. and Weiss, B.,** Beta-adrenergic receptors in aged rat brain: reduced number and capacity of pineal gland to develop supersensitivity, *Science,* 201, 61, 1978.

70. **Schocken, D. D. and Roth, G. S.,** Reduced beta-adrenergic concentrations in aging man, *Nature (London),* 267, 856, 1977.

71. **Pointon, S. E. and Banerjee, S. P.,** Beta-adrenergic and muscarinic cholinergic receptors in rat submaxillar glands: effect of thyroidectomy, *Biochim. Biophys. Acta,* 583, 129, 1979.

72. **Mukherjee, C., Caron, M. G., and Lefkowitz, R. J.,** Catecholamine-induced subsensitivity of adenylatecyclase associated with loss of B-adrenergic receptor binding sites, *Proc. Natl. Acad. Sci. U.S.A.,* 72, 1945, 1975.

73. **Mano, K., Akbarzadeh, A., and Townley, R. G.,** Effect of hydrocortisone on beta-adrenergic receptors in lung membrane, *Life Sci.,* 25, 1925, 1979.

74. **Bach, M. A. and Beaurain, G.,** Respective influence of extrinsic and intrinsic factors on the age-related decrease of thymic secretion, *J. Immunol.,* 122, 2505, 1979.

75. **Timiras, P. S.,** Decline in homeostatic regulation in development, in *Physiology and Aging,* Timiras, P. S., Ed. MacMillan, New York, 1972, 542.

76. **Fabris, N. and Muzzioli, M.,** Recovery of age-dependent immunological deterioration in Balb/c mice by short-term treatment with L-thyroxine, *Mech. Ageing Dev.,* in press.

77. **Besedovsky, H. O., Sorkin, E., Keller, M., and Muller, J.,** Changes in blood hormone levels during the immune response, *Proc. Soc. Exp. Biol. Med.,* 150, 466, 1975.

Chapter 9

MEASUREMENT OF BRAIN AGE:
CONCEPTUAL ISSUES AND NEUROBIOLOGICAL INDICES

Philip W. Landfield

TABLE OF CONTENTS

I. INTRODUCTION

Alterations in brain function are increasingly thought to play a role in the impaired regulation of endocrine-autonomic systems during the aging process.[1-3] Such age-dependent endocrine imbalances, in turn, have been suggested gradually to induce widespread physiological decline in peripheral organ systems. Support for this view of the brain as a "pacemaker" of aging derives from findings which show that age-related changes occur in neuroendocrine regulatory mechanisms[1,2] as well as in peripheral endocrine functions.[1,4,5] Thus, current evidence indicates that the study of altered brain mechanisms should prove of major importance in attempts to understand the causes and implications of hormonal changes during mammalian aging.

Apart from its involvement in hormonal regulation, moreover, brain aging is of course a significant research problem in its own right. That is, it appears to reflect the operation of fundamental biological phenomena, and it is clearly relevant to major human health and social issues.

Despite its importance as a scientific issue, and although considerable research progress has already been made in the description of brain aging, the investigation of brain aging mechanisms is still at a relatively early stage of development. Very little is known, for example, about the etiological factors that modulate rate of brain change over time, and our understanding of the effects of brain aging on peripheral phenomena is also extremely limited. Additionally, there are few definitive data to indicate which of the many brain correlates of aging are directly linked to functional (e.g., behavioral, endocrinologic regulatory) impairment. The resolution of these highly complex questions, then, will clearly require further intensive research efforts in which state-of-the-art neurobiological techniques and a recognition of some of the special methodological issues associated with aging research seem likely to be particularly important.

The present paper addresses one of these special methodologic problems which is, simply, how the degree of neurobiologic (as opposed to chronologic) age can be more accurately measured. Obviously, the chances for success in studies attempting to determine whether brain aging is related to peripheral endocrine (or other physiologic and behavioral) variables will be enhanced if the ability to assess subtle variations in the process of brain aging can be refined.

Although there have been many quantitative studies of age-dependent changes in individual brain variables (as summarized in later sections), the measurement of brain age, as a general process continues to pose some difficult problems for researchers. Primary among these, perhaps, is the fact that no single variable is currently known to be a direct and reliable correlate of the underlying brain aging process. Instead, the term "brain aging" operationally refers to a wide collection of neural variables which correlate roughly with age, but which are not consistently linked with one another, which differ across species, and which vary considerably among individuals within a species. Further, the temporal and quantitative relations of individual variables to underlying aging processes are only beginning to be understood. Lipofuscin granules, for example, appear to accumulate in neuronal cytoplasm as an approximately linear function of age, but other correlates of brain age (e.g., neuronal loss, glial reactivity) may increase more rapidly and, perhaps, exponentially in late life. Which of these, then, if any, is the best index of the underlying brain aging process? In fact, these observations suggest that there may be more than one underlying causal mechanism of "brain aging" and that these several mechanisms may proceed at varying rates.

Another problem, related to that noted above, is that many of the reported correlates of brain aging are undoubtedly secondary or tertiary responses to preceding brain changes or to peripheral alterations which feed back on the brain, rather than being

direct consequences of primary brain aging mechanisms (cf. Reference 6 for discussion of hierarchical mechanisms in aging). Thus, many observed correlates may not be relevant to impaired function, or may be only remotely related to fundamental brain processes.

Additionally, many forms of brain pathology that are not related to age can induce patterns of brain change which are overtly similar to those seen with normal brain aging. Therefore, there is a chance that measures of brain age may be confounded by the presence of unrelated pathology (particularly since aged subjects are more susceptible to a wide variety of diseases). The difficulty in measuring brain aging is further compounded by the fact that aging is an extremely gradual process. As a consequence, there is some overlap between populations of considerably different ages on most individual correlates of brain aging.

During the past few years, the author and collaborators have conducted studies in which the endocrine-physiologic states of aging rats are experimentally manipulated for prolonged periods of time (e.g., 6 to 10 months), in order to investigate the possibility that such factors modulate the rate of brain aging.[7-9] In earlier work, evidence was also found that the level of adrenal corticoid activity was correlated with at least one measure of brain aging in rats (astroglial hypertrophy in hippocampus).[10] Experiments of this kind rely heavily on the ability to detect what can, at best, be expected to be moderate degrees of difference in brain age (i.e., among animals of the same chronologic age that have been subjected to different experimental conditions). Therefore, the author's laboratory has been particularly interested in developing a systematic approach for dealing with the problems noted above and, concomitantly, in developing increasingly sensitive methods for measuring neurobiologic age.

In the following sections, some of the conceptual issues which have seemed important in attempts to improve measurement techniques are briefly considered, and a number of potential neurobiologic and behavioral indices of brain age are reviewed in the context of these considerations. The present survey, however, is selective, and some important neural correlates of age are not discussed. In particular, most of the correlates of brain aging reviewed here are those which bear some clear relevance to measurements in rodents as well as in larger species (as will be seen). A greater emphasis is also placed on neuromorphologic than on other neural correlates, since a large background literature is available in this discipline and since such methods are highly suitable for concurrent processing of brain tissues from large numbers of subjects. The discussions of behavioral, neurophysiological, and neurochemical correlates of age are limited to a few areas in which there is a relatively well-developed literature and/or which seem to provide good illustrative examples from which to generalize to other potentially valuable indices.

II. CONCEPTUAL ISSUES IN MEASURING BRAIN AGE

The major concern in selecting measures of brain aging, of course, is whether or not a particular variable correlates with age. That is, a brain variable must obviously be measurably different in aged subjects vs. young-mature subjects if it is to be used to assess brain age. Moreover, the more discrimination between age groups that it provides (i.e., the less overlap) the more useful it is presumed to be. (See Reference 11 for a discussion of the effect of variance and population size on the measurement of aging.) It is also often assumed that the earlier in life at which an aging correlate can be detected, the more valuable it is. However, this latter assumption may not be completely valid since, as noted above, all correlates of brain aging may not be directly linked, and some may proceed independently of others. Conceivably, therefore, some later

appearing correlates may be of greater relevance to, for example, functional decline. Nevertheless, since brain aging appears to begin by mid-life, age-correlated variables that can be detected early in mature life seem of potential interest in terms of assessing "primary" mechanisms.

Apart from the obvious point of correlation with age, the criteria emphasized in selecting indices for the measurement of brain age in rats are

1. Can the measure be generalized across species (i.e., is it universal among mammals)?
2. Is the overall procedure suitable for measuring multiple variables?
3. Are some of the variables clearly relevant to brain function?
4. Are some of the measures used sensitive to age correlates that begin to change relatively early in adult life?
5. Can the method(s) be applied with sufficient ease to be useful for measuring large quantities of material (i.e., can it be routinely utilized)?

The rationales behind these particular criteria will be discussed.

A. Generality Across Species

The temporal patterns and many qualitative and quantitative aspects of reproductive and general physiological senescence appear to be analogous across all higher vertebrate species; moreover, aging phenomena are apparently found in all multicellular animals.[12] Thus, aging appears to be an extremely fundamental aspect of the biology of vertebrates. Presumably, therefore, the underlying mechanisms of aging are also approximately similar across mammalian species. If aging of the brain is among the underlying mechanisms that govern the general mammalian aging process, as is currently suggested by numerous investigators, it also seems reasonable that at least some aspects of brain aging would be similar across mammalian species. The overt patterns of brain aging can be expected to differ somewhat among species, since the interaction of a common underlying aging mechanism with divergent, species-specific neural adaptations would have likely produced varied patterns of manifestation, and since different species may have evolved some relatively unique brain aging mechanisms. Nevertheless, it also seems probable that at least some aspects of brain aging (if the latter does in fact represent a fundamental aging component) would be relatively similar across species, as are other basic aspects of the aging process. Current evidence suggests that a number of brain variables do in fact show similar patterns of age-dependent change across species (e.g., neuronal density, glial reactivity, lipofuscin, and synaptic degeneration), while other variables exhibit significant species differences (as will be seen, also see discussion in Reference 13).

The use of indices that can be generalized across species, then, appears to increase the probability that the measures more directly reflect the operation of brain aging mechanisms common to all mammals. The study of such common mechanisms should facilitate the eventual generalization of findings from animal experiments to human studies.

Because of these considerations, many of the brain aging indices discussed in the present survey are considered in the context of this point of view.

B. Composite Indices of Multiple Variables

A primary aspect of the rationale for using an index comprised of multiple variables is that, because of extreme individual variability and limitations in measurement procedures, there is often considerable overlap between age groups on any single variable.

Part of the overlap is undoubtedly due to experimental error and lack of refinement or sensitivity in the still imperfect measurement techniques of neurobiology. In addition, however, there appears to be some "true" overlap between groups of aged and young subjects on most variables, even assuming completely accurate measurement. This is likely due, in part, to substantial individual variance in the rate of decline in any single process, as well as to differences in the initial levels from which the gradual decline begins. However, since some aged subjects appear to overlap with younger subjects on one or another but not all variables, a composite score derived from summing or averaging each subjects' values across a battery of multiple indices may considerably reduce total overlap by, presumably, canceling out the effect of experimental or individual variance across variables (and summing the variance due to actual age differences). The author and colleagues recently employed a composite index of this kind, which appeared to reduce overlap between groups.[9]

Another significant reason for using multiple indices is that they should reduce the likelihood of confounding measures of brain aging with those of unrelated pathologies that mimic some, but not all, correlates of brain aging. For example, it is now clear that brain aging is accompanied by reactive changes in astroglia, microglia, and oligodendroglia (as will be seen). However, many forms of unrelated neural trauma including degenerative disease, stroke, edema, epilepsy, renal or hepatic disease, hydroencephalus, blows to the head, etc., can also induce glial reactivity which mimics aspects of that seen with normal aging. Nevertheless, it seems less likely that an unrelated disease or trauma will mimic the pattern of changes across multiple correlates seen in normal brain aging than that it will mimic one or two correlates (senile dementia of the Alzheimer's type appears qualitatively to mimic essentially the entire range of normal brain aging changes,[14] but it remains unclear whether senile dementia is an age-correlated pathology unrelated to normal aging, or whether it is an extreme form of normal brain aging). Thus, in a probabilistic sense, the chances that an abnormal pathological alteration will be confounded with normal aging changes appear to be lessened as the number of variables examined is increased and if the overall pattern of alteration is considered.

As noted earlier, a third reason for using multiple variables to measure aging is that all correlates of brain aging may not proceed in "lock-step." Although primary aging mechanisms may be universal and fundamentally analogous, many of the known correlates of brain aging are presumably secondary, tertiary, or later events in the complex causal chain or normal age-related decline. And each stage of causality may well interact differently with species-specific or individual physiologies, or be subject to different etiological factors. (In this regard, evidence has recently been found that various correlates of brain aging can be experimentally manipulated independently of others.[9])

Thus, it seems beneficial to utilize a profile of scores on multiple age-dependent variables for at least three reasons:

1. To reduce variability of measurement.
2. To avoid confounding of normal brain aging by abnormal pathologies which superficially mimic some correlates.
3. To control for the possibility that rate of change in different age correlates may vary independently and may reflect different underlying mechanisms.

C. Functional Relevance of Some Variables

It is widely suspected that some, perhaps many, neurobiological correlates of brain aging may not be relevant to brain function in the intact animal; i.e., such correlates may either be secondary consequences of earlier and more critical alterations or may be basic age changes which induce little or no impairment of cellular function, at least within the species' normal life span. The latter for example, may be the case for lipofuscin granules.[15] Similarly, a number of age changes may be observed only under a specific set of experimental conditions and may not affect function under physiological conditions. Thus, in order to ensure that some measurements of aging be relevant to the animals' health, survival, or reproduction, one or more measures of normal brain function should seemingly be a component of any index of brain aging. Examples of functional measures include many behavioral, endocrine, autonomic, or neurophysiological measures which bear clear relevance to brain performance.

D. Early Changes

Aged animals are more susceptible to disease of many kinds. The possibility exists, therefore, that many putative measures of "normal" aging may in fact be manifestations of the sequelae of disease. During the past few years, in particular, this possibility has been of growing concern to researchers in aging.[13] That is, while all mammals may be subject to increased susceptibility to disease with aging, the actual diseases to which individual aging mammals succumb are widely varied and the biological alterations they induce are not necessarily analogous to those induced by aging processes common to the species (e.g., the susceptibility to pneumonia, but not the disease itself, is a consistent correlate of normal aging). Thus, animals from a long-term colony infected by respiratory illness, or animals exhibiting evidence of advanced pathology which could influence physiology in many systems, have been excluded from most recent analyses of normal aging changes. (However, these extreme forms of disease should not be confused with the declining function and reserve capacity that occurs in essentially all physiological systems and which are also often viewed as forms of pathology or disease. As noted by Wisniewski and Terry,[14] there is no clear break along the continuum between normal aging and the latter kinds of age-related "normal disease.")

One method of separating measures of normal brain aging from alterations induced by advanced pathology or infectious disease, seemingly, is to utilize at least some correlates of brain aging which exhibit an early age of onset and a gradual rate of age-dependent change. As noted, many age-related changes in physiology and brain function are detectable prior to the midpoint of the life span in humans. However, secondary diseases are presumably more likely to develop late in life and to progress rapidly. The use of brain aging correlates that develop early in mature life may also provide a means for studying primary etiological mechanisms since, by definition, such mechanisms must be operative at the onset of brain aging (at least for some components of the brain aging syndrome).

E. Ease of Measurement

The ease with which brain tissue can be analyzed is a major practical concern if large groups are to be studied. And experiments on the relations of brain aging to endocrine, other physiologic, or behavioral processes often require large groups in order to deal with the variability found in many correlates of brain age. Further, experimental variance is generally reduced if all animals can be concurrently processed or examined.

As previously discussed, there appear to be major advantages to measuring multiple correlates of brain age, and therefore this is also an important consideration in selecting methodological approaches. Many anatomical, behavioral, chemical, and neurophysiological methods are suitable for measuring only one or two major variables. Electron microscopy is of course highly valuable for the detailed assessment of multiple variables, but it is difficult to apply these procedures to large groups of animals. Epon®-embedded, semithin sections (e.g., 0.5 to 2 μm thick) have been increasingly utilized in neuroanatomical studies (see Reference 16 for methods and many references), and a number of investigators have also applied these techniques to the study of the aging brain.[17–22]

The author and colleagues have found that semithin sections are also very useful for the simultaneous analysis of neuronal and glial variables in the aging brain,[8,23] and have recently described and quantified the appearance of multiple neuronal and glial hippocampal correlates of aging in semithin sections in some detail.[9,24] Of course, other light microscopic techniques and methods in disciplines other than anatomy are applicable to, or can be modified for, the analysis of multiple correlates of brain aging.

III. CORRELATES OF BRAIN AGING

In the following sections, potential indices of brain aging from major neurobiologic disciplines are selectively surveyed within the context of some of the points noted earlier. At the end of each major section, a discussion of a few key methodological control problems relevant to that discipline is included.

A. Neuromorphology
1. Neuronal Density

An extensive and detailed study by Brody was the first major analysis to provide quantitative evidence of a decrease in neuronal density in human cerebral cortex during aging.[25] Since then, several investigators, including Brody and collaborators, have confirmed and extended this finding.[15] The human cerebellum has also been shown to undergo neuronal density decreases with age,[26] as does, apparently, the rat cerebellum.[27] On the other hand, brainstem nuclei appear to maintain stable neuronal populations with age.[15] Exceptions to the latter statement, however, include the pigmented catecholaminergic subcortical nuclei, the substantia nigra,[28] and the locus coeruleus,[29] which appear to lose substantial numbers of neurons with aging in humans. However, neuronal density has been reported to remain constant in the locus coeruleus of aging rats.[30] The hippocampus also exhibits decreased neuronal density during aging in humans[31] and monkeys.[32]

Although it now seems well established that there is an age-related decrease in neuronal density in some cortical structures of primates, initial studies with Long-Evans rats did not find clear neocortical cell loss.[33] As previously noted, this is an important point in determining whether decreased cortical cell density is a generalized correlate of mammalian brain aging or is, instead, limited to one or a few species. However, several recent studies indicate that decreased neuronal density during aging does occur in cortical structures of at least some strains or species of rodents. For example, a decreased intensity of staining was found in hippocampal pyramidal neuronal layers, as was a decrease in stained neocortical cells (by gold chloride), in aging Fischer rats.[34] Brizzee and Ordy[35] reported neuronal pyramidal cell decreases of about 15% in hippocampus of aged rats, using a Nissl stain procedure. In recent quantitative studies of semithin sections, the author and colleagues found decreases in pyramidal cell density of approximately 25% in the CA1[9] and CA3[24] hippocampal fields of aged Fischer rats. However, other investigators have reported no age-related decrease of dentate gyrus granule cell density in Fischer rats.[22]

With regard to other brain structures, a decrease in olfactory bulb mitral cell density was also found in 27-month-old rats in a study which showed that volumetric changes in the olfactory bulb could not account for the decrease.[20]

These observations, taken together, suggest that a decrease in neuronal density in some structures (including neocortex, hippocampus, and cerebellum and possibly ol-

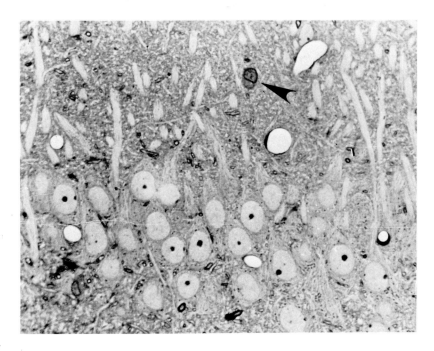

A

FIGURE 1. Comparison of neuronal cell density in hippocampus of young-mature and aged rats in semithin (1.5 μm) sections. (A) Pyramidal cell layer in field CA1 of the hippocampus of a young-mature Fischer rat. Pyramidal cell nuclei (light) are organized in a narrow band (stratum pyradmidale). Nucleoli are darkly staining. The large, apical dendritic shafts are seen projecting into the stratum radiatum from the pyramidal somal layer. Darker cells seen among the neuronal processes are microglia and oligodendrocytes (arrowheads). Small dark circles or ovoids are myelinated axons sectioned transversely or obliquely. Larger circular or eliptical holes in the tissue are sites of blood vessels. (B) Pyramidal cells from CA1 of an aged rat. Note reduced neuronal density with some relatively large "gaps" in the somal layer. Dark glia (arrowheads) can be seen in close apposition to large, translucent astroglial processes ("glial clusters" seen below) in several regions of the basal dendrites of the pyramidal cells (stratum oriens). Several lucent astroglial nuclei are also scattered throughout field. (Magnification × 620.)

factory bulb) is a correlate of aging in several mammalian species that have been carefully examined, and thus, such decreased density may well prove to be a general mammalian correlate of brain aging. Figure 1 (A and B) is an example of this decrease, as seen in semithin sections of pyramidal cells from the hippocampal CA1 regions of specific pathogen-free Fischer male rats.

2. Glial Reactivity

A number of early anatomical studies observed what seemed to be increases in glial cells in neural tissues from aged humans or animals, but only in relatively recent years has the application of quantitative analyses, specific metallic stains, and electron microscopy clearly characterized the nature of age-related glial changes. One of the first quantitative studies of glia as a function of age found increased glial cell density in cerebral cortex of aged rats,[33] although it was not completely clear which kind of glial cells were increased. An extensive electron microscopic analysis by Vaughan and Pe-

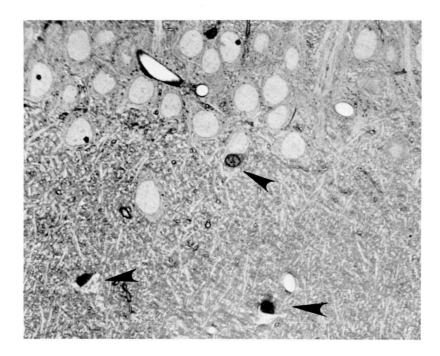

FIGURE 1B

ters,[36] however, showed that it is an increase in microglia (many transformed into reactive "gitter" cells) that is primarily responsible for the enhanced glial density in rat neocortex during aging; moreover, these latter researchers described in some detail the increased inclusions found in the three main glial species during aging. These inclusions, which differed among the glial types, seemed in some cases to include phagocytosed synaptic elements. Hasan and Glees[37] also described ultrastructural glial changes in aged rats (hippocampus), and noted increases in glial satellitosis and glial inclusions, but their descriptions were quite brief. They reported little change in hippocampal astrocytes with age. On the other hand, Sturrock[38] reported an increase in astroglial density in gray matter of aged rodents. Using Cajal's gold sublimate stain for astrocytes, however, the author and colleagues found that hippocampal astrocytes were substantially hypertrophied during aging in specific pathogen-free Fischer rats.[34] It was also found that this astrocyte hypertrophy begins as early as midlife, is most pronounced in dense synaptic terminal fields, but is not accompanied by proliferation of astrocytes.[39] These observations were confirmed in electron microscopic studies,[7,23,40] and such observations have also been extended to monkeys.[41] Gold chloride appears to stain the filaments associated with reactive astroglial hypertrophy, and such glial filaments are readily observed in electron microscopic studies of astroglial profiles in aged brain (Figure 2).

Electron microscopic studies of senile plaques in the brains of aged humans, monkeys, and dogs have also found that reactive glial cells and processes are present on the fringes of the clusters of degenerating synapses at the center of the plaque.[14,17,42] Since senile (or neuritic) plaques are seen in normal brain aging[14,43] as well as in senile dementia, the glial reactions in plaques may be partially analogous to the glial changes found in aging rat brain, because the latter also seem to "cluster" (cf. References 24 and 34). Golgi studies of brains from subjects with advanced senile dementia have also found evidence of massive astrogliosis.[44]

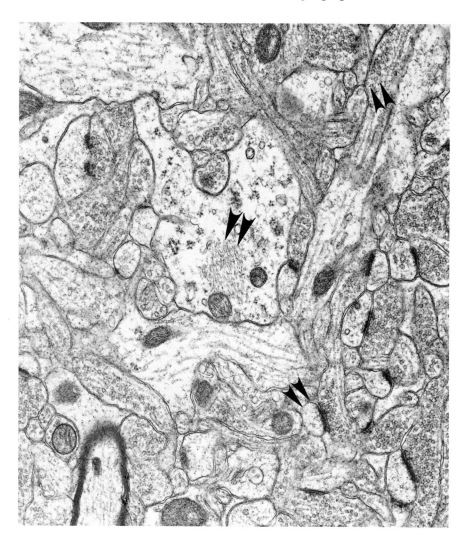

FIGURE 2. Ultrastructural profile of an astroglial process from the Schaffer-commissural axon terminal field in CA1 of the hippocampus of an aged rat. Bundles of filaments (double arrowheads) can be seen in the glial cytoplasm along with glycogen granules. Schaffer collateral en passant terminations (smaller arrowheads) are also seen in this field. (Magnification × 22,800.)

In recent quantitative studies of glial cells in semithin sections from hippocampus of rats, the author and colleagues found an age-related increase in a glial cell population that they termed "dark glia" (in contrast to the light staining astrocytes in semithin sections).[9,23,24] This dark glial population is comprised of both "dark oligodendrocytes" and microglia which are difficult to separately categorize in 1.5-μm-thick semithin sections. By several criteria,[16,36] however, a majority of the dark glia appear to be microglia, which generally confirms the report of an increase in neocortical microglia[36] and extends the result to hippocampus. This dark glia index, however, is one which can sometimes exhibit considerable overlap between young and aged animals, and its potential utility as a sensitive measure of brain aging is therefore not yet established. Nevertheless, several other indices of glial reactivity appear to be suitable for analyses in semithin sections. It was recently observed[9,24] that astrocytes (or large astrocytic processes) are more frequently observed to be in close membrane apposition to dark glial cells in hippocampus of aged animals (Figures 3A and B). These heterogeneous ''glial clusters'' may conceivably be analogous to the clusters of reactive glia found in primate senile plaques. An index of glial clusters may therefore prove of particular interest in quantifying rat brain aging. Additionally, the author and collaborators[9,23,24] and others[21] found that the age-dependent astrocyte inclusions that have been described at the electron microscopic level[36] can be readily quantified in semithin sections (Figures 4A and B), and measures of these inclusions are therefore also utilized to quantify brain aging at the light microscopic level.

3. Synaptic Deterioration

Congophilic senile plaques have been observed for many years in autopsied brains of elderly humans, particularly in those with senile dementia. In recent years, however, the application of electron microscopic (EM) techniques to brain material from humans, monkeys, and dogs has substantially clarified the underlying nature of these plaques.[17,42] It is now clear that these plaques are primarily comprised of clusters of degenerating synaptic terminals and dendritic spines, and are surrounded by reactive glial elements. In later stages, extracellular amyloid fibrils are prominent. The degeneration of the synaptic elements appears to be the initial step in plaque development.[45] Plaques have been reported in humans, monkeys, and dogs, and are most common in neocortex and hippocampus.[17,43] While found in normal elderly humans, the density of plaques is greatly increased in senile dements.[43]

Although spontaneous plaques as such have not been seen in rodents, somewhat analogous processes of synaptic deterioration do apparently occur. Decreases in the Golgi staining of small dendritic spines, and in the dendritic tree in general, in aging rats or mice have been reported in several studies.[18–20] A decreased density of axon terminals at the ultrastructural level was also seen in some analyses.[18] In a series of quantitative EM studies, a decreased density of terminals[22] and dendritic volume[46] have been reported in dentate gyrus of aging Fischer rats. The author and colleagues have also found that there is a decreased density of synapses in field CA1 of hippocampus (in preparation). However, clusters of degenerating synapses, such as are found in plaques in aged humans, monkeys, and dogs,[17,42] have not yet been seen in aged rat brain.

In summary, a decrease in synaptic density appears to be widespread among mammalian species although the topographical patterns of this process apparently differ across species. Additionally, it seems likely that synaptic changes are closely related to observed glial alterations, either as cause or effect (i.e., increased glial reactivity may of course be a reaction to neuronal degeneration, but it could, alternatively, precede neuronal changes, and ''choke off'' synaptic function).

4. Lipofuscin

The accumulation of lipofuscin granules in neuronal cytoplasm was among the earliest morphological brain correlates of aging to be recognized.[47] Neuronal lipofuscin appears to accumulate in a relatively linear fashion in humans,[15] monkeys,[48] and rodents.[49,50] In rats, hippocampal pyramidal cells, cerebellar Purkinje cells, and neocortical neurons are notably affected,[49] although many other regions show accumulation. In larger (e.g., pyramidal) cells, the lipofuscin tends to aggregate at the base of the apical dendrites.[15,48–50] Figure 5 shows examples of lipofuscin granules at the electron microscopic level.

Lipofuscin granules apparently begin to accumulate shortly after birth and, therefore, certainly meet the previously discussed criterion of gradual and early change. Moreover, their presence appears universal, even being found in the tissues of invertebrates.

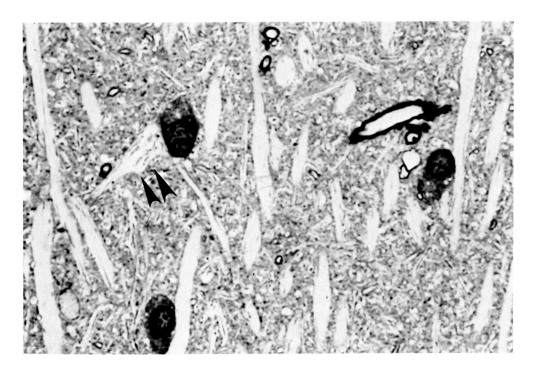

FIGURE 3A. Dark glia (microglia and dark oligodendrocytes) are seen among the apical dendrites of CA1 pyramidal cells from an aged Fischer rat. Adjacent to one of the dark glial cells is a large astrocytic process (arrowheads), forming a "glial cluster." (Magnification × 1550).

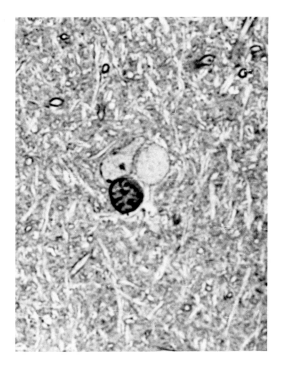

FIGURE 3B. Glial cluster from stratum oriens of an aged rat comprised of dark glial cell, two astroglial nuclei, and astroglial cytoplasm (containing several inclusion granules). (Magnification × 1550.)

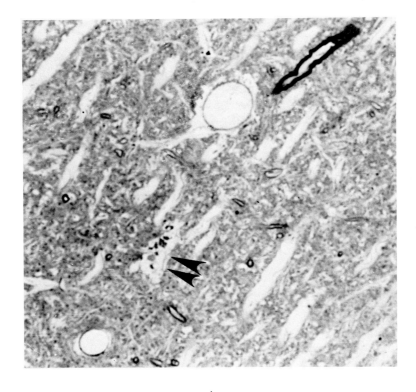

A

FIGURE 4. Astrocyte in hippocampus of aged rat as seen in two serial semithin sections. (A) large astrocyte process containing inclusion granules (arrowheads) is seen near to astroglial nucleus. (B) Serial section shows that process arises from the glial soma. Granules are found in approximately same area of process in both sections. (Magnification × 1550.)

Lipofuscin appears to be comprised of combined lysosomal and lipid fragments, although the exact origin of the pigment remains to be clarified.

Although lipofuscin granules might appear to be a "perfect" brain aging measure, they possess one unfortunate property: it has yet to be clearly shown that lipofuscin is in any way associated with declining cellular function. In fact, the inferior olivary nucleus, in which the cells appear to accumulate more lipofuscin than most, is among those brain nuclei that do not lose cells with age.[15,29]

As noted, this survey focuses on a few main correlates which may be applicable to rodents as well as other species and, therefore, two major correlates of human brain aging, neurofibrillary tangles and granulovacuolar degeneration, are not discussed here. The latter two age changes appear to be largely confined to human brain aging and spontaneous animal analogues have not been observed. However, these phenomena are of considerable importance to the human pattern of brain aging and relevant data are reviewed in depth in several sources. Moreover, a number of other morphologic correlates of brain age, for which the degree of species generality is still unclear, are discussed in several reviews of age-related brain changes.[15,17,42]

5. Specific Methodological Problems

In much of the preceding discussion the term "neuronal density decreases," as opposed to "neuronal loss," was used because, in rats, it is still not fully clear that the

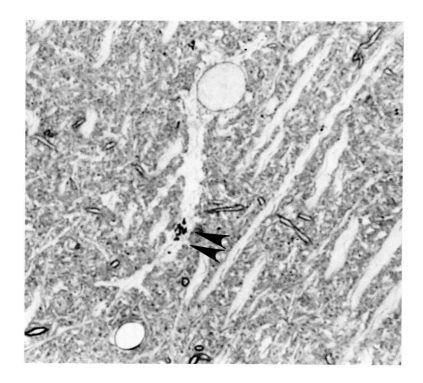

FIGURE 4B

reduced neuronal density in hippocampus during aging is due to neuronal loss rather than to expansion of hippocampal volume. That is, it has been reported that the volume of the hippocampus[51] and the olfactory bulb[20] increases with age in rats. In several studies, strong trends in this direction were also observed.[39] It seems highly possible that increases in hippocampal volume are partly a function of the increase in hippocampal astrocyte volume, which is consistently seen in normally aging rats (and in other species). However, human cerebral cortex and other regions appear, if anything, to decrease in volume with age.[15,26,47] It seems likely, then, that the loss of neurons in certain specific regions is a consistent correlate of normal brain aging. Nevertheless, the relationship of neuronal density to alteration of brain region size with aging, at least in rodents, seems deserving of further clarification.

A well recognized problem in counting cell density in aging subjects is the possibility that the size of the counted unit differs with age. If the counted unit (soma, nucleus, or nucleolus) is decreased in size with age, there is of course a reduced probability of counting the unit in brain sections. Since there is some evidence that somal or nuclear diameter may be decreased with age,[18,52,53] counts may be affected by such size differences. This problem, termed "split-cell error," has been addressed by many investigators over the past several decades and a series of correction factors have been developed. These have been extensively reviewed elsewhere[54,55] and will not be considered further in this survey. It should perhaps be noted, however, that most investigations rely on nucleolar counts in cell counting studies, and it has been found that nucleolar diameter does not appear to be altered as a function of age in hippocampal neurons of rats.[9] Thus, split-nucleolar error does not seem to be a major factor in studies of hippocampal neuronal density in aging rats.

A problem relevant to essentially all morphometric studies of brain aging is the possibility that fixation or preparation artifacts affect the aged tissue differently from

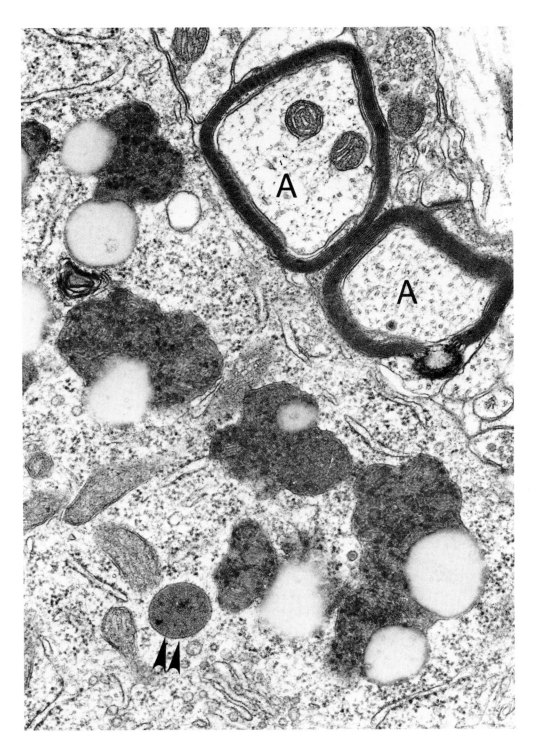

FIGURE 5. Lipofuscin granules in somal cytoplasm of a pyramidal neuron in hippocampus of an aged rat. Note dispersal of endoplasmic reticulum in the region of the lipofuscin accumulation. Granules exhibit typical pattern of vesiculated opaque material in combination with translucent vacuoles. Lysosomes (double arrowheads) are believed to be component of lipofuscin. Myelinated axons (A) are seen just exterior to somal membrane. (Magnification × 38,000.)

young.[47] One of the most effective practical means of dealing with this problem is to use several different methods for studying the same process. For example, the author and others have confirmed the initial observations on hippocampal astrocyte reactivity, made with gold chloride staining,[34] in subsequent analyses at the electron microscopic level. Additionally, observations on hippocampal neuronal density in gold chloride studies were confirmed in semithin sections.[9] The initial findings with the gold chloride could simply have reflected different affinities of aged cells for gold staining, rather than an actual increase in reactivity or decrease in neuronal density. Similarly, several other laboratories have used semithin sections or EM to confirm their Golgi observations on dendritic atrophy with age.[18-20] It has also been suggested that neurons from aged animals may be less intensely stained by Nissl stains. Bondareff[47] has reviewed many of the earlier papers in the area of brain morphology and aging from the point of view of such possible staining or preparation artifacts.

B. Behavior

As noted, a functional index of brain aging could conceivably select from a wide range of behavioral, autonomic, or neuroendocrine regulatory variables, so long as the index assessed activity of the brain by methods that were in some way relevant to normal physiological conditions. These cannot be comprehensively reviewed here, and the following discussion is limited to a brief consideration of altered performance on learning and memory tasks during aging. (See Reference 56 for comprehensive behavioral reviews.)

Because of a particular emphasis on neurobiological aging of the hippocampus, the author's laboratory assesses functional brain aging using a series of maze learning-retention tasks known to be affected by hippocampal lesions. Clearly, the observation that aging animals are impaired on some of the same tasks as are hippocampally-lesioned animals[57] does not directly demonstrate that age-related hippocampal pathology is responsible for the behavioral deficits found in aged animals. However, such observations are at least consistent with predictions arising from the hypothesis that age-related behavioral change is, in part, affected by hippocampal change.[34,57]

Considerable evidence indicates that memory and learning performance is impaired in aged humans[58] and monkeys.[59] With regard to the present emphasis on phenomena which can be generalized across mammalian species, it seems of interest that many other studies also suggest that brain "plasticity" functions may be impaired in rodents with age.[60-63] Much of this work has been recently reviewed.[58,60,61]

Doty[64] found that aging rats exhibit impaired performance on a maze task when trials were massed, but not when distributed. Goodrick,[63] however, found essentially the opposite effect, but there were major procedural differences between the studies.

A number of investigators have pointed to task difficulty as a key factor in age-related performance impairment in rats.[62] Although virtually all investigators agree that no age differences are found in the acquisition of a simple two-choice discrimination task (e.g., T-maze) by rats, tasks with additional choice points (e.g., four-choice discrimination mazes) consistently demonstrate age differences.[60,62]

Reversal learning tasks are known to be impaired by large hippocampal lesions, but there is some disagreement as to whether or not reversal is impaired in aged animals. In some studies, no impairment of reversal was seen, while in others, reversal learning was impaired.[58,60,63] Again, however, evidence of impairment in some reversal tasks appeared to depend on the degree of task difficulty.[58,60,62]

Recent studies have also utilized spatial maze tasks for the assessment of age-related performance. Performance of aging rats on such tasks was found to be deficient.[65,66] However, Wallace et al.[66] suggested that a visual acuity deficit might be one factor influencing the reduced performance of aged Fischer rats. These investigators also studied short-term memory in an operant conditioning task, but found no aging deficit.[66]

In attempts to find a task that could assess age-related impairments in complex information processing or storage systems, the author and colleagues first employed a paradigm incorporating tests of active avoidance in a simple Y-maze avoidance. Several 2-min retention tests on which no foot-shocks were given were also interspersed with the foot-shock training trials.[57] In more recent studies with a similar task, however, it was found (in agreement with research of others) that performance impairment can be more consistently observed when a reversal paradigm is included. Aged animals exhibit fewer correct choices and higher latencies on reversal trials, although they often perform as well as young animals on the initial training or test trials.[9] Recent studies in the author's laboratory (unpublished) found evidence that this deficit on reversal tests may depend upon a memory impairment (i.e., more forgetting seems to occur between trials even though acquisition appears normal). These findings are therefore consistent with those of Gold and McGaugh[61] who reported more rapid forgetting in aged Fischer rats on both a one-trial passive avoidance task and on a discriminated active avoidance task.

However, one factor that is often overlooked in studies on animal learning (and not solely in aging studies), is that differences in task difficulty are usually present between tasks that are being compared on some dimension of their design other than difficulty. Reversal learning, for example, is not simply a paradigm involving inhibition of prior tendencies. It also requires that more information be processed and compared than is the case for the original learning (i.e., the new information to be acquired, and the relations of this to the previously acquired information, must be dealt with in reversal tasks). Similarly, spatial mazes probably require that a great deal more information be learned than do most other tasks, since correct choice depends upon memory of the relations between, for example, all eight arms of a radial maze. Operant conditioning, on the other hand, appears to be a relatively simple task that is typically also associated with considerable overtraining. Thus, task difficulty may well be a serious confounding factor in attempting to compare performance across tasks which are thought to differ primarily on factors other than difficulty.

Differences between results from various laboratories on learning tasks, then, may be due to a wide variety of factors including subtle differences in task difficulty, trial spacing, or in physiological age. As an example of the latter, inbred Fischer 344 rats maintained in somewhat different environments and on different diets have been found to exhibit quite different mean life spans and mean body weights.[13]

Obviously, simply because a task requires learning and memory for its performance does not mean that relative performance in that task is determined solely, or even primarily, by differences in learning-memory mechanisms. Numerous factors affect maze learning performance in animals, including motivation, activity levels, sensory perception, motor abilities, reaction speed, arousal levels, and inhibitory mechanisms, as well as the "plasticity" mechanisms which directly participate in the acquisition, storage, or retrieval of information. Aging animals, for example, have been found to undergo alterations in appetitive motivational systems, in foot-shock thresholds, and are well known to show reduced reaction speeds. Further, visual and auditory acuity declines and olfactory function, running wheel activity, and motor functions and strength are substantially changed, as is open field exploratory activity.[56,58,60] All of these age-related phenomena, and others, must be controlled for in attempting to assess brain information processing and storage systems in aged animals.

Thus, the measurement of behavioral plasticity during aging requires that considerable attention be given to experimental design. Many alternative interpretations can be controlled for, however, if it can be shown that the aged animals can perform the task normally and are only impaired if certain specific conditions are introduced (e.g., a delay in testing, a reversal procedure, etc.). There are, of course, similarly extensive control problems that must be considered in the assessment of other complex functional measures.

C. Neurophysiology

There is a relatively small literature on the use of electrophysiological methods to assess brain aging and, therefore, serious problems arise in attempting to relate animal studies to findings in humans. Although human research has yielded several consistent EEG[67] and evoked potential[68] correlates of aging, there have been few animal studies on age-related EEG changes, and those few [69] have not found clear-cut EEG changes as a function of age. Nevertheless, the human and rat EEGs exhibit major differences (e.g., no alpha rhythms in rats) and, in any case, there have been far too few EEG studies in aging animals to determine at this point whether or not consistent age differences can be found. Further research however, should be able to clarify this question.

In elderly humans, alpha rhythm mean frequency is consistently slowed;[67] there is an increase in EEG fast activity and an increased incidence of focal slow activity.[70] Moreover, several investigators have found significant correlations between measures of intellectual function and EEG changes with age.[71,72] Studies of evoked potentials also indicate that evoked electrical activity may provide useful correlations with age-dependent behavioral change.[73] Some data suggest that EEG changes, at least in senile dementia, may be correlated with altered cerebral blood flow.[74]

There have been relatively few microelectrode investigations of age changes in neural function, and most of these have been conducted in peripheral or spinal systems.[75–77] In an ongoing series of studies, however, the author and co-workers have been examining the synaptic physiology of a well-defined brain pathway (Schaffer-commissural monosynaptic projection to field CA1 of hippocampus) in both intact aging animals[78] and in the in vitro hippocampal slice.[79] The results indicate that age differences in synaptic physiology are relatively subtle below the mean longevity age of Fischer rats (e.g., 27 to 28 months), and their detection, therefore, is facilitated by administering "challenging" stimulation. In response to single stimulation pulses, for example, the postsynaptic responses (EPSP and spike) of hippocampal neurons are often found to be only slightly modified. However, if repetitive stimulation is administered (e.g., 4 to 15 Hz), hippocampal synapses in aged rats do not exhibit as large a frequency potentiation of postsynaptic response as do synapses in young rats, and/or exhibit a more rapid depression.[78,79]

Other physiological experiments suggest that neurotransmitter mobilization or stores may be deficient in the hippocampus of aging animals.[80,81] Additionally, the author and colleagues found that the degree of this impairment in hippocampal frequency potentiation was significantly correlated with degree of active avoidance deficit in aged rats,[57] suggesting that these synaptic phenomena may be functionally relevant.

Barnes[65] has recently utilized a somewhat similar paradigm in the dentate gyrus (which exhibits properties of potentiation similar to those of hippocampus), but instead studied very long-term potentiation in chronically implanted animals, aged 27 to 34 months. In that study, reduced extracellular EPSP amplitude to single pulses was observed and very long-term potentiation (e.g., 3 weeks) decayed more rapidly in aging animals (but LTP was not different in initial levels). This decay was correlated with impairment on a spatial maze.

Smith[82] using a neuromuscular junction preparation from aged rats, found synaptic deficits during repetitive stimulation that were similar to those Landfield and colleagues observed in the brain; i.e., neuromuscular junction transmission fails more rapidly in aged animals during repetitive stimulation, and the deficit appears to be due to transmitter depletion. Some years ago, Wayner and Emmers[76] reported that spinal synaptic delay is increased in aged rats, which also suggests that the synapse is an important site of age-dependent physiological change.

Clearly, it will be some time before measures such as these can be routinely applied to assess degree of neurobiologic age, and such methods obviously cannot be employed in humans. However, as further progress is made, it may well prove to be possible to compare cortically or skull-recorded potentials from humans to electrophysiological correlates of brain aging in laboratory animals.

Among the major control and interpretative problems in neurophysiological research are possible disruptive effects of peripheral disease on extracellular-intracellular electrolyte ratios, possible altered responses of aging animals to anesthesia, and the reported decreases in synaptic and cellular density.[57] Problems of disturbed electrolyte balance can perhaps best be circumvented by using healthy aging animals or by employing in vitro neurophysiological procedures in which the extracellular ionic environment is controlled by the investigator. With regard to the use of anesthesia in acute neurophysiological studies, it is clear that aging animals metabolize drugs differently, exhibit altered concentrations of receptors, and are less able to effectively maintain body temperature during anesthesia.[13] Both chronic and in vitro preparations allow this difficulty to be avoided. However when anesthetized preparations are used, careful regulation of temperature is important. The decline in synaptic and cellular density is important to the interpretation of any age differences that may be found in the amplitude of electrical responses, since such differences could be due to lesser numbers of underlying neural elements or to each element producing a lesser response. However, several neurophysiological paradigms are suitable for separating the effects of a reduced population of responding elements from the effects of a reduced response in individual elements (cf. Reference 57).

D. Neurochemistry

This section very briefly considers two aspects of neurochemistry and aging (i.e., neurotransmission and energy metabolism) in which it is becoming increasingly possible to compare findings from human and animal studies.

Among the most consistent findings to date is evidence that brain catecholaminergic systems in rodents exhibit either reduced turnover or reduced content.[83–86] Further, presumed functions of catecholaminergic systems appear to be impaired (e.g., in the regulation of hormonal systems and in the control of some motor behaviors).[83,85,87,88] In humans, deficiencies in catecholamine-related enzymatic systems are also present.[89,90] Catecholamine binding to brain receptors is decreased in aging animals.[91–93] Further, a variety of specific brain receptors may be reduced, since it was previously shown that glucocorticoid binding is decreased in aged rat brain.[95] Decreased catecholamines in human caudate nucleus and hypothalamus could well be related to the earlier-mentioned cell loss in substantia nigra and in locus coeruleus, respectively.

Cholinergic systems also appear to exhibit major alterations with age, particularly in senile dementia.[95–97] Additionally, there is increasing evidence that such alterations in septo-hippocampal systems may be related to impaired memory functions in aged humans, monkeys, and rodents.[98–100] Alterations in amino acids have also been detected in aging neural tissue.[101] That the deficits may not be limited to transmitter-receptor interactions, moreover, is suggested by evidence that second messenger systems are changed in brains of aging animals.[102–104]

These chemical changes in systems believed to be involved in synaptic transmission, then, possess obvious potential relevance to the alterations in synaptic physiology and morphology noted above.

Several studies have found that cerebral metabolism is also decreased in aging rodents, particularly when the brain is "challenged."[105–107] Cerebral metabolism, in addition, is altered in elderly humans, but it is still not known whether this effect is limited to those with senile dementia or whether it also affects the normal elderly (to lesser degrees).[74]

It should also be noted that there are of course many other important aspects of neurochemistry and aging that were not considered here, including factors related to axonal transport and microtubular assembly, trophic factors, RNA and protein synthesis, phosphorylation of enzymes, membrane permeability changes, genetic regulation, etc., which will undoubtedly prove to be of fundamental significance in the eventual analysis of underlying mechanisms and, in all likelihood, in the measurement of brain aging changes.

Several special control problems appear relevant to the large majority of neurochemical studies on brain aging (also see discussion in Reference 108). These include age-related decline in synaptic and cellular density, altered glia to neuronal ratios, and possible disturbances in cerebral vasculature and energy metabolism. That is, it is difficult to pinpoint the basis of an observed age-dependent change in the concentration of some molecular species (e.g., neurotransmitter) since either an alteration in the synthesis (or metabolism) of that substance, or an alteration in the density of the elements (e.g., synapses) which synthesize or store the substance, could yield similar results. However, normalizing the substance in relation to some other specific (e.g., synaptic) marker molecule, or using morphometric analyses of synaptic density seem to be among possible effective control procedures for this problem. Similarly, distinguishing changes due to altered glial activity or size from changes due to altered neuronal function is extremely difficult in the aged brain. Again, however, specific marker enzymes, morphometric methods, or cell separation techniques may be of use in controlling for these problems. Alterations in extracellular space, glial activity, cerebral metabolism, or vascular function may all affect precursor distribution and uptake in aged brain and thus, precursor availability is a critical design consideration in many neurochemical studies of aging.

IV. CONCLUSIONS

Selected aspects of neurobiology and aging have been briefly summarized and considered in terms of present and potential contributions to the measurement of brain aging. More comparative information currently exists for morphometric and behavioral measures of brain aging and, therefore, indices from these disciplines currently appear to be among the more useful for the routine measurement of brain age. However, neurophysiological and neurochemical techniques provide new approaches for basic analyses of brain aging mechanisms, and, in the near future, seem likely to provide accurate and reliable indices for the assessment of normal brain aging. It is suggested here, however, that neurobiologic-behavioral aging correlates used to measure brain age should meet several criteria. That is, at least some of the correlates should exhibit an early onset and gradual progression, should assess functional brain change during aging, and should be compatible with inclusion in a composite index of multiple variables.

ACKNOWLEDGMENTS

Studies described in this paper are supported in part by research grants AG 01552 and AG 01737. The author thanks Teresa Horton and Stephanie Burgoyne for excellent clerical and editorial contributions.

REFERENCES

1. **Finch, C. E.**, The regulation of physiological changes during mammalian aging, *Q. Rev. Biol.*, 51, 49, 1976.
2. **Meites, J., Huang, H. H., and Simpkins, J. W.**, Recent studies on neuroendocrine control of reproductive senescence in rats, in *The Aging Reproductive System*, Schneider, E. L., Ed., Raven Press, New York, 1978, 213.
3. **Shock, N. W.**, Physiological aspects of aging in man, *Ann. Rev. Physiol.*, 23, 97, 1974.
4. **Andres, R. and Tobin, J. D.**, Endocrine systems, in *Handbook of the Biology of Aging*, Finch, C. E. and Hayflick, L., Eds., Van Nostrand-Reinhold, New York, 1977, 357.
5. **Wexler, B. C.**, Comparative aspects of hyperadrenocroticism and aging, in *Hypothalamus Pituitary and Aging*, Everitt, A. F. and Burgess, J. A., Eds., Charles C Thomas, Springfield, Ill., 1976, p 333.
6. **Landfield, P. W.**, Adrenocortical hypotheses of brain and somatic aging, in *Biological Mechanisms of Aging*, NIH Publ. No. 81-2194, Schimke, R., Ed., National Institutes of Health, Washington, D.C., 1981, 658.
7. **Landfield, P. W.**, An endocrine hypothesis of brain aging and studies of brain-endocrine correlations and monosynaptic neurophysiology during aging, in *Parkinson's Disease II. Aging and Neuroendocrine Relationships*, Finch, C., Potter, D., and Kenny, A., Eds., Plenum Press, New York, 1978, 179.
8. **Landfield, P. W., Wurtz, C., Lindsey, J. D., and Lynch, G.**, Long-term adrenalectomy reduces some morphological correlates of brain aging, *Soc. Neurosci. Abstr.*, 5, 20, 1979.
9. **Landfield, P. W., Baskin, R. K., and Pitler, T. A.**, Brain aging correlates: retardation by hormonal-pharmacological treatments, *Science*, 214, 581, 1981.
10. **Landfield, P. W., Waymire, J. C., and Lynch, G.**, Hippocampal aging and adrenocorticoids: quantitative correlations, *Science*, 202, 1098, 1978.
11. **Ludwig, F. C. and Smoke, M. E.**, The measurement of biological age, *Exp. Aging Res.*, 6, 497, 1980.
12. **Strehler, B. L.**, *Time, Cells and Aging*, 2nd ed., Academic Press, New York, 1977.
13. NAS Committee on Animal Models of Aging, *Mammalian Models for Research on Aging*, National Academy Press, Washington, D.C., 1981.
14. **Wisniewski, H. M. and Terry, R. D.**, Neuropathology of the aging brain, in *Neurobiology of Aging*, Terry, R. D., and Gershon, S., Eds., Raven Press, New York, 1976.
15. **Brody, H. and Vijayashankar, N.**, Anatomical changes in the nervous system, in *Handbook of the Biology of Aging*, Finch, C. E. and Hayflick, L., Eds., Van Nostrand-Reinhold, New York, 1977, 241.
16. **Ling, E. A., Paterson, J. A., Privat, A., Mori, S., and Leblond, C. P.**, Investigation of glial cells in semithin sections. I. Identification of glial cells in the brain of young rats, *J. Comp. Neurol.*, 149, 43, 1973.
17. **Wisniewski, H. M. and Terry, R. D.**, Morphology of the aging brain, human and animal, *Prog. Brain Res.*, 40, 167, 1973.
18. **Feldman, M. L.**, Aging changes in the morphology of cortical dendrites, in *Neurobiology of Aging*, Terry, R. D. and Gershon, S., Eds., Raven Press, New York, 1976, 211.
19. **Vaughan, D. W.**, Age-related deterioration of pyramidal cell basal dendrites in rat auditory cortex, *J. Comp. Neurol.*, 171, 501, 1977.
20. **Hinds, J. W. and Mcnelly, N. A.**, Aging of the rat olfactory bulb: growth and atrophy of constituent layers and changes in size and number of mitral cells, *J. Comp. Neurol.*, 171, 345, 1977.
21. **Brawer, J. R., Schipper, H., and Naftolin, F.**, Ovary-dependent degeneration in the hypothalamic arcuate nucleus, *Endocrinology*, 107, 274, 1980.
22. **Geinisman, Y., Bondareff, W., and Dodge, J. T.**, Partial deafferentation of neurons in the dentate gyrus of the senescent rat, *Brain Res.*, 134, 541, 1977.
23. **Landfield, P. W., Lindsey, J. D., Braun, L., Wurtz, C., Maxwell, M., and Lynch, G.**, Quantitative E.M. and semithin studies on synaptic vesicles and degeneration, astrocyte reactivity, microglia, lipofuscin and displaced nucleoli in hippocampal neurons of rats during aging, *Proc. Gerontol. Soc.*, 31, 92, 1978.
24. **Landfield, P. W., Braun, L., Lindsey, J. D., Pitler, T. A., and Lynch, G.**, Hippocampal aging in rats: a morphometric study of multiple variables in semithin sections, *Neurobiol. Aging*, 2, 265, 1981.

25. **Brody, H.,** Organization of cerebral cortex. III. A study of aging in the human cerebral cortex, *J. Comp. Neurol.,* 102, 511, 1955.

26. **Corsellis, J. A. N.,** Some observations on the Purkinje cell population and on brain volume in human aging, in *Neurobiology of Aging,* Terry, R. D. and Gershon, S., Eds., Raven Press, New York, 1976, 205.

27. **Rogers, J., Silver, M. A., Shoemaker, W. J., and Bloom, F. E.,** Senescent changes in a neurobiological model system: cerebellar Purkinje cell electrophysiology and correlative anatomy, *Neurobiol. Aging,* 1, 3, 1980.

28. **McGeer, P. L., McGeer, E. G., and Suzuki, J. S.,** Aging and extrapyramidal function, *Arch. Neurol.,* 34, 33, 1977.

29. **Brody, H.,** An examination of cerebral cortex and brain-stem aging, in *Neurobiology of Aging,* Terry, R. D. and Gershon, S., Eds., Raven Press, New York, 1976, 171.

30. **Goldman, G. and Coleman, P. D.,** Neuron numbers in locus coeruleus do not change with age in Fischer 344 rat, *Neurobiol. Aging,* 2, 33, 1981.

31. **Ball, M. J.,** Neuronal loss, neurofibrillary tangles and granulovacuolar degeneration in the hippocampus with aging and dementia: a quantitative study, *Acta Neuropathol.,* 37, 111, 1977.

32. **Brizzee, K. R., Ordy, J. M., and Bartus, R. T.,** Localization of cellular changes within multimodal sensory regions in aged monkey brain: possible implications for age-related cognitive loss, *Neurobiol. Aging,* 1, 45, 1980.

33. **Brizzee, K. R., Sherwood, N., and Timiras, P. S.,** A comparison of cell populations at various depth levels in cerebral cortex of young adult and aged Long-Evans rats, *J. Gerontol.,* 23, 289, 1968.

34. **Landfield, P. W., Rose, G., Sandles, L., Wohlstadter, T., and Lynch, G.,** Patterns of astroglial hypertrophy and neuronal degeneration in the hippocampus of aged, memory-deficient rats, *J. Gerontol.,* 32, 3, 1977.

35. **Brizzee, K. R. and Ordy, J. M.,** Age pigments, cell loss and hippocampal function, *Mech. Aging Develop.,* 9, 143, 1979.

36. **Vaughan, D. W. and Peters, A.,** Neuroglial cells in the cerebral cortex of rats from young adulthood to old age: an electron microscope study, *J. Neurocytol.,* 3, 405, 1974.

37. **Hasan, M. and Glees, P.,** Ultrastructural age changes in hippocampal neurons, synapses and neuroglia, *Exp. Gerontol.,* 8, 75, 1973.

38. **Sturrock, R. R.,** Quantitative morphological changes in neurons and neuroglia in the indusium griseum of aging mice, *J. Gerontol.,* 32, 647, 1977.

39. **Lindsey, J. D., Landfield, P. W., and Lynch, G.,** Early onset and topographical distribution of hypertrophied astrocytes in hippocampus of aging rats: a quantitative study, *J. Gerontol.,* 34, 661, 1979.

40. **Geinisman, Y., Bondareff, W., and Dodge, J. T.,** Hypertrophy of astroglial processes in the dentate gyrus of the senescent rat, *Am. J. Anat.,* 153, 537, 1978.

41. **Knox, C. A., Jirge, S. K., Brizzee, K. R., Ordy, J. M., and Bartus, R. T.,** Quantitative analysis of synaptic junctions, axon preterminals and astroglial processes in the hippocampus of young and old rhesus monkeys, *Soc. Neurosci. Abstr.,* 5, 18, 1979.

42. **Terry, R. D. and Wisniewski, H. M.,** Ultrastructure of senile dementia and of experimental analogs, in *Aging and the Brain,* Gaitz C. M., Ed., Plenum Press, New York, 1972, 89.

43. **Tomlinson, B. E. and Henderson, G.,** Some quantitative cerebral findings in normal and demented old people in *Neurobiology of Aging,* Terry, R. D. and Gershon, S., Eds., Raven Press, New York, 1976, 183.

44. **Scheibel, M. E. and Scheibel, A. B.,** Structural changes in the aging brain, in *Aging I,* Brody, H., Harmon, D., and Ordy, J. M., Eds., Raven Press, New York, 1975, 11.

45. **Wisniewski, H. M., Ghetti, B., and Terry, R. D.,** Neuritic (senile) plaques and filamentous changes in aged rhesus monkeys, *J. Neuropath. Exp. Neurol.,* 32, 566, 1973.

46. **Geinisman, Y., Bondareff, W., and Dodge, J. T.,** Dendritic atrophy in the dentate gyrus of the senescent rat, *Am. J. Anat.,* 152, 321, 1978.

47. **Bondareff, W.,** Morphology of the aging nervous system, in *Handbook of Aging and the Individual,* Birren, J. E., Ed., University of Chicago Press, Chicago, Ill., 1959, 136.

48. **Brizzee, K. R., Ordy, J. M., and Kaack, B.,** Early appearance and regional differences in intra-neuronal and extraneuronal lipofuscin accumulation with age in the brain of a nonhuman primate, *J. Gerontol.,* 29, 366, 1974.

49. **Reichel, W., Hollander, J., Clark, J. H., and Strehler, B.,** Lipofuscin pigment accumulation as a function of age and distribution in rodent brain, *J. Gerontol.,* 23, 71, 1968.

50. **Samorajski, T., Ordy, J. M., and Keefe, J. R.,** The fine structure of lipofuscin age pigment in the nervous system of aged mice, *J. Cell Biol.,* 26, 779, 1965.

51. **Diamond, M. C., Johnson, R. E., and Ingham, C.,** The development, adult and aging patterns of the cerebral cortex, hippocampus and diencephalon, *Behav. Biol.,* 14, 163, 1975.

52. **Lin, K. H., Peng, Y. M., Peng, M. T., and Tseng, T. M.,** Changes in the nuclear volume of rat hypothalamic neurons in old age, *Neuroendocrinology,* 21, 247, 1976.

53. **Vaughan, D. W. and Vincent, J. M.,** Ultrastructure of neurons in the auditory cortex of ageing rats: a morphometric study, *J. Neurocytol.,* 9, 215, 1979.

54. **Konigsmark, B. W.** Methods for counting of neurons, in *Contemporary Research Methods in Neuroanatomy,* Nauta, W. and Ebbesson, S. O., Eds., Springer-Verlag, Berlin, 1970, 315.

55. **Ebbesson, S. O. E. and Tang, D.,** A method for estimating the number of cells in histological sections, *J. Royal Micros. Soc.,* 84, 449, 1965.

56. **Birren, J. E. and Schaie, K. W., eds.,** Handbook of the Psychology of Aging, Van Nostrand-Reinhold, New York, 1977.

57. **Landfield, P. W.,** Correlative studies of brain neurophysiology and behavior during aging, in *Psychobiology of Aging,* Stein, D., Ed., Elsevier, New York, 1980, 227.

58. **Arenberg, D. and Robertson-Tchabo, E. A.,** Learning, in *Handbook of the Psychology of Aging,* Birren, J. E. and Schaie, K. W., Van Nostrand-Reinhold, New York, 1977, 421.

59. **Bartus, T. R.,** Physostigmine and recent memory: effects in young and aged nonhuman primates, *Science,* 206, 1087, 1979.

60. **Elias, P. K. and Elias, M. F.,** Effects of age on learning ability: contributions from the animal literature, *Exp. Aging Res.,* 2, 165, 1976.

61. **Gold, P. E. and McGaugh, J. L.,** Changes in learning and memory during aging, in *Neurobiology of Aging,* Ordy, J. M. and Brizzee, K. R., Eds., Plenum Press, New York, 1975, 145.

62. **Botwinick, J., Brinley, J. F., and Robbin, J. S.,** Learning and reversing a four-choice multiple Y-maze by rats of three ages, *J. Gerontol.,* 18, 179, 1963.

63. **Goodrick, C. L.,** Learning, retention and extinction of a complex maze habit for mature-young and senescent Wistar albino rats, *J. Gerontol.,* 23, 198, 1968.

64. **Doty, B. A.,** Age and avoidance conditioning in rats, *J. Gerontol.,* 21, 287, 1966.

65. **Barnes, C. A.,** Memory deficits associated with senescence: a neurophysiological and behavioral study in the rat, *J. Comp. Physiol.,* 93, 74, 1979.

66. **Wallace, J. E., Krauter, E. E., and Campbell, B. A.,** Animal models of declining memory in the aged: Short-term and spatial memory in the aged rat, *J. Gerontol.,* 35, 355, 1980.

67. **Busse, E. W. and Obrist, W. D.,** Pre-senescent electroencephalographic changes in normal subjects, *J. Gerontol.,* 20, 315, 1965.

68. **Thompson, L. W., Michalewski, H. J., and Saul, R. E.,** Age differences in cortical evoked potentials: a comparison of normal and older adults and individuals with CNS disorders, in *Senile Dementia: a Biomedical Approach,* Nandy, K., Ed., Elsevier, Amsterdam, 1978, 139.

69. **Zepelin, H., Whitehead, E. E., and Rechtschaffen, A.,** Aging and sleep in the albino rat, *Behav. Biol.,* 7, 65, 1972.

70. **Busse, E. W. and Obrist, W. D.,** Significance of focal electroencephalographic changes in the elderly, *Postgrad. Med.,* 34, 179, 1963.

71. **Wang, H. S., Obrist, W. D., and Busse, E. W.,** Neurophysiological correlates of the intellectual function of elderly persons living in the community, *Am. J. Psychiatr.,* 126, 1205, 1970.

72. **Busse, E. W., Barnes, R. H., Friedmen, E. L., and Kelty, E. J.,** Psychological functioning of aged individuals with normal and abnormal electroencephalograms: I. A study of non-hospitalized community volunteers, *J. Nerv. Ment. Dis.,* 124, 135, 1956.

73. **Thompson, L. W. and Wilson, S.,** Electrocortical reactivity and learning in the elderly, *J. Gerontol.,* 21, 45, 1966.

74. **Obrist, W. D., Sokoloff, L., Lassen, N. A., Lane, M. H., Butler, R. N., and Feinberg, I.,** Relation of EEG to cerebral blood flow and metabolism in old age, *Electroencephalogr. Clin. Neurophysiol.,* 15, 610, 1963.

75. **Birren, J. E. and Wall, P. D.,** Age changes in conduction velocity, refractory period, number of fibers, connective tissue space and blood vessels in sciatic nerves of rats, *J. Comp. Neurol.,* 104, 1, 1956.

76. **Wayner, M. J. and Emmers, R.,** Spinal synaptic delay in young and aged rats, *Am. J. Physiol.,* 194, 403, 1958.

77. **Vyskocil, F. and Gutmann, E.,** Spontaneous transmitter release from nerve endings and contractile properties in the soleus and diaphragm muscles of senile rats, *Experientia,* 28, 280, 1972.

78. **Landfield, P. W., McGaugh, J. L., and Lynch, G.,** Impaired synaptic potentiation processes in the hippocampus of aged, memory-deficient rats, *Brain Res.,* 150, 85, 1978.

79. **Landfield, P. W. and Lynch, G.,** Impaired monosynaptic potentiation in in vitro hippocampal slices from aged, memory-deficient rats, *J. Gerontol.,* 32, 523, 1977.

80. **Landfield, P. W., Wurtz, C., and Lindsey, J. D.,** Quantification of synaptic vesicles in hippocampus of aging rats and initial studies of possible relations to neurophysiology, *Brain Res. Bull.,* 4, 757, 1979.

81. **Landfield, P. W.,** Age-related impairment of hippocampal frequency potentiation: evidence of an underlying deficit in transmitter release from studies of magnesium-bathed hippocampal slices, *Soc. Neurosci. Abstr.,* 7, 371, 1981.

82. **Smith, D. O.,** Reduced capabilities of synaptic transmission in aged rats, *Exp. Neurol.,* 66, 650, 1979.

83. **Finch, C. E.,** Age-related changes in brain catecholamines: a synopsis of findings in C57BJ/6J mice and other rodent models, in *Parkinson's Disease II. Aging and Neuroendocrine Relationships,* Finch, C. E., Potter, D. E., and Kenny, A. D., Eds., Plenum Press, New York, 1978, 15.

84. **Riegle, G. E. and Miller, A. E.,** Aging effects on the hypothalamic-hypophyseal-gonadal control system in the rat, in *The Aging Reproductive System,* Schneider, E. L., Ed., Raven Press, New York, 1978, 159.

85. **Clemens, J. A. and Bennett, D. R.,** Do aging changes in the preoptic area contribute to loss of cyclic endocrine function? *J. Gerontol.,* 32, 19, 1977.

86. **Simpkins, J. W., Mueller, G. P., Huang, H. H., and Meites, J.,** Evidence for depressed catecholamine and enhanced serotonin metabolism in aging male rats: possible relation to gonadotropin secretion, *Endocrinology,* 100, 1672, 1977.

87. **Joseph, J. A., Berger, R. C., Engel, B. T., and Roth, G. S.,** Age-related changes in the nigrostriatum: a behavioral and biochemical analysis, *J. Gerontol.,* 33, 643, 1978.

88. **Marshall, J. F. and Berrios, N.,** Movement disorders of aged rats: reversal by dopamine receptor stimulation, *Science,* 206, 477, 1979.

89. **Carlsson, A.,** Age-dependent changes in brain monoamines, in *Parkinson's Disease II. Aging and Neuroendocrine Relationships,* Finch, C. E., Potter, D. E., and Kenny, A. D., Eds., Plenum Press, New York, 1978, 1.

90. **McGeer, P. L. and McGeer, E. G.,** Aging and neurotransmitter systems, in *Parkinson's Disease II. Aging and Neuroendocrine Relationships,* Finch, C. E., Potter, D. E., and Kenny, A. D., Eds., Plenum Press, New York, 1978, 41.

91. **Greenberg, L. H. and Weiss, B.,** β-adrenergic receptors in aged rat brain: reduced number and capability of pineal gland to develop supersensitivity, *Science,* 201, 61, 1978.

92. **Severson, J. A. and Finch, C. E.,** Reduced dopaminergic binding during aging in the rodent striatum, *Brain Res.,* 192, 147, 1980.

93. **Makman, M. H., Ahn, H. S., Thal, L. J., Dvorkin, B., Horowitz, S. G., Sharpless, N. S., and Rosenfeld, N.,** Biogenic amine-stimulated adenylate cyclase and spiroperidol-binding sites in rabbit brain: evidence for selective loss of receptors with aging, in *Parkinson's Disease II. Aging and Neuroendocrine Relationships,* Finch, C. E., Potter, D. E., and Kenny, A. D., Eds., Plenum Press, New York, 1978, 211.

94. **Roth, G. S.,** Reduced glucocorticoid binding site concentration in cortical neuronal perikarya from senescent rats, *Brain Res.,* 107, 345, 1976.

95. **Davies, P. and Verth, A. H.,** Regional distribution of muscarinic acetylcholine receptor in normal and Alzheimer-type dementia brains, *Brain Res.,* 138, 385, 1978.

96. **Reisine, T. D., Yamamura, H. I., Bird, E. D., Spokes, E., and Enna, S. J.,** Pre- and postsynaptic neurochemical alterations in Alzheimer's disease, *Brain Res.,* 159, 477, 1978.

97. **James, T. C. and Kanungo, M. S.,** Alterations in atropine sites of the brain of rats as a function of age, *Biochem. Biophys. Res. Commun.,* 72, 170, 1976.

98. **Drachman, D. A. and Leavitt, J.,** Human memory and the cholinergic system: a relationship to aging, *Arch. Neurol.,* 27, 783, 1977.

99. **Lippa, A., Pelham, R. W., Beer, B., Citchert, D. J., Dean, R. L., and Bartus, R. T.,** Brain cholinergic dysfunction and memory in aged rats, *Neurobiol. Aging,* 1, 13, 1980.

100. **Ingram, D. K., London, E. D., and Goodrick, C. L.,** Age and neurochemical correlates of radial maze performance in rats, *Neurobiol. Aging,* 2, 41, 1981.

101. **Timiras, P. A., Hudson, D. B., and Oklund, S.,** Changes in central nervous system free amino acids with development and aging, *Prog. Brain Res.,* 40, 267, 1973.

102. **Schmidt, M. J. and Thornberry, J. F.,** Cyclic AMP and cyclic GMP accumulation in vitro in brain regions of young, old and aged rats, *Brain Res.,* 193, 169, 1978.

103. **Berg, A. and Zimmerman, I. D.,** Effects of electrical stimulation and noepinephrine on cyclic-AMP levels in the cerebral cortex of the aging rat, *Mech. Aging Develop.,* 4, 377, 1975.

104. **Walker, J. P. and Boas-Walker, J.,** Properties of adenyl cyclase from senescent rat brain, *Brain Res.,* 554, 391, 1973.

105. **Haining, J., Turner, M. D., and Pantall, R. M.,** Local cerebral blood flow in young and old rats during hypoxia and hypercapnia, *Am. J. Physiol.,* 218, 1020, 1970.
106. **Patel, M. S.,** Age-dependent changes in the oxidative metabolism of rat brain, *J. Gerontol.,* 32, 643, 1977.
107. **Sylvia, A. L. and Rosenthal, M.,** Effects of age on brain oxidative metabolism in vivo, *Brain Res.,* 165, 235, 1979.
108. **Appel, S. H.,** Brain macromolecular synthesis and aging, in *Survey Report on the Aging Nervous System,* DHEW Publ. No. 74-296, Maletta, G. J., Ed., U.S. Department of Health, Education and Welfare, Washington, D.C., 1974.

INDEX

A

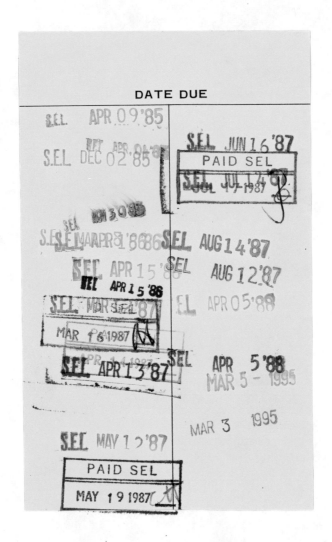